# Head and Neck Critical Illness

# Head and Neck Critical Illness: Basic and Clinical Research Implications

Editor

**Hiroyuki Tomita**

MDPI • Basel • Beijing • Wuhan • Barcelona • Belgrade • Manchester • Tokyo • Cluj • Tianjin

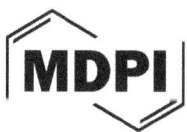

*Editor*
Hiroyuki Tomita
Gifu University School of Medicine
Japan

*Editorial Office*
MDPI
St. Alban-Anlage 66
4052 Basel, Switzerland

This is a reprint of articles from the Special Issue published online in the open access journal *Journal of Clinical Medicine* (ISSN 2077-0383) (available at: https://www.mdpi.com/journal/jcm/special_issues/head_neck_malignancies).

For citation purposes, cite each article independently as indicated on the article page online and as indicated below:

LastName, A.A.; LastName, B.B.; LastName, C.C. Article Title. *Journal Name* **Year**, *Article Number*, Page Range.

**ISBN 978-3-03943-563-0 (Hbk)**
**ISBN 978-3-03943-564-7 (PDF)**

© 2020 by the authors. Articles in this book are Open Access and distributed under the Creative Commons Attribution (CC BY) license, which allows users to download, copy and build upon published articles, as long as the author and publisher are properly credited, which ensures maximum dissemination and a wider impact of our publications.

The book as a whole is distributed by MDPI under the terms and conditions of the Creative Commons license CC BY-NC-ND.

# Contents

**About the Editor** .................................................. vii

**Hiroyuki Tomita**
Comment from the Editor on the Special Issue "Head and Neck Critical Illness: Basic and Clinical Research Implications"
Reprinted from: *J. Clin. Med.* **2019**, *8*, 1905, doi:10.3390/jcm8111905 .................. 1

**Cecilia Salom, Saúl Álvarez-Teijeiro, M. Pilar Fernández, Reginald O. Morgan, Eva Allonca, Aitana Vallina, Corina Lorz, Lucas de Villalaín, M. Soledad Fernández-García, Juan P. Rodrigo and Juana M. García-Pedrero**
Frequent Alteration of Annexin A9 and A10 in HPV-Negative Head and Neck Squamous Cell Carcinomas: Correlation with the Histopathological Differentiation Grade
Reprinted from: *J. Clin. Med.* **2019**, *8*, 229, doi:10.3390/jcm8020229 .................... 3

**Nadège Kindt, Géraldine Descamps, Jérôme R. Lechien, Myriam Remmelink, Jean-Marie Colet, Ruddy Wattiez, Guy Berchem, Fabrice Journe and Sven Saussez**
Involvement of HPV Infection in the Release of Macrophage Migration Inhibitory Factor in Head and Neck Squamous Cell Carcinoma
Reprinted from: *J. Clin. Med.* **2019**, *8*, 75, doi:10.3390/jcm8010075 ..................... 15

**Thomas Senghore, Huei-Tzu Chien, Wen-Chang Wang, You-Xin Chen, Chi-Kuang Young, Shiang-Fu Huang and Chih-Ching Yeh**
Polymorphisms in *ERCC5* rs17655 and *ERCC1* rs735482 Genes Associated with the Survival of Male Patients with Postoperative Oral Squamous Cell Carcinoma Treated with Adjuvant Concurrent Chemoradiotherapy
Reprinted from: *J. Clin. Med.* **2019**, *8*, 33, doi:10.3390/jcm8010033 ..................... 33

**Julián Suarez-Canto, Faustino Julián Suárez-Sánchez, Francisco Domínguez-Iglesias, Gonzalo Hernández-Vallejo, Juana M. García-Pedrero and Juan C. de Vicente**
Distinct Expression and Clinical Significance of Zinc Finger AN-1-Type Containing 4 in Oral Squamous Cell Carcinomas
Reprinted from: *J. Clin. Med.* **2018**, *7*, 534, doi:10.3390/jcm7120534 .................... 47

**Yeona Cho, Jun Won Kim, Hong In Yoon, Chang Geol Lee, Ki Chang Keum and Ik Jae Lee**
The Prognostic Significance of Neutrophil-to-Lymphocyte Ratio in Head and Neck Cancer Patients Treated with Radiotherapy
Reprinted from: *J. Clin. Med.* **2018**, *7*, 512, doi:10.3390/jcm7120512 .................... 59

**Francisco Hermida-Prado, Sofía T. Menéndez, Pablo Albornoz-Afanasiev, Rocío Granda-Diaz, Saúl Álvarez-Teijeiro, M. Ángeles Villaronga, Eva Allonca, Laura Alonso-Durán, Xavier León, Laia Alemany, Marisa Mena, Nagore del-Rio-Ibisate, Aurora Astudillo, René Rodríguez, Juan P. Rodrigo and Juana M. García-Pedrero**
Distinctive Expression and Amplification of Genes at 11q13 in Relation to HPV Status with Impact on Survival in Head and Neck Cancer Patients
Reprinted from: *J. Clin. Med.* **2018**, *7*, 501, doi:10.3390/jcm7120501 .................... 73

**Yen-Hao Chen, Chih-Yen Chien, Fu-Min Fang, Tai-Lin Huang, Yan-Ye Su, Sheng-Dean Luo, Chao-Cheng Huang, Wei-Che Lin and Shau-Hsuan Li**
Nox4 Overexpression as a Poor Prognostic Factor in Patients with Oral Tongue Squamous Cell Carcinoma Receiving Surgical Resection
Reprinted from: *J. Clin. Med.* **2018**, *7*, 497, doi:10.3390/jcm7120497 .................... 87

Pei-Feng Liu, Hsueh-Wei Chang, Jin-Shiung Cheng, Huai-Pao Lee, Ching-Yu Yen, Wei-Lun Tsai, Jiin-Tsuey Cheng, Yi-Jing Li, Wei-Chieh Huang, Cheng-Hsin Lee, Luo-Pin Ger and Chih-Wen Shu
Map1lc3b and Sqstm1 Modulated Autophagy for Tumorigenesis and Prognosis in Certain Subsites of Oral Squamous Cell Carcinoma
Reprinted from: *J. Clin. Med.* **2018**, 7, 478, doi:10.3390/jcm7120478 . . . . . . . . . . . . . . . . . 99

Geng-He Chang, Meng-Chang Ding, Yao-Hsu Yang, Yung-Hsiang Lin, Chia-Yen Liu, Meng-Hung Lin, Ching-Yuan Wu, Cheng-Ming Hsu and Ming-Shao Tsai
High Risk of Deep Neck Infection in Patients with Type 1 Diabetes Mellitus: A Nationwide Population-Based Cohort Study
Reprinted from: *J. Clin. Med.* **2018**, 7, 385, doi:10.3390/jcm7110385 . . . . . . . . . . . . . . . . . 119

Shian-Ren Lin and Ching-Feng Weng
PG-Priming Enhances Doxorubicin Influx to Trigger Necrotic and Autophagic Cell Death in Oral Squamous Cell Carcinoma
Reprinted from: *J. Clin. Med.* **2018**, 7, 375, doi:10.3390/jcm7100375 . . . . . . . . . . . . . . . . . 131

Miao-Fen Chen, Ming-Shao Tsai, Wen-Cheng Chen and Ping-Tsung Chen
Predictive Value of the Pretreatment Neutrophil-to-Lymphocyte Ratio in Head and Neck Squamous Cell Carcinoma
Reprinted from: *J. Clin. Med.* **2018**, 7, 294, doi:10.3390/jcm7100294 . . . . . . . . . . . . . . . . . 149

Lutfi Kanmaz and Erdal Karavas
The Role of Diffusion-Weighted Magnetic Resonance Imaging in the Differentiation of Head and Neck Masses
Reprinted from: *J. Clin. Med.* **2018**, 7, 130, doi:10.3390/jcm7060130 . . . . . . . . . . . . . . . . . 165

Paolo Brusini, Claudia Tosoni and Marco Zeppieri
Canaloplasty in Corticosteroid-Induced Glaucoma. Preliminary Results
Reprinted from: *J. Clin. Med.* **2018**, 7, 31, doi:10.3390/jcm7020031 . . . . . . . . . . . . . . . . . 175

Jessica K. Miller, Siné McDougall, Sarah Thomas and Jan Wiener
The Impact of the Brain-Derived Neurotrophic Factor Gene on Trauma and Spatial Processing
Reprinted from: *J. Clin. Med.* **2017**, 6, 108, doi:10.3390/jcm6120108 . . . . . . . . . . . . . . . . . 183

Kazuhiro Kobayashi, Kenji Hisamatsu, Natsuko Suzui, Akira Hara, Hiroyuki Tomita and Tatsuhiko Miyazaki
A Review of HPV-Related Head and Neck Cancer
Reprinted from: *J. Clin. Med.* **2018**, 7, 241, doi:10.3390/jcm7090241 . . . . . . . . . . . . . . . . . 197

Dimitrios Velissaris, Martina Pintea, Nikolaos Pantzaris, Eirini Spatha, Vassilios Karamouzos, Charalampos Pierrakos and Menelaos Karanikolas
The Role of Procalcitonin in the Diagnosis of Meningitis: A Literature Review
Reprinted from: *J. Clin. Med.* **2018**, 7, 148, doi:10.3390/jcm7060148 . . . . . . . . . . . . . . . . . 209

Masaya Kawaguchi, Hiroki Kato, Hiroyuki Tomita, Keisuke Mizuta, Mitsuhiro Aoki, Akira Hara and Masayuki Matsuo
Imaging Characteristics of Malignant Sinonasal Tumors
Reprinted from: *J. Clin. Med.* **2017**, 6, 116, doi:10.3390/jcm6120116 . . . . . . . . . . . . . . . . . 225

Surinder S. Moonga, Kenneth Liang and Burke A. Cunha
Acute Encephalitis in an Adult with Diffuse Large B-Cell Lymphoma with Secondary Involvement of the Central Nervous System: Infectious or Non-Infectious Etiology?
Reprinted from: *J. Clin. Med.* **2017**, 6, 117, doi:10.3390/jcm6120117 . . . . . . . . . . . . . . . . . 241

# About the Editor

**Hiroyuki Tomita** (MD, Ph.D., Associate Professor) specializes in pathology, oncology and laboratory animal science with genetically modified animals. In particular, he has published numerous papers on the mechanisms of carcinogenesis and the tumor microenvironment of oral and digestive cancers using mice models. He is also a board-certified specialist of the Japanese Society of Pathology and performs diagnostic pathology (https://www.researchgate.net/profile/Hiroyuki_Tomita).

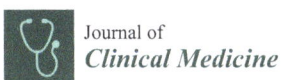 

*Editorial*

# Comment from the Editor on the Special Issue "Head and Neck Critical Illness: Basic and Clinical Research Implications"

### Hiroyuki Tomita

Department of Tumor Pathology, Gifu University Graduate School of Medicine, 1-1 Yanagido, Gifu 501-1194, Japan; h_tomita@gifu-u.ac.jp

Received: 5 November 2019; Accepted: 5 November 2019; Published: 7 November 2019

**Abstract:** While oncogenic mutations of head and neck squamous cell carcinomas (HNSCC) in head and neck malignancies are uncommon, analysis using next-generation sequencing (NGS) technologies is growing. Further, single-cell analysis is being developed to overcome cancer cell heterogeneity and improve the poor survival of patients. However, it is important for researchers to know how to use this information to improve patients' survival.

**Keywords:** head and neck cancer; NGS; squamous cell carcinoma

---

Among head and neck malignancies, head and neck squamous cell carcinomas (HNSCC) comprise a heterogeneous group of malignant neoplasms arising from the squamous cell epithelium of the upper aerodigestive tract. The sites of the HNSCC development include the oral cavity, nasopharynx, oropharynx, hypopharynx, and larynx. Squamous cell carcinomas arising from these sites account for the sixth most common malignancy worldwide [1]. The 5-year survival rates for HNSCCs have remained at approximately 50% for the past 40 years [2].

The understanding of the molecular and genetic alterations leading to oncogenesis in head and neck cancers, including HNSCC, has dramatically increased in the past decade. Initial steps taken to grasp the genetic pathogenesis of head and neck cancer paid attention to cytogenetic studies. The development of microarray technology has made it possible to classify HNSCCs into distinct types based on various gene expression patterns. Recently, next-generation sequencing (NGS) technologies have enabled many researchers to sequence a large number of cancers to identify novel gene abnormalities (i.e., mutations, translocations, and fusions). An underlying motivation for genomic profiling studies by these researchers was to gain a more radical understanding of the molecular alterations in head and neck cancer for the establishment of novel targeting therapeutics.

Conventional methods that have been used to study gene expression and chemotherapeutic responses in cancer molecular assays are performed on whole cell populations in tumor tissue. Therefore, the results from these methods average the differences between individual cells in tumor tissue [3]. This approach oversimplifies the complexity of the various genetic profiles existing in the tumor microenvironment (TME) and distorts results relating to the proportion and identity of cancer stem cells.

On the contrary, single-cell genomic profiling by single-cell sequencing is performed independent of pooled samples or cell populations, permitting a higher fidelity representation of intra- and intertumoral cell heterogeneity in the TME [4,5]. Using single-cell sequencing means that each unique head and neck cancer cell type can be identified and elucidated. Further, a more profound discrimination of intra- and intertumoral differences is critical in developing novel therapeutic strategies targeted at increasing tumor-specific antigen responses [3].

Oncogenic mutations in HNSCC are uncommon. Targeting these alterations may require investigating comprehensive fatal approaches against cancer cells [5]. Moreover, oncogenic signaling pathways can be activated by various non-genetic mechanisms that are not detected by genomic efforts. It is necessary to challenge how we use the information obtained from NGS to develop and improve diagnostic and therapeutic modalities.

**Conflicts of Interest:** The authors declare no competing financial interests.

## References

1. Fitzmaurice, C.; Allen, C.; Barber, R.M.; Barregard, L.; Bhutta, Z.A.; Brenner, H.; Dicker, D.J.; Chimed-Orchir, O.; Dandona, R.; Dandona, L.; et al. Global, Regional, and National Cancer Incidence, Mortality, Years of Life Lost, Years Lived With Disability, and Disability-Adjusted Life-years for 32 Cancer Groups, 1990 to 2015: A Systematic Analysis for the Global Burden of Disease Study. *JAMA Oncol.* **2017**, *3*, 524–548. [PubMed]
2. Siegel, R.L.; Miller, K.D.; Jemal, A. Cancer Statistics, 2017. *CA Cancer J. Clin.* **2017**, *67*, 7–30. [CrossRef] [PubMed]
3. Pai, S.I.; Westra, W.H. Molecular pathology of head and neck cancer: implications for diagnosis, prognosis, and treatment. *Annu. Rev. Pathol.* **2009**, *4*, 49–70. [CrossRef] [PubMed]
4. Agrawal, N.; Frederick, M.J.; Pickering, C.R.; Bettegowda, C.; Chang, K.; Li, R.J.; Fakhry, C.; Xie, T.X.; Zhang, J.; Wang, J.; et al. Exome sequencing of head and neck squamous cell carcinoma reveals inactivating mutations in NOTCH1. *Science* **2011**, *333*, 1154–1157. [CrossRef]
5. Stransky, N.; Egloff, A.M.; Tward, A.D.; Kostic, A.D.; Cibulskis, K.; Sivachenko, A.; Kryukov, G.V.; Lawrence, M.S.; Sougnez, C.; McKenna, A.; et al. The mutational landscape of head and neck squamous cell carcinoma. *Science* **2011**, *333*, 1157–1160. [CrossRef] [PubMed]

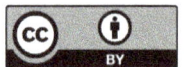

© 2019 by the author. Licensee MDPI, Basel, Switzerland. This article is an open access article distributed under the terms and conditions of the Creative Commons Attribution (CC BY) license (http://creativecommons.org/licenses/by/4.0/).

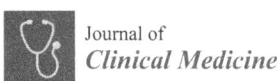 

Article

# Frequent Alteration of Annexin A9 and A10 in HPV-Negative Head and Neck Squamous Cell Carcinomas: Correlation with the Histopathological Differentiation Grade

Cecilia Salom [1,†], Saúl Álvarez-Teijeiro [1,2,†], M. Pilar Fernández [3], Reginald O. Morgan [3], Eva Allonca [1,2], Aitana Vallina [4], Corina Lorz [2,5], Lucas de Villalaín [6], M. Soledad Fernández-García [4], Juan P. Rodrigo [1,2,*] and Juana M. García-Pedrero [1,2,*]

1. Department of Otolaryngology, Hospital Universitario Central de Asturias and Instituto de Investigación Sanitaria del Principado de Asturias, Instituto Universitario de Oncología del Principado de Asturias, University of Oviedo, Avda. Roma, 33011 Oviedo, Spain; mariaceciliasalom@gmail.com (C.S.); saul.teijeiro@gmail.com (S.Á.-T.); ynkc1@hotmail.com (E.A.)
2. CIBERONC, Av. Monforte de Lemos 3-5, 28029 Madrid, Spain; clorz@ciemat.es
3. Department of Biochemistry and Molecular Biology and Institute of Biotechnology of Asturias, University of Oviedo, Julian Clavería, 33006 Oviedo, Spain; pfernandez@uniovi.es (M.P.F.); morganreginald@uniovi.es (R.O.M.)
4. Department of Pathology, Hospital Universitario Central de Asturias and Instituto Universitario de Oncología del Principado de Asturias, University of Oviedo, Avda. Roma, 33011 Oviedo, Spain; alaicla@hotmail.es (A.V.); solefghdr@hotmail.com (M.S.F.-G.)
5. Molecular Oncology Unit, CIEMAT (ed 70A), Av. Complutense 40, 28040 Madrid, Spain
6. Department of Oral Surgery, Hospital Universitario Central de Asturias and Instituto de Investigación Sanitaria del Principado de Asturias, Instituto Universitario de Oncología del Principado de Asturias, University of Oviedo, Avda. Roma, 33011 Oviedo, Spain; lvillalain@hotmail.com
* Correspondence: jprodrigo@uniovi.es (J.P.R.); juanagp.finba@gmail.com (J.M.G.-P.); Tel.: +34-985-108-000 (J.P.R.); +34-985-107-937 (J.M.G.-P.)
† These authors contributed equally to this work.

Received: 3 December 2018; Accepted: 4 February 2019; Published: 10 February 2019

**Abstract:** The annexin protein superfamily has been implicated in multiple physiological and pathological processes, including carcinogenesis. Altered expression of various annexins has frequently been observed and linked to the development and progression of various human malignancies. However, information is lacking on the expression and clinical significance of annexin A9 (ANXA9) and A10 (ANXA10) in head and neck squamous cell carcinomas (HNSCC). ANXA9 and ANXA10 expression was evaluated in a large cohort of 372 surgically treated HPV-negative HNSCC patients and correlated with the clinicopathologic parameters and disease outcomes. Down-regulation of ANXA9 expression was found in 42% of HNSCC tissue samples, compared to normal epithelia. ANXA9 expression in tumors was significantly associated with oropharyngeal location and histological differentiation grade ($p < 0.001$). In marked contrast, ANXA10 expression was absent in normal epithelium, but variably detected in the cytoplasm of cancer cells. Positive ANXA10 expression was found in 64% of tumors, and was significantly associated with differentiation grade ($p < 0.001$), being also more frequent in oropharyngeal tumors ($p = 0.019$). These results reveal that the expression of both ANXA9 and ANXA10 is frequently altered in HNSCC and associated to the tumor differentiation grade, suggesting that they could be implicated in the pathogenesis of these cancers.

**Keywords:** annexin A9; annexin A10; head and neck squamous cell carcinoma; differentiation grade; immunohistochemistry

---

## 1. Introduction

Twelve annexins comprise a ubiquitous, multigene family in vertebrates with properties that enable binding interactions with calcium and cell membrane components, including anionic phospholipids, cytoskeletal proteins and extracellular matrix glycoproteins. Annexin-knockdown or annexin-knockout models have provided limited insight into the biological functions of different annexin proteins [1] and there are only indirect links based on statistical association with genetic diseases. They have been implicated in a variety of biological processes, including membrane organization, vesicle trafficking, calcium metabolism, cell adhesion, subcellular transport, growth and differentiation, and wound healing [2,3], many of which are relevant to cancer progression.

Annexins are characterized structurally by a conserved C-terminal core that consists of a tetrad of homologous annexin (ANX) domains, each 68–69 amino acids long, harboring ligands that can coordinate calcium ions in conjunction with membrane phospholipids, or bind to other proteins and carbohydrate-containing biomolecules. The binding properties and targets of each annexin are distinct, exemplified by the apparent calcium-independence of annexins A9 and A10 [4]. The N-terminal region of each annexin is unique, with a variable length and amino acid sequence that contributes to annexin conformation, protein interactions and non-overlapping functional specificity in the biological activity of different annexins [5,6].

More than 4000 annexins have been reported in different species, widely distributed among eukaryotes and prevalent in different forms of prokaryotes and unicellular eukaryotes [1,4]. The twelve annexins common to vertebrates are referred to as annexins A1–A13 (ANXA1–ANXA13) with ANXA12 remaining unassigned. There are 13 human annexin genes, including a unique duplication of ANXA8, ranging in size from 15 kb (ANXA9) to 96 kb (ANXA10) and spread throughout the genome on chromosomes 1, 2, 4, 5, 8, 9, 10 and 15 [1,7].

The expression pattern and tissue distribution of annexins vary widely. While annexins A1, A2, A4, A5, A6, A7 and A11 are ubiquitously expressed, others exhibit very restrictive expression such as ANXA3 in neutrophils, ANXA8 in placenta and skin, ANXA9 in the tongue, ANXA10 in the stomach and ANXA13 in the small intestine [7]. The promoter regulation of annexin A9 has been partially characterized [8], but distal DNA elements, regulatory RNAs and epigenetic changes are under current study in high-throughput experiments, so the molecular basis of its expression remains incomplete.

The term annexinopathy has been used to define those human diseases in which abnormal levels and pleiotropic effects of annexins contribute to the pathogenesis [9,10]. Although direct involvement of these proteins in the etiology of any genetic disease has not been demonstrated, they have been implicated in various pathologies such as diabetes, cardiovascular and autoimmune diseases, infection and cancer [10,11]. Mounting evidence shows that several annexins are frequently altered in cancers, suggesting a possible role in the process of tumorigenesis. Some annexins have been found overexpressed in specific types of tumors, while others consistently show loss of expression [9–11]. Emerging mechanistic studies are helping to relate annexin expression changes to tumor cell function, particularly tumor growth, invasion and metastasis, angiogenesis and drug resistance. The expression of individual annexins is associated with particular cancer types hence annexins could also be useful biomarkers in the clinic [10,11]. More precise localization of these proteins in different tissues could deepen our understanding of their pathophysiological functions, which continues to be a key area of investigation.

The overall goal of this study was to investigate the expression pattern and clinical significance of ANXA9 and ANXA10, specifically in head and neck squamous cell carcinomas (HNSCC). ANXA9 shows generally restricted tissue expression but is known to exhibit altered expression in breast cancer [12], colorectal cancer [13] and cutaneous melanoma [14]. It was also shown to be overexpressed in differentiating keratinocytes in pemphigus [15] and binds to other cytoskeletal proteins [16]. Several studies have been published to date on the expression ANXA10 in gastrointestinal cancers, and its overexpression in oral cancer is correlated with cell proliferation [17]. We focused our study on the expression and clinical significance of ANXA9 and ANXA10 specifically in HNSCC using immunohistochemistry techniques in a large homogeneous cohort of 372 surgically treated, HPV-negative, HNSCC patients.

## 2. Materials and Method

### 2.1. Patients and Tissue Specimens

Surgical tissue specimens from 372 patients with HPV-negative HNSCC who underwent resection of their tumors at the Hospital Universitario Central de Asturias between 1990 and 2009 were retrospectively collected, in accordance to approved institutional review board guidelines. All experimental protocols were approved by the Institutional Ethics Committee of the Hospital Universitario Central de Asturias and by the Regional CEIC (Comité Ético de Investigación Clínica) from Principado de Asturias (approval number: 81/2013 for the project PI13/00259). Informed consent was obtained from all patients. Representative tissue sections were obtained from archival, paraffin-embedded blocks and the histological diagnosis was confirmed by an experienced pathologist (M.S.F.-G.).

All patients had a single primary tumor, microscopically clear surgical margins and received no treatment prior to surgery. Only fourteen patients were women, and the mean age was 58.6 years (range 30 to 86 years). All but twelve patients were habitual tobacco smokers, 198 moderate (1–50 pack-year) and 153 heavy (>50 pack-year), and 335 were alcohol drinkers. The stage of the tumors was determined according to the TNM system of the International Union Against Cancer (7th Edition). Two hundred and thirty (62%) of 372 patients received postoperative radiotherapy. Patients were followed-up for a minimum of 36 months. The mean follow-up for the whole series was 34.6 months (median, 21.5 months); for the patients without recurrence, 71 months (median, 67 months); and for the patients dead by the tumor, 18 months (median, 13.5 months). Recurrence was defined as relapse of the tumor in the five first years after treatment at any site: local recurrence, nodal metastasis, or distant metastasis. Information on HPV status was available for all the patients. HPV status was analyzed using p16-immunohistochemistry, high-risk HPV DNA detection by in situ hybridization and genotyping by GP5+/6+-PCR, as previously reported [18,19]. The characteristics of the studied cases are shown in Table 1.

### 2.2. Tissue Microarray (TMA) Construction

Three morphologically representative areas were selected from each individual tumor paraffin block. Subsequently, three 1 mm cylinders were taken to construct TMA blocks, as described previously [20,21], containing a total of 372 HNSCC (134 tonsillar, 107 base of tongue, 64 hypopharyngeal and 67 laryngeal carcinomas). In addition, each TMA included three cores of normal epithelium as an internal negative control. The normal epithelium was obtained from adult male, non-smokers and non-drinkers, patients that were operated from tonsillectomy due to chronic tonsillitis, and patients operated from benign vocal cord lesions (e.g., polyps, cysts).

Table 1. Clinicopathologic characteristics of the tumors studied.

| Characteristic | No. Cases (%) |
|---|---|
| Age, mean (range) | 58.6 (30–86 years) |
| Location | |
| Oropharynx | 241 (65) |
| Hypopharynx | 64 (17) |
| Larynx | 67 (18) |
| pathologic T classification | |
| T1 | 38 (10) |
| T2 | 77 (21) |
| T3 | 125 (34) |
| T4 | 132 (35) |
| pathologic N classification | |
| N0 | 103 (28) |
| N1 | 46 (12) |
| N2 | 183 (49) |
| N3 | 40 (11) |
| Stage | |
| I | 20 (5) |
| II | 24 (6) |
| III | 64 (17) |
| IV | 264 (71) |
| Degree of differentiation | |
| Well-differentiated | 147 (39) |
| Moderately-differentiated | 148 (40) |
| Poorly-differentiated | 77 (21) |
| Total | 372 |

*2.3. Immunohistochemical Study*

The formalin-fixed, paraffin-embedded tissue samples were cut into 3-μm sections and dried on Flex IHC microscope slides (Dako, Glostrup, Denmark). The sections were deparaffinized with standard xylene and hydrated through graded alcohols into water. Antigen retrieval was performed with proteinase K and the samples were placed for 15 min in hydrogen peroxide at 3%. Staining was done at room temperature on an automatic staining workstation (Dako Autostainer Plus) using the following primary antibodies (developed by Dr. MP Fernández, Department of Biochemistry, University of Oviedo [4]) and conditions: Anti-ANXA9 at a concentration of 1:100 for 30 min and anti-ANXA10 at a concentration of 1:100 for 45 min. Immunodetection was carried out with the Dako EnVision Flex + Visualization System (Dako Autostainer), using diaminobenzidine as a chromogen. Counterstaining with hematoxylin for 7 min was the final step.

After staining, the sections were dehydrated and set up in a slide in a standard medium. Negative controls were carried out without the primary antibody. The vascular endothelium, in which the expression of both annexins had previously been shown, was used as a positive control.

Since staining showed a homogeneous distribution, a semiquantitative scoring system based on staining intensity was applied. Immunostaining was scored blinded to clinical data by two independent observers as negative (0), weak to moderately (1+), and strongly positive (2+) based on staining intensity. Scores $\geq 1$ were considered as positive expression.

## 3. Results

*3.1. Expression of ANXA9 and ANX10 in Normal Epithelia*

Non-keratinized stratified squamous epithelium showed different expression patterns for the two annexins studied. ANXA9 expression was absent in basal and parabasal cells, while expression increased towards the most differentiated layers of the epithelium (Figure 1A). Contrasting this, negative ANXA10 expression was detected in all cell layers of normal epithelium (Figure 1D).

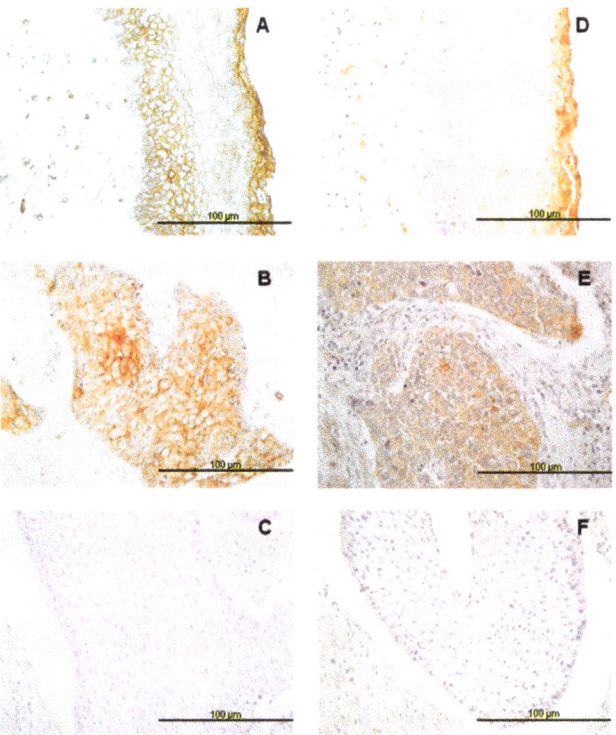

**Figure 1.** Immunohistochemical analysis of annexins A9 (ANXA9) and A10 (ANXA10) expression in head and neck squamous cell carcinomas (HNSCC) tissue specimens. Representative examples of ANXA9 (**A**) and ANXA10 (**D**) expression in normal epithelium, positive ANXA9 (**B**) and ANXA10 (**E**) expression in carcinomas, and negative ANXA9 (**C**) and ANXA10 (**F**) expression in carcinomas. Original magnification ×40.

### 3.2. Expression of ANXA9 in HNSCC Tissue Specimens

Immunohistochemical analysis of ANXA9 expression was successfully evaluated in 346 of 372 tumor samples. Two-hundred of them (58%) showed positive ANXA9 expression predominantly with a membranous pattern, although cytoplasmic expression was also observed in some cases (Figure 1B,C). The relationship between the expression of ANXA9 and clinicopathologic characteristics is shown in Table 2. Positive ANXA9 expression was strongly and significantly associated with the degree of differentiation of the tumors ($p < 0.001$). Thus, ANXA9 expression was mainly found in well-differentiated tumors whereas expression was reduced in moderately and poorly differentiated tumors (Figure 2A,C). We also observed differences in ANXA9 expression between the different HNSCC subsites, with ANXA9 expression being significantly higher in oropharyngeal tumors ($p < 0.001$).

**Table 2.** Relationship between ANXA9 and ANXA10 expression and clinicopathological parameters.

| Characteristic | No. Cases for ANXA9 | Positive ANXA9 Expression (%) | p | No. Cases for ANXA10 | Positive ANXA10 Expression (%) | p |
|---|---|---|---|---|---|---|
| Location | | | | | | |
| Oropharynx | 234 | 166 (71) | | 231 | 160 (69) | |
| Hypopharynx | 58 | 17 (29) | 0.000 # | 55 | 28 (51) | 0.019 # |
| Larynx | 54 | 17 (31) | | 54 | 31 (57) | |
| pT Classification | | | | | | |
| T1-T2 | 100 | 52 (52) | | 95 | 58 (61) | |
| T3 | 120 | 73 (61) | 0.377 # | 119 | 75 (63) | 0.591 # |
| T4 | 126 | 73 (59) | | 123 | 83 (67) | |
| pN Classification | | | | | | |
| N0 | 87 | 48 (55) | 0.616 † | 87 | 53 (61) | 0.439 † |
| N1-3 | 259 | 152 (59) | | 253 | 166 (66) | |
| Stage | | | | | | |
| I-II | 33 | 14 (42) | | 32 | 19 (59) | |
| III | 61 | 39 (64) | 0.124 # | 60 | 39 (65) | 0.822 # |
| IV | 252 | 147 (58) | | 248 | 161 (65) | |
| Degree of differentiation | | | | | | |
| Well-differentiated | 136 | 98 (72) | | 134 | 103 (77) | |
| Moderately-differentiated | 137 | 73 (53) | 0.000 # | 137 | 85 (62) | 0.000 # |
| Poorly-differentiated | 73 | 29 (40) | | 69 | 31 (45) | |
| Recurrence | | | | | | |
| No | 132 | 77 (58) | 0.91 † | 132 | 80 (61) | 0.248 † |
| Yes | 214 | 123 (57) | | 208 | 139 (67) | |
| Total | 346 | 200 (58) | | 340 | 219 (64) | |

# Chi-square and † Fisher's exact tests.

No associations were found between ANXA9 expression and T and N classifications or tumor recurrence ($p = 0.91$). In addition, ANXA9 expression was not associated with disease-specific survival (log rank $p = 0.497$) nor overall survival (log rank $p = 0.406$) (data not shown).

### 3.3. Expression of ANXA10 in HNSCC Specimens

Immunohistochemical ANXA10 expression was successfully evaluated in 340 of 372 tumor samples. Positive ANXA10 expression was observed in a total of 219 (64%) cases, mainly detected in the cytoplasm of cancer cells (Figure 1E,F). Furthermore, ANXA9 and ANXA10 expression were significantly correlated (Spearman correlation coefficient 0.459, $p < 0.001$).

Similar to ANXA9, ANXA10 expression was significantly higher in oropharyngeal tumors ($p = 0.019$). Also, ANXA10 expression was significantly associated with the degree of differentiation of the tumors (decreased expression with dedifferentiation, $p < 0.001$, Figure 2B,D). No associations were observed with T and N classifications, disease stage, or tumor recurrence (Table 2). In addition, ANXA10 expression was not associated with either disease-specific (log rank $p = 0.077$) or overall survival (log rank $p = 0.167$).

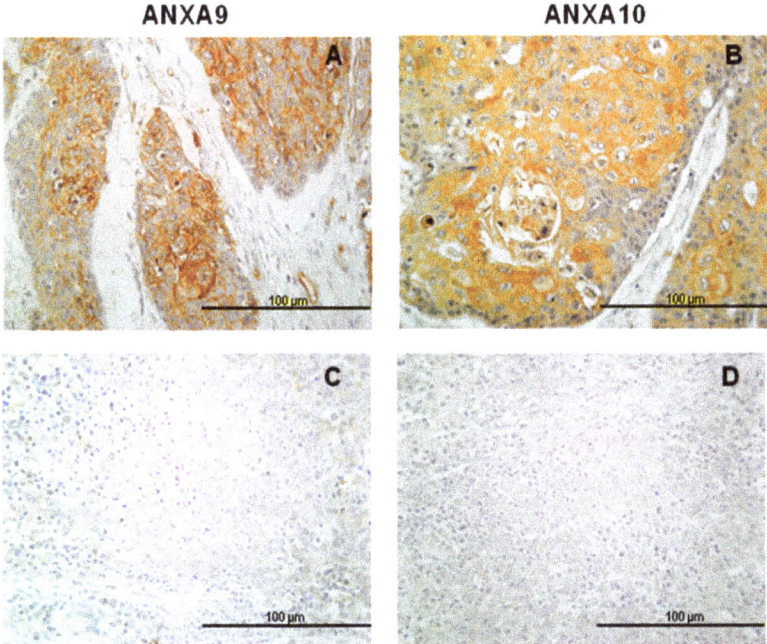

**Figure 2.** ANXA9 and ANXA10 protein expression in HNSCC specimens according to the degree of differentiation. Representative examples of well-differentiated tumors showing positive expression of ANXA9 (**A**) and ANXA10 (**B**), and poorly differentiated tumors showing negative expression of ANXA9 (**C**) and ANXA10 (**D**) expression in carcinomas. Original magnification ×40.

*3.4. In Silico Analysis of ANXA9 and ANXA10 mRNA Expression Using The Cancer Genome Atlas (TCGA) HNSCC Data*

In order to extend and confirm our results, we also performed analysis of the transcriptome data from the TCGA HNSCC cohort accessed via the original publication [22], or using the platform cBioPortal for Cancer Genomics (http://cbioportal.org/) [23] and the UALCAN web tools (http://ualcan.path.uab.edu/) [24]. Thus, ANXA9 mRNA levels were found to be significantly decreased in primary tumors compared to normal tissue samples ($p < 0.001$; Figure 3A), whilst ANXA10 mRNA levels increased in tumors versus normal tissue ($p < 0.001$; Figure 3B). These results are in good agreement with our observations at the protein level. In addition, possible correlations between ANXA9 and ANXA10 mRNA expression and the tumor grade were assessed using a homogeneous cohort of 243 HPV-negative HNSCC patients. We found that ANXA9 mRNA levels inversely and significantly correlated with the degree of histological differentiation (Spearman correlation coefficient $-0.244$, $p < 0.001$; Figure 3C). Consistent with our IHC protein data, ANXA9 mRNA levels were higher in well-differentiated tumors than in moderately and poorly differentiated tumors. However, ANXA10 mRNA levels did not significantly correlate with the tumor grade ($p = 0.605$; Figure 3D).

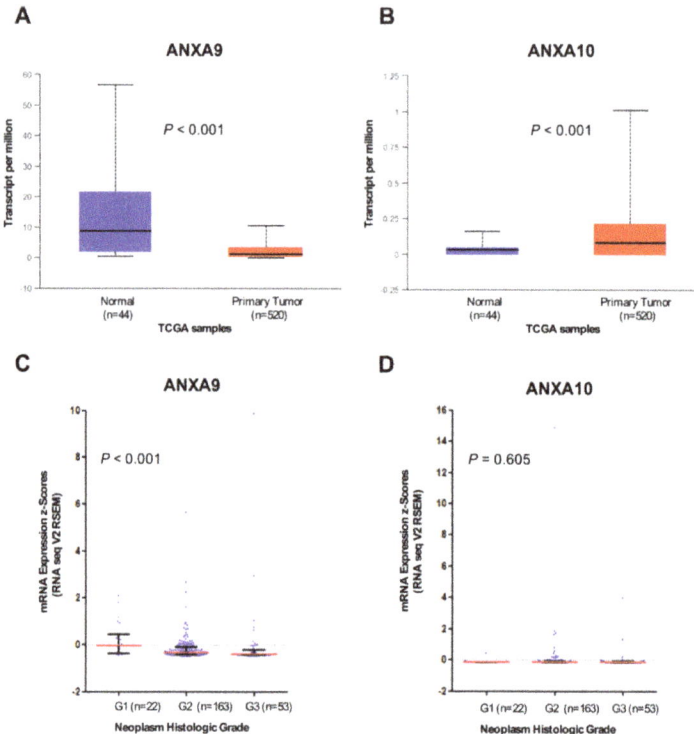

**Figure 3.** Analysis of ANXA9 and ANXA10 mRNA expression using RNAseq data from the TCGA HNSCC cohorts. Box plots comparing the mRNA expression levels of ANXA9 (**A**) and ANXA10 (**B**) in primary tumors (in red) versus normal tissue (in blue) using UALCAN online resources (http://ualcan.path.uab.edu/). The median, quartiles and range of values are shown. ANXA9 (**C**) and ANXA10 (**D**) expression (RNA seq V2 RSEM, z-score threshold ±2) was analyzed in relation to the tumor grade, categorized as well-differentiated (G1), moderately differentiated (G2) and poorly differentiated (G3) using the TCGA HPV-negative HNSCC cohort ($n$ = 243). Horizontal lines (in red) represent the median values, with interquartile range. Sigma (two-tailed) $p$-values.

## 4. Discussion

Annexins are commonly altered in cancers [9,25]. ANXA9 is a unique member of the annexin family whose intracellular activity does not appear to be regulated by calcium [10,26]. Its closest evolutionary relatives are ANXA1 and ANXA2 [1,4] and members of this clade are thought to function in the organization and regulation of membrane/cytoskeleton linkages [4,27]. As both ANXA1 and ANXA2 have been found down-regulated in head and neck squamous cell carcinoma [28–30], it was of special interest to determine whether ANXA9 showed a similar pattern of expression as this might relate to common features in the evolution, structure and function of these clade members.

We observed a weak membranous ANXA9 expression in the most differentiated cells in normal epithelium. In tumor cells, the expression is mainly membranous, similar to that observed for ANXA2 [28] and the expression of ANXA9 is mainly associated with the degree of differentiation of the tumor, with higher expression in well differentiated cases. This is consistent with elevated ANXA9 observed in differentiating keratinocytes [15]. However, ANXA9 expression was not associated with any other clinical and pathological parameter or with the prognosis in head and neck carcinomas. Analogous findings were obtained by analyzing RNAseq data from the available TCGA HNSCC cohorts. Accordingly, ANXA9 down-regulation was frequently detected in HNSCC at both mRNA and protein levels. Moreover, ANXA9 mRNA expression in tumors was inversely correlated with the histological differentiation grade, thus confirming our IHC protein data. Hence, together these results reflect that transcriptional regulatory mechanisms contribute to the loss of ANXA9 expression in HNSCC, as we previously demonstrated for the functionally and evolutionary-related members ANXA1 and ANXA2 [29,30].

Few studies have analyzed the expression of ANXA9 in cancers. One study showed that *ANXA9* gene expression is associated with bone metastasis in breast cancer [31]. In colorectal cancer, patients with high *ANXA9* gene expression also had lower overall survival [32]. ANXA9 protein expression in colorectal cancer was higher than in normal mucosa, and associated with invasion and lymphatic metastasis and, consequently, a worse prognosis [13]. These studies suggest a role for ANXA9 in invasion and metastasis, but this role could not be confirmed in head and neck cancers.

Several studies have identified ANXA10 as a tumor suppressor, diagnostic marker, potential therapeutic target, or prognostic factor in various malignancies, including bladder cancer, hepatocellular carcinoma, acute myeloid leukemia, gastric carcinoma, oral squamous cell carcinoma, pancreatobiliary adenocarcinoma, and urothelial carcinoma [33–37]. Studies have shown that ANXA10 was down-regulated in hepatocellular carcinoma and was associated with a poor prognosis [34,35]. ANXA10 has recently been identified as a marker with high specificity for the serrated histology of colorectal cancer [33,38]. The physiological importance of abundant ANXA10 expression specific to the stomach mucosa and intestinal M-cells is currently unknown.

Only one previous study has analyzed ANXA10 in head and neck cancer; Shimizu et al. [17] showed that ANXA10 is overexpressed frequently in oral squamous cell carcinomas and that this overexpression is associated with tumor size. They suggested that ANXA10 expression may be associated with tumor progression by promoting cell-cycle progression in the G1 phase through activation of the ERK/MAPK signaling pathway, leading to decreased expression of cyclin-dependent kinase inhibitors (CDKIs). While further studies are needed to study the interaction of ANXA10 and the ERK/MAPK signaling pathway, these data suggested that ANXA10 plays an important role in cellular proliferation.

We also observed that ANXA10 was not visibly expressed in normal epithelium, while it was variably expressed in the cytoplasm of cancer cells. Consistent with this, analysis of the transcriptome data from the TCGA HNSCC also demonstrated the up-regulation of ANXA10 mRNA expression in tumors compared to the corresponding normal tissue. In addition, we found that ANXA10 expression, as ANXA9, was lower in poorly differentiated tumors, but it was not related to other clinicopathologic parameters or prognosis. However, we were unable to confirm the correlation of ANXA10 protein expression with the histological grade using RNAseq data. Nevertheless, these apparently contradictory results may reflect the contribution of additional regulatory mechanisms (e.g., translational or post-translational) leading to the frequent up-regulation of ANXA10 protein in over 60% of tumor samples.

## 5. Conclusions

These original results indicate that the expression of annexins A9 and A10 is frequently altered in HNSCC at both mRNA and protein level, suggesting that they could be implicated in the pathogenesis or compensatory mechanisms of these cancers. Additional studies are ongoing to establish the pathogenic roles of these proteins in the progression of squamous cell carcinomas of the head and neck and especially, to determine whether their altered expression is a cause or consequence of the cancerous state. The association of ANXA9 with pathogenic prognosis in colorectal cancer [13] contrasts with a proposed tumor suppressor role for ANXA10 in gastric cancer [36]. The unique, calcium-independent actions of these two annexins may also contribute to a better understanding of their underlying mechanisms. Since these particular annexins are poorly expressed in general but exhibit highly tissue-specific expression, it will undoubtedly be important to explore the role of epigenetic regulatory changes responsible for their selective expression in normal versus cancer tissues.

**Author Contributions:** Conceptualization, J.P.R. and J.M.G.-P.; formal analysis, C.L. and J.P.R.; funding acquisition, J.P.R. and J.M.G.-P.; Investigation, C.S., S.Á.-T., E.A., L.d.V. and M.S.F.-G.; methodology, M.P.F., R.O.M., E.A. and A.V.; project administration, J.M.G.-P.; resources, M.P.F., R.O.M. and A.V.; supervision, J.M.G.-P.; visualization, J.P.R.; writing—original draft, C.S.; writing—review and editing, M.P.F., R.O.M., C.L., J.P.R. and J.M.G.-P.

**Funding:** This study was supported by grants from the Plan Nacional de I+D+I 2013-2016 ISCIII (PI13/00259), RD12/0036/0015 of Red Temática de Investigación Cooperativa en Cáncer (RTICC), PI16/00280 and CIBERONC (CB16/12/00390 and CB16/12/00228), the Instituto de Investigación Sanitaria del Principado de Asturias (ISPA), PCTI-Asturias (GRUPIN14-003), Fundación Bancaria Caja de Ahorros de Asturias-IUOPA and the FEDER Funding Program from the European Union.

**Acknowledgments:** We thank the samples and technical assistance kindly provided by the Principado de Asturias BioBank (PT13/0010/0046), financed jointly by Servicio de Salud del Principado de Asturias, Instituto de Salud Carlos III and Fundación Bancaria Cajastur and integrated in the Spanish National Biobanks Network.

**Conflicts of Interest:** The authors declare no conflict of interest.

## References

1. Moss, S.E.; Morgan, R.O. The annexins. *Genome Biol.* **2004**, *5*, 219. [CrossRef] [PubMed]
2. Gerke, V.; Moss, S.E. Annexins: From Structure to Function. *Physiol. Rev.* **2002**, *82*, 331–371. [CrossRef] [PubMed]
3. Jimenez, A.J.; Perez, F. Plasma membrane repair: The adaptable cell life-insurance. *Curr. Opin. Cell Biol.* **2017**, *47*, 99–107. [CrossRef] [PubMed]
4. Fernandez, M.P.; Garcia, M.; Martin-Almedina, S.; Morgan, R.O. Novel domain architectures and functional determinants in atypical annexins revealed by phylogenomic analysis. *Biol. Chem.* **2017**, *398*, 751–763. [CrossRef] [PubMed]
5. Rescher, U.; Gerke, V. Annexins—Unique membrane binding proteins with diverse functions. *J. Cell Sci.* **2004**, *117*, 2631–2639. [CrossRef] [PubMed]
6. Clark, G.B.; Morgan, R.O.; Fernandez, M.P.; Roux, S.J. Evolutionary adaptation of plant annexins has diversified their molecular structures; interactions and functional roles. *New Phytol.* **2012**, *196*, 695–712. [CrossRef] [PubMed]
7. Mirsaeidi, M.; Gidfar, S.; Vu, A.; Schraufnagel, D. Annexins family: Insights into their functions and potential role in pathogenesis of sarcoidosis. *J. Transl. Med.* **2016**, *14*, 89. [CrossRef]
8. Chlystun, M.; Markoff, A.; Gerke, V. Structural and functional characterisation of the mouse annexin A9 promoter. *Biochim. Biophys. Acta* **2004**, *1742*, 141–149. [CrossRef]
9. Rand, J.H. The annexinopathies: A new category of diseases. *Biochim. Biophys. Acta* **2000**, *149*, 169–173. [CrossRef]
10. Mussunoor, S.; Murray, G.I. The role of annexins in tumour development and progression. *J. Pathol.* **2008**, *216*, 131–140. [CrossRef]
11. Hayes, M.J.; Longbottom, R.E.; Evans, M.A.; Moss, S.E. Annexinopathies. *Subcell Biochem.* **2007**, *45*, 1–28.
12. Cosphiadi, I.; Atmakusumah, T.D.; Siregar, N.C.; Muthalib, A.; Harahap, A.; Mansyur, M. Bone metastasis in advanced breast cancer: Analysis of gene expression microarray. *Clin. Breast Cancer* **2018**, *17*, 30777. [CrossRef] [PubMed]
13. Yu, S.; Bian, H.; Gao, X.; Gui, L. Annexin A9 promotes invasion and metastasis of colorectal cancer and predicts poor prognosis. *Int. J. Mol. Med.* **2018**, *41*, 2185–2192. [CrossRef] [PubMed]
14. Amos, C.I.; Wang, L.E.; Lee, J.E.; Gershenwald, J.E.; Chen, W.V.; Fang, S.; Kosoy, R.; Zhang, M.; Qureshi, A.A.; Vattathil, S.; et al. Genome-wide association study identifies novel loci predisposing to cutaneous melanoma. *Hum. Mol. Genet.* **2011**, *20*, 5012–5023. [CrossRef] [PubMed]
15. Nguyen, V.T.; Ndoye, A.; Grando, S.A. Pemphigus vulgaris antibody identifies pemphaxin. A novel keratinocyte annexin-like molecule binding acetylcholine. *J. Biol. Chem.* **2000**, *275*, 29466–29476. [CrossRef] [PubMed]
16. Boczonadi, V.; Määttä, A. Annexin A9 is a periplakin interacting partner in membrane-targeted cytoskeletal linker protein complexes. *FEBS Lett.* **2012**, *586*, 3090–3096. [CrossRef] [PubMed]
17. Shimizu, T.; Kasamatsu, A.; Yamamoto, A.; Koike, K.; Ishige, S.; Takatori, H.; Sakamoto, Y.; Ogawara, K.; Shiiba, M.; Tanzawa, H.; et al. Annexin A10 in Human Oral Cancer: Biomarker for Tumoral Growth via G1/S Transition by Targeting MAPK Signaling Pathways. *PLoS ONE* **2012**, *7*, e45510. [CrossRef]

18. Rodrigo, J.P.; Heideman, D.A.; García-Pedrero, J.M.; Fresno, M.F.; Brakenhoff, R.H.; Díaz Molina, J.P.; Snijders, P.J.; Hermsen, M.A. Time trends in the prevalence of HPV in oropharyngeal squamous cell carcinomas in northern Spain (1990–2009). *Int. J. Cancer* **2014**, *134*, 487–492. [CrossRef]
19. Rodrigo, J.P.; Hermsen, M.A.; Fresno, M.F.; Brakenhoff, R.H.; García-Velasco, F.; Snijders, P.J.; Heideman, D.A.; García-Pedrero, J.M. Prevalence of human papillomavirus in laryngeal and hypopharyngeal squamous cell carcinomas in northern Spain. *Cancer Epidemiol.* **2015**, *39*, 37–41. [CrossRef]
20. Menéndez, S.T.; Rodrigo, J.P.; Alvarez-Teijeiro, S.; Villaronga, M.Á.; Allonca, E.; Vallina, A.; Astudillo, A.; Barros, F.; Suárez, C.; García-Pedrero, J.M. Role of HERG1 potassium channel in both malignant transformation and disease progression in head and neck carcinomas. *Mod. Pathol.* **2012**, *25*, 1069–1078. [CrossRef]
21. Rodrigo, J.P.; Menéndez, S.T.; Hermida-Prado, F.; Álvarez-Teijeiro, S.; Villaronga, M.Á.; Alonso-Durán, L.; Vallina, A.; Martínez-Camblor, P.; Astudillo, A.; Suárez, C.; et al. Clinical significance of Anoctamin-1 gene at 11q13 in the development and progression of head and neck squamous cell carcinomas. *Sci. Rep.* **2015**, *5*, 15698. [CrossRef] [PubMed]
22. Cancer Genome Atlas Network. Comprehensive genomic characterization of head and neck squamous cell carcinomas. *Nature* **2015**, *517*, 576–582. [CrossRef]
23. Cerami, E.; Gao, J.; Dogrusoz, U.; Gross, B.E.; Sumer, S.O.; Aksoy, B.A.; Jacobsen, A.; Byrne, C.J.; Heuer, M.L.; Larsson, E.; et al. The cBio cancer genomics portal: An open platform for exploring multidimensional cancer genomics data. *Cancer Discov.* **2012**, *2*, 401–404. [CrossRef] [PubMed]
24. Chandrashekar, D.S.; Bashel, B.; Balasubramanya, S.A.H.; Creighton, C.J.; Rodriguez, I.P.; Chakravarthi, B.V.S.K.; Varambally, S. UALCAN: A portal for facilitating tumor subgroup gene expression and survival analyses. *Neoplasia* **2017**, *19*, 649–658. [CrossRef] [PubMed]
25. Fatimathas, L.; Moss, S.E. Annexins as disease modifiers. *Histol. Histopathol.* **2010**, *25*, 527–532. [CrossRef] [PubMed]
26. Goebeler, V.; Ruhe, D.; Gerke, V.; Rescher, U. Atypical properties displayed by annexin A9; a novel member of the annexin family of $Ca^{2+}$ and lipid binding proteins. *FEBS Lett.* **2003**, *546*, 359–364. [CrossRef]
27. Morgan, R.O.; Martin-Almedina, S.; Iglesias, J.M.; Gonzalez-Florez, M.I.; Fernandez, M.P. Evolutionary perspective on annexin calcium-binding domains. *Biochim. Biophys. Acta* **2004**, *1742*, 133–140. [CrossRef]
28. Garcia-Pedrero, J.M.; Fernandez, M.P.; Morgan, R.O.; Herrero Zapatero, A.; Gonzalez, M.V.; Suarez Nieto, C.; Rodrigo, J.P. Annexin A1 down-regulation in head and neck cancer is associated with epithelial differentiation status. *Am. J. Pathol.* **2004**, *164*, 73–79. [CrossRef]
29. Álvarez-Teijeiro, S.; Menéndez, S.T.; Villaronga, M.A.; Pena-Alonso, E.; Rodrigo, J.P.; Morgan, R.O.; Granda-Díaz, R.; Salom, C.; Fernandez, M.P.; García-Pedrero, J.M. Annexin A1 down-regulation in head and neck squamous cell carcinoma is mediated via transcriptional control with direct involvement of miR-196a/b. *Sci. Rep.* **2017**, *7*, 67–90. [CrossRef]
30. Pena-Alonso, E.; Rodrigo, J.P.; Parra, I.C.; Pedrero, J.M.; Meana, M.V.; Nieto, C.S.; Fresno, M.F.; Morgan, R.O.; Fernandez, M.P. Annexin A2 localizes to the basal epithelial layer and is down-regulated in dysplasia and head and neck squamous cell carcinoma. *Cancer Lett.* **2008**, *263*, 89–98. [CrossRef]
31. Smid, M.; Wang, Y.; Klijn, J.G.; Sieuwerts, A.M.; Zhang, Y.; Atkins, D.; Martens, J.W.; Foekens, J.A. Genes associated with breast cancer metastatic to bone. *J. Clin. Oncol.* **2006**, *24*, 2261–2267. [CrossRef]
32. Miyoshi, N.; Yamamoto, H.; Mimori, K.; Yamashita, S.; Miyazaki, S.; Nakagawa, S.; Ishii, H.; Noura, S.; Ohue, M.; Yano, M.; et al. Anxa9 gene expression in colorectal cancer: A novel marker for prognosis. *Oncol. Lett.* **2014**, *8*, 2313–2317. [CrossRef] [PubMed]
33. Kim, J.H.; Rhee, Y.Y.; Kim, K.J.; Cho, N.Y.; Lee, H.S.; Kang, G.H. Annexin A10 expression correlates with serrated pathway features in colorectal carcinoma with microsatellite instability. *Apmis* **2014**, *122*, 1187–1195. [CrossRef] [PubMed]
34. Liu, S.H.; Lin, C.Y.; Peng, S.Y.; Jeng, Y.M.; Pan, H.W.; Lai, P.L.; Liu, C.L.; Hsu, H.C. Down-regulation of annexin A10 in hepatocellular carcinoma is associated with vascular invasion; early recurrence; and poor prognosis in synergy with p53 mutation. *Am. J. Pathol.* **2002**, *160*, 1831–1837. [CrossRef]
35. Peng, S.Y.; Ou, Y.H.; Chen, W.J.; Li, H.Y.; Liu, S.H.; Pan, H.W.; Lai, P.L.; Jeng, Y.M.; Chen, D.C.; Hsu, H.C. Aberrant expressions of annexin A10 short isoform; osteopontin and alpha-fetoprotein at chromosome 4q cooperatively contribute to progression and poor prognosis of hepatocellular carcinoma. *Int. J. Oncol.* **2005**, *26*, 1053–1061. [PubMed]

36. Kim, J.K.; Kim, P.J.; Jung, K.H.; Noh, J.H.; Eun, J.W.; Bae, H.J.; Xie, H.J.; Shan, J.M.; Ping, W.Y.; Park, W.S.; et al. Decreased expression of annexin A10 in gastric cancer and its overexpression in tumor cell growth suppression. *Oncol. Rep.* **2010**, *24*, 607–612. [CrossRef] [PubMed]
37. Munksgaard, P.P.; Mansilla, F.; Brems Eskildsen, A.S.; Fristrup, N.; Birkenkamp-Demtröder, K.; Ulhøi, B.P.; Borre, M.; Agerbæk, M.; Hermann, G.G.; Orntoft, T.F.; et al. Low ANXA10 expression is associated with disease aggressiveness in bladder cancer. *Br. J. Cancer* **2011**, *105*, 1379–1387. [CrossRef] [PubMed]
38. Sajanti, S.A.; Väyrynen, J.P.; Sirniö, P.; Klintrup, K.; Mäkelä, J.; Tuomisto, A.; Mäkinen, M.J. Annexin A10 is a marker for the serrated pathway of colorectal carcinoma. *Virchows Arch.* **2015**, *466*, 5–12. [CrossRef] [PubMed]

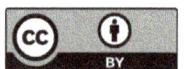

© 2019 by the authors. Licensee MDPI, Basel, Switzerland. This article is an open access article distributed under the terms and conditions of the Creative Commons Attribution (CC BY) license (http://creativecommons.org/licenses/by/4.0/).

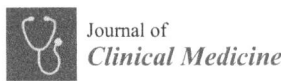 

Article

# Involvement of HPV Infection in the Release of Macrophage Migration Inhibitory Factor in Head and Neck Squamous Cell Carcinoma

Nadège Kindt [1], Géraldine Descamps [1], Jérôme R. Lechien [2], Myriam Remmelink [3], Jean-Marie Colet [4], Ruddy Wattiez [5], Guy Berchem [6], Fabrice Journe [1,7] and Sven Saussez [1,2,*]

[1] Department of Human Anatomy and Experimental Oncology, Université de Mons (UMons), Research Institute for Health Sciences and Technology, 7000 Mons, Belgium; nadege.kindt@umons.ac.be (N.K.); geraldine.descamps@umons.ac.be (G.D.); fabrice.journe@umons.ac.be (F.J.)
[2] Department of Oto-Rhino-Laryngology, Université Libre de Bruxelles (ULB), CHU Saint-Pierre, 1000 Brussels, Belgium; jerome.lechien@umons.ac.be
[3] Department of Pathology, Université Libre de Bruxelles (ULB), Erasme Hospital, 1070 Brussels, Belgium; myriam.remmelink@erasme.ulb.ac.be
[4] Department of Human Biology & Toxicology, Université de Mons (UMons), Research Institute for Health Sciences and Technology, 7000 Mons, Belgium; jean-marie.colet@umons.ac.be
[5] Laboratory of Proteomics and Microbiology, Research Institute for Biosciences, Université de Mons (UMons), 7000 Mons, Belgium; ruddy.wattiez@umons.ac.be
[6] Laboratory of Experimental Cancer Research, Luxembourg Institute of Health (LIH), 1526 Luxembourg, Luxembourg; guy.berchem@lih.lu
[7] Laboratory of Oncology and Experimental Surgery, Institut Jules Bordet, Université Libre de Bruxelles (ULB), 1000 Brussels, Belgium
* Correspondence: sven.saussez@umons.ac.be; Tel.: +32-6537-3556

Received: 5 December 2018; Accepted: 6 January 2019; Published: 10 January 2019

**Abstract:** Human papilloma virus (HPV) infection has been well-established as a risk factor in head and neck squamous cell carcinoma (HNSCC). The carcinogenic effect of HPV is mainly due to the E6 and E7 oncoproteins, which inhibit the functions of p53 and pRB, respectively. These oncoproteins could also play a role in the Warburg effect, thus favoring tumor immune escape. Here, we demonstrated that the pro-inflammatory cytokine macrophage migration inhibitory factor (MIF) is expressed at higher levels in HPV-negative patients than in HPV-positive patients. However, the secretion of MIF is higher in HPV-positive human HNSCC cell lines, than in HPV-negative cell lines. In-HPV positive cells, the half inhibitory concentration ($IC_{50}$) of MIF inhibitor (4-iodo-6-phenylpyrimidine (4-IPP)) is higher than that in HPV-negative cells. This result was confirmed in vitro and in vivo by the use of murine SCCVII cell lines expressing either E6 or E7, or both E6 and E7. Finally, to examine the mechanism of MIF secretion, we conducted proton nuclear magnetic resonance ($^1$H-NMR) experiments, and observed that lactate production is increased in both the intracellular and conditioned media of HPV-positive cells. In conclusion, our data suggest that the stimulation of enzymes participating in the Warburg effect by E6 and E7 oncoproteins increases lactate production and hypoxia inducible factor 1α (HIF-1α) expression, and finally induces MIF secretion.

**Keywords:** HNSCC; HPV; MIF; 4-IPP; metabolism

## 1. Introduction

Head and neck squamous cell carcinomas (HNSCC) are frequent in both men and women worldwide, with approximately 550,000 new cases annually [1]. It has long been recognized that tobacco and alcohol are the two main risk factors for these cancers, but a few years ago, human papilloma virus (HPV) was identified as an additional contributor leading to the development of a new subgroup of HNSCC, mainly associated with HPV-16 and HPV-18 types [2,3]. The impact of HPV infection remains controversial concerning the prognostic values of HNSCC, but recent studies put to light a new blood test that contributes to the detection of circulating tumor HPV DNA (notably HPV-16) and that can predict cancer recurrence [4,5]. It should be noted that differences throughout the world; for example, the prevalence of HPV-16 infection in oropharyngeal cancer, is nearly 60% in North America, whereas it is approximately 30% in Europe (Samples from Germany, United Kingdom and Italy) [6]. However, in the county of Stockholm, researchers have observed an increase of HPV prevalence in tonsil carcinoma by over 90% of cases until 2006 and 2007 [7]. Moreover, a large amount of evidence supports the idea that two HPV-positive cancer subpopulations may be distinguished. The first population is mainly composed of younger adults, primarily Caucasians and nonsmokers, with a favorable prognosis; while the second group includes patients who smoke and use alcohol, and these patients have a poorer prognosis [6,8–10].

Macrophage migration inhibitory factor (MIF) is an ubiquitous pro-inflammatory cytokine discovered in 1966 by Bloom and Bennett [11]. This cytokine has been investigated in many clinical and experimental studies in both inflammatory diseases and cancer. Indeed, MIF is involved in cancer progression through different pathways leading to cell proliferation, cell invasion, angiogenesis and tumor immune escape [12]. Implications for MIF in HNSCC have already been reported in several studies, which have established that MIF leads to cancer progression and poorer prognosis, notably in laryngeal carcinoma [13]. Indeed, our previous study has shown that mice that receive a murine squamous carcinoma cells underexpressing MIF and are treated with cisplatin or 5-fluouracil have a better prognosis than mice receiving control cells [13].

The objective of our research is to assess MIF production in HNSCC regarding HPV infection. Indeed, MIF regulation has been studied in several virus-induced cancers, but it has never been examined in HPV-infected carcinomas. Thus, we have evaluated MIF expression in a series of 156 clinical samples including oral cavity and oropharyngeal carcinomas. Moreover, MIF secretion was investigated in vitro and in vivo by using three HPV-negative and three HPV-positive HNSCC human cell lines, as well as murine SCCVII cell lines expressing the E6 and/or E7 HPV oncoproteins. Finally, proton nuclear magnetic resonance ($^1$H-NMR) experiments were conducted to examine the mechanism involved in HPV-dependent MIF secretion in HNSCC.

## 2. Materials and Methods

### 2.1. Clinical Characteristics

Formalin-fixed paraffin-embedded oral cavity and oropharyngeal cancer specimens were obtained from 156 patients who underwent curative surgery at Saint-Pierre Hospital (Brussels, Belgium), EpiCURA Baudour Hospital (Baudour, Belgium) and Erasme hospital (Brussels, Belgium) during the years from 1996–2008. The clinical characteristics of the patients are outlined in Tables 1 and 2, which presents information concerning the patients' age, gender, tumor localization, tumor histopathological grade, Tumor Node Metastasis (TNM) stage, risk factors, tumor recurrence, and clinical follow-up. This retrospective study was approved by the Institutional Review Board of Jules Bordet Institute (CE2319). All patients included in this study have received information regarding the use of residual human corporal materials for clinical research, and written informed consent was obtained from the patients.

### 2.2. DNA Extraction

The formalin-fixed, paraffin-embedded tissue samples were sectioned, deparaffinized, and digested with proteinase K by overnight incubation at 56 °C. DNA was purified using a QIAamp DNA Mini Kit (Qiagen, Benelux, Belgium), as previously described [14].

## 2.3. Detection of HPV by Polymerase Chain Reaction (PCR) Amplification

HPV DNA detection was performed using PCR with GP5+/GP6+ primers (synthesized by Eurogentec, Liege, Belgium) that amplified a consensus region located within the L1 region of the HPV genome, as previously described [14].

## 2.4. Real-time PCR Amplification of HPV Type-Specific DNA

All DNA extracts were tested for the presence of 18 different HPV genotypes using TaqMan-based real-time quantitative PCR that targeted type-specific sequences of the viral genes, as previously described [14].

## 2.5. RNA Extraction

After five days of cell culture, total RNA was collected in RLT buffer supplemented with β-mercaptoethanol (RNeasy Mini Kit, Qiagen, Venlo, The Netherlands) at 4 °C, and the sample were then centrifuged in RNeasy spin columns. After the wash steps, RNA was collected in RNase-free water, and subjected to DNase treatment as described by the manufacturer. The RNA concentration was evaluated using a NanoDropTM 1000 spectrophotometer (Thermo Scientific, Wilmington, DE, USA). RNA quality was assessed, based on the RNA profile generated by a Bioanalyzer 2100 (Agilent Technologies, Santa Clara, CA, USA).

## 2.6. Real-Time PCR for MIF mRNA Quantification

MIF mRNA expression was quantified by real-time PCR. Complementary DNA (cDNA) was synthesized using a standard reverse transcription method (qScript cDNA SuperMix, Quanta Biosciences, Gaithersburg, MD, USA). Real-time PCR reactions were performed using the SYBR Green PCR Master Mix (Applied Biosystems, Foster City, CA, USA) and sequence-specific primer sets designed with PrimerBank [15] for MIF (forward: 5'-GCAGAACCGCTCCTACAGCA-3', reverse: 5'-GGCTCTTAGGCGAAGGTGGA-3) and for 18S (forward: 5'-GCGGCGGAAAATAGCCTTTG-3', reverse: 5'-GATCACACGTTCCACCTCATC-3') (Life Technologies, Ghent, Belgium). The amplification was performed on a LightCycler 480 System (Roche Diagnostics GmbH, Mannheim, Germany) using an initial activation step (95 °C for 10 min) followed by 40 cycles of amplification (95 °C for 15 s and 60 °C for 60 s). Melting curves from 60 °C to 99 °C were assessed to evaluate PCR specificity. A preliminary analysis demonstrated linear and similar amplification efficacies. Relative quantification was determined by normalizing the cycle threshold (CT) of MIF with the CT of β-actin (loading control) using the $2-\Delta CT$ method.

## 2.7. Immunohistochemistry of p16

Each HPV-positive case was further immunohistochemically evaluated for p16 expression, using the recommended mouse monoclonal antibody (CINtec p16, Ventana, Tucson, USA) [16], and an automated immunostaining protocol (Bond-Max, Leica Microsystems, Wetzlar, Germany). Immunohistochemistry was performed as previously described [9].

## 2.8. Immunohistochemistry for MIF Protein Detection

MIF expression was detected by immunohistochemistry in tumor samples, and was performed on paraffin-embedded sections, as previously detailed [17].

## 2.9. Computer-Assisted Morphometry

A morphological examination of immunostained tissue sections was carried out on a Zeiss Axioplan microscope equipped with a color change-couple device (CCD) camera (ProgRes C10plus, Jenoptik, Jena, Germany). Morphometric analysis was performed using KS 400 imaging software (Carl Zeiss Vision, Hallbergmoos, Germany), as described previously [13].

## 2.10. LC MS/MS Analysis and Data Processing

Protein identification and quantification were performed using a label-free strategy on an UHPLC-HRMS platform (Eksigent 2D Ultra and AB SCIEX TripleTOF 5600). The peptides (2 μg) were separated on a 25 cm C18 column (Acclaim PepMap100, 3 μm, Dionex, Thermo Scientific, Wilmington, DE, USA) using a linear gradient (5–35% over 120 min) of acetonitrile (ACN) in water containing 0.1% formic acid at a flow rate of 300 nL min$^{-1}$. To obtain the highest possible retention time stability, which is required for label-free quantification, the column was equilibrated with a 10× volume of 5% ACN before each injection. Mass spectra (MS) were acquired across a 400–1500 m/z range in high-resolution mode with a 500 ms accumulation time. The precursor selection parameters were as follows: 200 cps intensity threshold, 50 precursor maximum per cycle, 50 ms accumulation time, and 15 s exclusion after one spectrum. These parameters led to a duty cycle of 3 s per cycle, ensuring that high-quality extracted ion chromatograms (XICs) were obtained for peptide quantification.

ProteinPilot Software (v4.1) was used to conduct a database search against the UniProt Trembl database (09/30/2011 version), which was restricted to Homo sapiens entries. The search parameters included differential amino acid mass shifts for carbamidomethyl cysteine, all biological modifications, amino acid substitutions, and missed trypsin cleavage.

For peptide quantification, PeakView was used to construct XICs for the top five peptides of each protein identified with a false discovery rate (FDR) of lower than 1%. Only unmodified and unshared peptides were used for quantification. Peptides were also excluded if their identification confidence as determined by ProteinPilot was below 0.99. A retention time window of 2 min, and a mass tolerance of 0.015 m/z were used. The calculated XICs were exported into MarkerView, and signals were normalized based on the summed area of the entire run. Only proteins presenting a fold-change of greater than/less than 1.5/0.6 with a p-value lower than 0.05 across the three biological replicates analyzed were accounted for in the metabolic characterization. Fold-changes were assessed by using a Student's t-test. Finally, proteins identified by one peptide were validated manually.

## 2.11. Cell Culture

UPCI-SCC-131, Detroit 562, UPCI-SCC-90, and UPCI-SCC-154 (DSMZ, Braunschweig, Germany) cell lines were grown in minimum essential medium (MEM, Gibco Life Technologies, Paisley, UK) supplemented with 10% fetal bovine serum, 2 mM L-glutamine, 1% penicillin/streptomycin, and 1% nonessential amino acids (Gibco Life Technologies, Paisley, UK). The FaDU and 93VU-147T cell lines were grown in Dulbecco's modified Eagle medium (DMEM, Lonza, Verviers, Belgium) supplemented with 10% fetal bovine serum (FBS), 2% L-glutamine, and 1% penicillin/streptomycin. The 93VU-174T cell line was obtained from Dr. de Winter (University Medical Center of Amsterdam, Amsterdam, The Netherlands).

Mouse SCCVII cells were transfected with three different vectors, to express either the HPV oncoproteins E6 or E7, or both E6 and E7 in the Radiation Oncology Department at the Université Catholique de Louvain (Prof. Vincent Grégoire), as previously described [18]. Cells were cultured in T-flasks containing minimum essential medium (MEM) supplemented with 10% FBS, 2 mM L-glutamine, 1% antibiotic/antimycotic mix, and 1% nonessential amino acids (Gibco Life Technologies, Paisley, UK).

A MIF knockdown (MIF-KD) cell line derived from SCCVII, as well as a matched control with normal MIF expression, was generated in the Department of Pediatrics at the Medical College of Wisconsin (Dr. Bryon Johnson). Knock-down of MIF expression in the SCCVII cell line was achieved by using the BLOCK-iT Lentiviral RNAi from Invitrogen (Thermo Scientific, Carlsbad, CA, USA), following a procedure detailed in a previous publication [19]. Cells were cultured as described previously [13].

Routine cell culture was carried out at 37 °C in a humidified cell incubator at 5% $CO_2$.

For the hypoxic condition, human HPV-negative and HPV-positive cell lines were maintained in a hypoxia chamber (InvivO2 400 Hypoxia Workstation, Ruskinn) in a humidified atmosphere containing 5% $CO_2$ and 0.1% $O_2$ at 37 °C for 48 h.

## 2.12. MIF Inhibitor

The MIF inhibitor 4-iodo-6-phenylpyrimidine (4-IPP) was purchased from Tocris Bioscience (Bristol, UK). Stock solutions of the compound were prepared in ethanol, stored at −20 °C, and used within one month.

## 2.13. Determination of MIF Concentrations

Concentrations of MIF in serum and conditioned medium were assayed by a sandwich enzyme-linked immunosorbent assay (ELISA) using a commercial kit (DuoSet ELISA Development kit, R&D Systems, Minneapolis, MN, USA). The assays were carried out according to the instructions provided by the supplier. MIF concentrations in samples of serum and conditioned medium were determined by interpolation from a reference curve established from increasing concentrations of recombinant human or mouse MIF.

## 2.14. IC50 Determination for the MIF Inhibitor by a Crystal Violet Stain Assay

Cells were seeded in 96-well plates. The following day, cells were fed fresh medium (DMEM or MEM, 10% FBS) with or without 4-IPP. After a 3-day exposure, the culture medium was discarded, and cells were fixed with 1% glutaraldehyde. Following fixation, cells were stained with 1% crystal violet. Destaining was performed under gently running tap water, and cell monolayers were lysed in 0.2% Triton X-100. The absorbance of cell lysates was measured at 570 nm using a LabSystems Multiskan MS microplate reader (ThermoScientific, Pittsburgh, PA, USA).

## 2.15. Western Blotting for the Evaluation of HIF-1α and MIF Expression

Human HPV-positive and HPV-negative cell lines and SCCVII CT, E6, E7, and E6/E7 murine cell lines were plated in Petri dishes, cultured for five days, and lysed using detergent solution (RIPA buffer) supplemented with protease and phosphatase inhibitors (All reagents from Pierce, Thermo Scientific, Pierce, Washington, USA). Protein concentrations were determined by a BCA protein assay (Pierce) using bovine serum albumin as the standard. Extracted proteins (40 µg) were loaded on 4–20% Mini-PROTEAN TGX gels (SDS) (Bio-Rad Laboratories, München, Germany) and were electrotransferred onto nitrocellulose membranes (iBlot®Dry Blotting System, Life Technologies-Invitrogen, Ghent, Belgium). Immunodetection was performed using an anti-HIF-1α antibody (1/600), an anti-MIF antibody (1/500), and an anti-actin antibody (1/500) (Pierce). A peroxidase-labeled anti-rabbit IgG antibody (1/5000) (Amersham Pharmacia Biotech, Roosendaal, The Netherlands) was used as the secondary antibody. Bound peroxidase activity was detected using the SuperSignal®West Pico Chemiluminescent Substrate (Pierce) following the manufacturer's instructions. The bands were visualized by exposing the membranes to photosensitive film (Hyperfilm ECL, Amersham Pharmacia Biotech). Bands intensities were quantified using ImageJTM software (a public domain image software developed by W. Rasband at the Research Services Branch of the National Institute of Mental Health, NIH, Bethesda, MD, USA).

## 2.16. Animal Study

Experiments were conducted on 40 female C3H/HeN mice (Charles River Laboratory, L'Arbresle, France). The animals were maintained and handled in compliance with the guidelines issued by the Belgian Ministry of Trade and Agriculture. SCCVII cells transfected with vectors expressing E6/E7 or with control vector (CT) were inoculated in the mylohyoid muscle following a procedure detailed in a previous publication [18]. Animals were checked for tumor onset, and were euthanized when they exhibited either a tumor diameter exceeding 15 mm, or a weight loss of more than 20%. Postmortem, blood samples were collected and processed for serum.

## 2.17. Cell Sample Preparation for NMR Analysis

Cells of each human cell line were seeded in six 150 mm cell culture dishes, and were maintained in complete MEM. After four days, the medium was replaced by MEM without FBS. After 48 h, the medium was harvested, centrifuged for 10 min at 1200 rpm and stored at −80 °C until NMR analysis. Then, the cells were washed twice with ice-cold Dubelcco's Phosphate Buffer Saline (DPBS). Then the cells were quenched using 3 mL of cold methanol, detached using a cell scraper and pipetted into a 15 mL centrifuge tube to which 702 µL of ice-cold distilled water was added. All cell extracts were vortexed and suspended in a solution of chloroform/methanol/water in a ratio of 4:3:2. After centrifugation for 30 min at 15000 g, the upper aqueous layer was extracted and used for further analysis; the organic phase was discarded. The aqueous phases from the samples were dried at 25 °C using a centrifugal vacuum concentrator (Eppendorf) and stored at −80 °C until NMR analysis.

## 2.18. H-NMR Sample Preparation and Spectroscopy

A total of 700 µL and 250 µL of phosphate buffer (0.04M $NaH_2PO_4$ and 0.2M $Na_2HPO_4$, pH 7.4) was added to dried samples and to 500 µL of media, respectively. Samples were then centrifuged for 10 min at 13,000 g, and 650 µL of each sample was transferred to a 5 mm NMR tube, to which 50 µL of 3.5 mM 3-(trimethylsilyl)-propionic-2,2,3,3-d4 acid (TSP) prepared in 100% $D_2O$, was added. The samples were analyzed on a Bruker Avance 500 spectrometer (11.8 T) operating at 500 MHz for proton observation with a 5 mm BBI 1H/D-probe. A one-dimensional spectrum was acquired at 297 °K, using a 1D-NOESY PRESAT pulse sequence. For each samples, 256 free induction decays (FID) were collected using a spectral width of 10,330.578 Hz, an acquisition time of 2.65 s, and a pulse recycle delay of 3 s. After 1H-NMR acquisition, the FID signal was imported into MestReNova 10.0 software (Mestrelab Research, Santiago de Compostela, Spain) for Fourier transformation. Then, the spectra were automatically phased and baseline-corrected, and calibrated against TSP. The resonance of the methyl groups in TSP was arbitrarily set to 0.00 ppm. The spectral region from 0.08–10.00 ppm was automatically reduced to 496 integrated regions (bins) of 0.02 ppm width each. The regions from 4.50–5.20 ppm containing the residual water signal were removed. Each integrated region was normalized to the total spectral area.

The integrated reduced data were imported into SIMCA-P+12 (Umetrics, Umea, Sweden) for PLS-DA. For the quantification of lactate, the resonance with the higher resolution was selected and fitted. An area under the curve (AUC) in arbitrary units was obtained (MestReNova software). This method allowed for statistical comparison between the cell lines.

## 2.19. Statistical Analyses

SigmaPlot® 11 software was used for statistical analyses. Parametric analyses were conducted with the Student's t-test or with analysis of variance for comparison among more than two groups, and pairwise comparisons were performed using the Holm–Sidak method. Nonparametric analyses were performed with the Mann-Whitney U test (two groups). A $p \leq 0.05$ was considered to indicate a statistically significant difference.

## 3. Results

### 3.1. Tissue MIF Expression is Decreased in the Oral Cavity and in Oropharyngeal Carcinomas Infected with HPV

The immunohistochemical staining of MIF was examined in two series of 117 cases of oral cavity, and 39 cases of oropharyngeal carcinomas. We did not find statistical correlations between MIF expression and age, gender, tumor localization, histological grade, tumor stage or alcohol and tobacco consumption in these series (Tables 1 and 2). However, a staining intensity analysis demonstrated that oropharyngeal and oral cavity cancer tissues infected with transcriptionally active HPV (p16+) showed a decrease in MIF expression compared to oropharyngeal and oral cavity cancer tissues not infected by HPV (n = 21 and n = 65 respectively) (Figure 1, $p = 0.001$ and $p = 0.004$ respectively, Kruskal-Wallis test).

**Table 1.** Oropharyngeal cancer patients' characteristics.

|  | Number of Cases |
|---|---|
| **Age (years)** |  |
| Median | 57 |
| Range | 44–90 |
| **Gender** |  |
| Male | 31 |
| Female | 8 |
| **Localization** |  |
| Tonsils | 13 |
| Soft palate | 11 |
| Base of tongue | 6 |
| Posterior wall | 3 |
| Unknown | 6 |
| **Histological grade** |  |
| Well differentiated | 14 |
| Moderately differentiated | 12 |
| Poorly differentiated | 6 |
| Unknown | 7 |
| **TNM stage** |  |
| T1-2 | 19 |
| T3-4 | 10 |
| Unknown | 10 |
| **Risk factors** |  |
| *Alcohol* |  |
| Non-drinker | 3 |
| Drinker | 24 |
| Unknown | 12 |
| *Tobacco* |  |
| Non-smoker | 2 |
| Smoker | 25 |
| Unknown | 12 |
| *HPV status* |  |
| HPV−ve | 21 |
| HPV+ve/p16+ | 3 |
| HPV+ve/p16− | 10 |
| HPV+ve/p16 unknown | 5 |
| **Recurrence** |  |
| Yes | 15 |
| None | 15 |
| Unknown | 9 |
| **Clinical follow-up (months)** |  |
| Median | 33 |
| Range | 1–121 |

**Table 2.** Oral cavity cancer patients' characteristics.

|  | Number of Cases |
|---|---|
| **Age (years)** |  |
| Median | 58 |
| Range | 23–87 |
| **Gender** |  |
| Male | 97 |
| Female | 20 |
| **Localization** |  |
| Tongue | 27 |
| Floor of the mouth | 35 |
| Gingivae | 12 |
| Buccal mucosa | 7 |
| Retromolar trigone | 3 |
| Lips | 2 |
| Hard palate | 1 |
| Unknown | 30 |
| **Histological grade** |  |
| Well differentiated | 44 |
| Moderately differentiated | 53 |
| Poorly differentiated | 19 |
| Unknown | 1 |
| **TNM stage** |  |
| T1-2 | 79 |
| T3-4 | 31 |
| Unknown | 7 |
| **Risk factors** |  |
| *Alcohol* |  |
| Non-drinker | 47 |
| Drinker | 49 |
| Unknown | 21 |
| *Tobacco* |  |
| Non-smoker | 40 |
| Smoker | 57 |
| Unknown | 20 |
| *HPV status* |  |
| HPV−ve | 65 |
| HPV+ve/p16+ | 6 |
| HPV+ve/p16- | 42 |
| HPV+ve/p16 unknown | 4 |
| **Recurrence** |  |
| Yes | 44 |
| None | 59 |
| Unknown | 14 |
| **Clinical follow-up (months)** |  |
| Median | 32 |
| Range | 1–188 |

This result was confirmed by a previous proteomic analysis comparing HPV+ve versus HPV−ve tumors, which indicated that the MIF expression was two-fold lower in an HPV+ve oral cavity cancer tissue as compared to a HPV−ve oral cavity cancer tissue ($p = 0.016$, Student's *t*-test, data not shown).

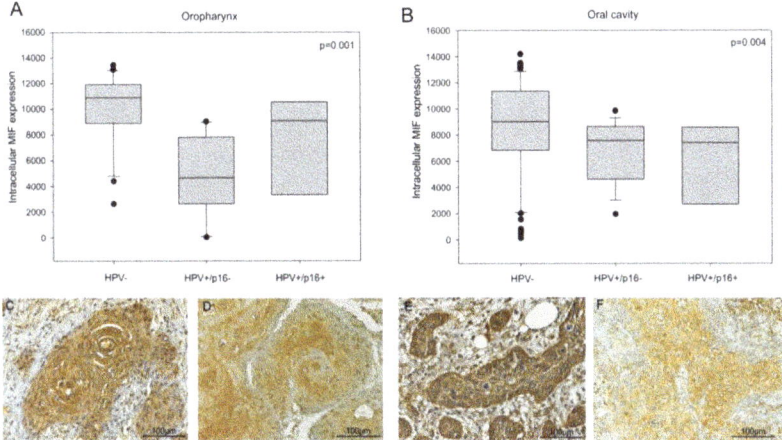

**Figure 1.** Intracellular migration inhibitory factor (MIF) expression in head and neck cancer patients. (**A**) Quantitative analysis of MIF expression in a series of 39 oropharyngeal cancer patients, including 21 Human Papilloma Virus negative (HPV-ve) cases and 18 HPV+ve cases ($p = 0.001$, Kruskal–Wallis test) and (**B**) 117 oral cavity cancer patients, including 65 HPV-ve cases and 52 HPV+ve cases ($p = 0.004$, Kruskal–Wallis test). (**C,D**) Immunohistochemistry of MIF in HPV-ve (**C**) and HPV+ve (**D**) oropharyngeal cancer cases and (**E,F**) in HPV-ve (**E**) and HPV+ve (**F**) oral cavity cancer cases.

## 3.2. MIF mRNA Synthesis and Protein Secretion is Increased in HPV-Infected Human Head and Neck Cancer Cell Lines

To evaluate the differential expression of MIF in HNSCC cells with regard to HPV status, we compared the MIF messenger RNA (mRNA) expression in three human HPV-negative (FaDu, UPCI-SCC-131 and Detroit 562) and three HPV-positive (UPCI-SCC090, UPCI-SCC154 and 93VU147T) cell lines. The quantitative analysis of the MIF mRNA expression by real-time PCR demonstrated that the MIF mRNA expression was three times greater in HPV-positive cell lines than in HPV-negative ones (Figure 2A, $p < 0.001$, Student's $t$-test), while the MIF protein expression was equally the same among all of the cell lines (Figure 2B).

Moreover, the concentration of MIF was examined in the culture supernatants of the HNSCC cell lines and the SCCVII MIF Knockdown (KD) and Scramble (sc). The conditioned medium from HPV-positive cell lines showed a significantly higher MIF level than the medium originating from HPV-negative cell lines (Figure 2C, $p = 0.04$, Student's $t$-test). As expected, the conditioned medium from SCCVII MIFKD exhibited a significantly lesser MIF level than the medium from SCCVII MIFsc cells (Figure 2E, $p = 0.045$, Student's $t$-test).

Finally, the use of 4-IPP, an inhibitor of MIF, in HPV-negative and HPV-positive HNSCC cell lines revealed that the concentrations required to achieve a 50% inhibition of cell proliferation were significantly higher in HPV-positive cell lines than in HPV-negative cell lines (Figure 2D, $p = 0.018$, Student's $t$-test). This result agrees with the observations that MIF was more highly secreted by HPV-positive cell lines and that higher concentrations of 4-IPP were required to block this higher level of MIF, and consequently to inhibit cell proliferation.

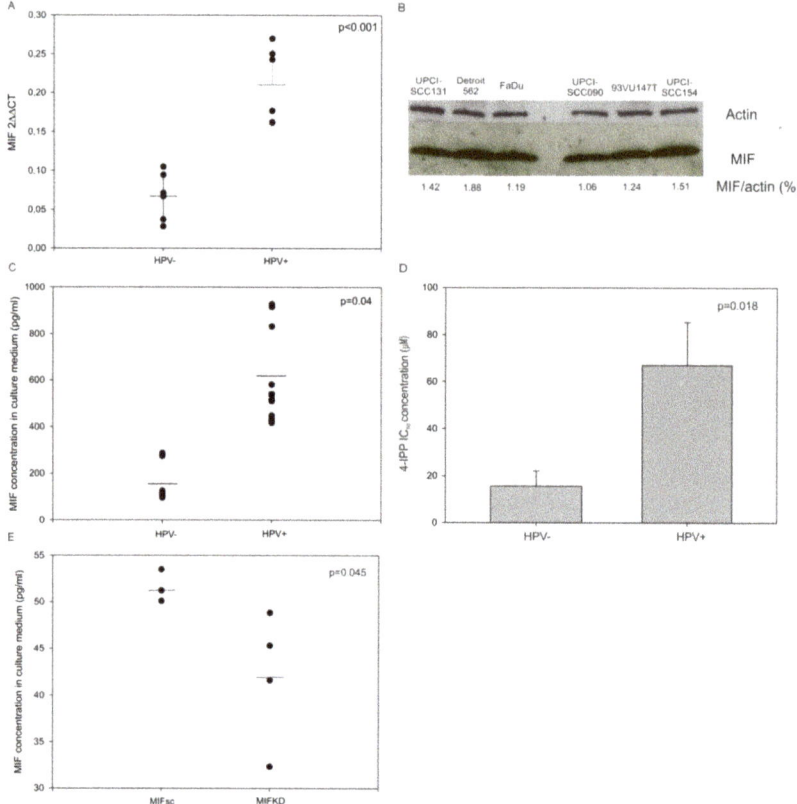

**Figure 2.** Relative MIF messenger RNA (mRNA), protein expression and macrophage migration inhibitory factor (MIF) concentration in culture medium from mouse and human culture cell lines and the response to MIF inhibitor. (**A**) Upregulation of MIF mRNA in human papilloma virus (HPV)-positive cell lines compared to the MIF expression in HPV-negative cell lines ($p < 0.001$, Student's $t$-test). (**B**) Western blot analysis showing the MIF expression in HPV-ve and +ve cell lines. (**C**) Increased MIF level in the culture medium of HPV+ve cells (n = 3) compared to the MIF level in the culture medium of HPV-ve cells (n = 3) ($p = 0.04$, Student's $t$-test). (**D**) Concentration of 4-iodo-6-phenylpyrimidine (4-IPP) required to achieve 50% inhibition of cell proliferation in human HPV-ve and HPV+ve cell lines ($p = 0.018$, Student's $t$-test). (**E**) Increased MIF levels in the culture medium of SCCVII MIFKD cells (n = 4) compared to the SCCVII MIFsc cells (n = 3) ($p = 0.045$, Student's $t$-test).

### 3.3. MIF Secretion is Increased in Murine Head and Neck Cancer Cell Lines Transfected with E6/E7 Oncoproteins In Vitro and In Vivo

To investigate the role of HPV oncoproteins in MIF secretion, we analyzed the concentrations of MIF in the cell culture medium of SCCVII CT, E6, E7, and E6/E7. This analysis showed that cells expressing HPV oncoproteins released more MIF than the control cells (Figure 3A, $p < 0.001$, one-way-analysis of variance (ANOVA) test). Furthermore, the murine SCCVII cell lines expressing the HPV oncoproteins E6 and/or E7 were exposed to 4-IPP for three days, to examine the resistance to 4-IPP, as measured by cell proliferation. The results showed that SCCVII E6, E7, and E6/E7 cells were all more resistant to the MIF inhibitor compared to the SCCVII CT cells, further demonstrating that E6 and E7 were involved in MIF secretion (Figure 3B, $p < 0.001$, one-way-ANOVA test). Finally, the in vitro data were validated using an orthotopic animal model to confirm that MIF was more highly secreted by cells expressing HPV oncoproteins. SCCVII E6/E7 or SCCVII CT cells were injected into the floor of the mouth of C3/Hen mice. As expected from in vitro data, mice receiving SCCVII E6/E7 cells presented higher serum MIF levels than mice receiving SCCVII CT cells (Figure 3C, $p = 0.013$, Mann-Whitney test).

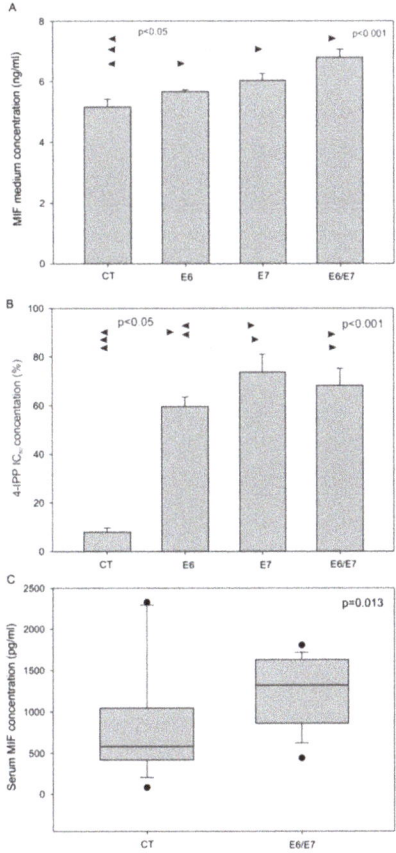

Figure 3. Macrophage migration inhibitory factor (MIF) secretion by murine cells in vitro and in vivo, and 4-IPP IC50 in murine cell lines. (A) Increase in the MIF concentration in the culture medium of SCCVII cells expressing HPV oncoproteins ($p <0.001$, one-way ANOVA). (B) Percentage of cell proliferation after exposure to 50 µM 4-iodo-6-phenylpyrimidine (4-IPP) in SCCVII CT, E6, E7 and E6/E7 cell lines ($p <0.001$, one-way ANOVA test). (C) Increase in the serum MIF levels of mice receiving SCCVII E6/E7 cells (n = 18), compared to the serum MIF levels of mice in the control group (CT) (n = 16) ($p = 0.013$, Mann–Whitney test).

### 3.4. Lactate Production and HIF-1α Expression are Increased in HPV-Positive Cell Lines

We hypothesized that MIF secretion may be affected by a Warburg effect involving E6 and E7 oncoproteins, as observed in lung cancer [20]. To assess this hypothesis, a nuclear magnetic resonance analysis was performed; the partial least-squares discriminant analysis (PLS-DA) allowed us to divide the HPV-positive cells from the HPV-negative ones (Figure 4A, CV-ANOVA, $p <0.001$). The loading plot showed that only lactate comes through the analysis (data not shown). Thus, we examined the lactate production in both the intracellular and extracellular compartments of HPV-negative and HPV-positive cells. The results displayed a significant increase in lactate production in the culture medium (Figure 4B, $p$ <0.001, Mann–Whitney test) as well as in the intracellular compartment (Figure 4C, $p$ = 0.024, Mann-Whitney test) of the HPV-positive cells compared to the lactate production in the culture medium and the intracellular compartment of the HPV-negative cells.

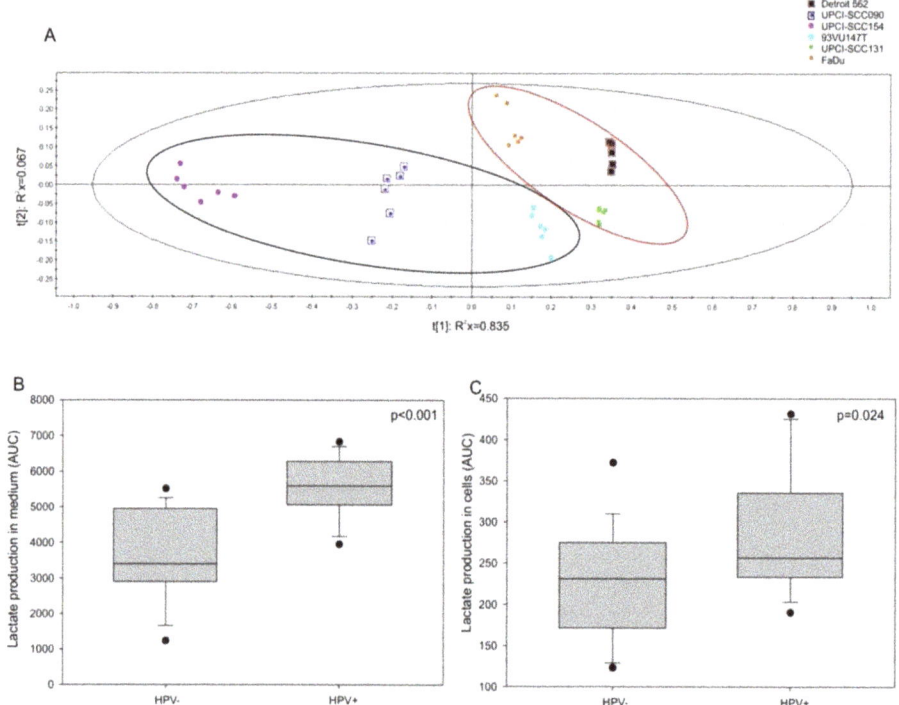

**Figure 4.** Lactate production in human cell lines. (**A**) Partial least-squares discriminant analysis (PLS-DA) for human papilloma virus (HPV)-positive and HPV-negative cell lines. Increase in lactate production in (**B**) the extracellular compartment ($p$ <0.001, Mann-Whitney test) and in (**C**) the intracellular compartment ($p$ = 0.024, Mann-Whitney test) of HPV-positive and HPV-negative cells.

Besides, it was reported that the induction of the Warburg effect by the HPV oncoproteins through the mTOR signaling pathway leads to the accumulation of HIF-1α [21]. To verify whether HPV oncoproteins play a role in the increase in HIF-1α in HNSCC, we analyzed HIF-1α expression by Western blotting in HPV-positive and HPV-negative human cell lines, as well as in SCCVII CT, E6, E7, and E6/E7 murine cell lines. The data in Figure 5A demonstrate that globally HPV-positive human cell lines and the SCCVII E6/E7 murine cell line expressed more HIF-1α than the HPV-negative human cell lines and the SCCVII CT murine cell line, respectively, under normoxic culture conditions. Additionally, under hypoxic conditions, which stimulate HIF-1α expression and activity, HPV-negative cell lines (FaDu, Detroit 562 and UPCI-SCC131) released more MIF in the culture medium (Figure 5B, $p$ <0.001, Student's $t$-test) than did the HPV-positive ones, thus demonstrating that the increase in HIF-1α led to the rise in MIF secretion. However, the data in Figure 5C show that, under hypoxia, HPV-positive cell lines (UPCI-SCC154, UPCI-SCC090 and 93VU147T) did not secrete significantly more MIF than they did under normoxia; this effect was potentially due to a high baseline level of HIF-1α expression and MIF secretion in these cells (Figure 5C, $p$ = N.S., Student's $t$-test).

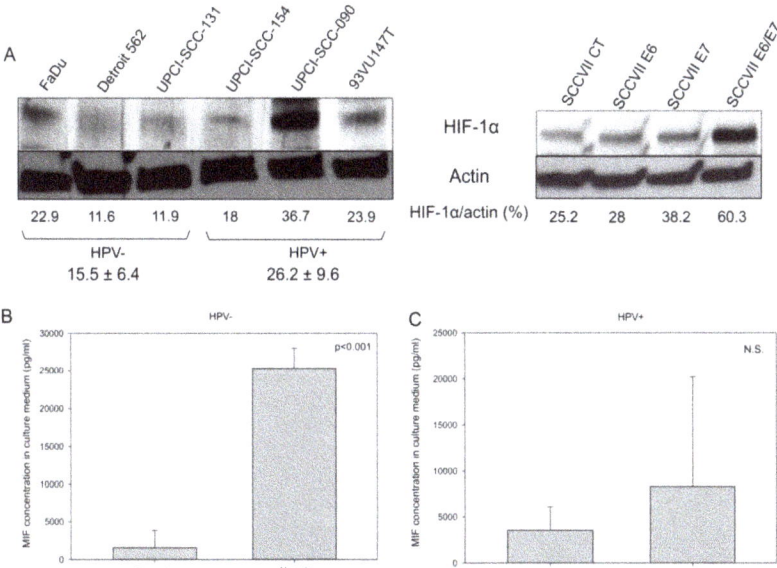

**Figure 5.** Hypoxia inducible factor 1α (HIF-1α) expression in human and murine cell lines. (**A**) Western blot analysis demonstrating the upregulation of HIF-1α in two human papilloma virus (HPV)-positive cell lines (UPCI-SCC-090 and 93VU147T) and in the murine SCCVII E6/E7 cell line. Concentration of macrophage migration inhibitory factor (MIF) in the culture medium of (**B**) human HPV-negative cell lines ($p <0.001$, Student's $t$-test), and (**C**) in human positive cell lines (N.S., Student's $t$-test) under normoxic and hypoxic conditions.

## 4. Discussion

As we have previously seen in oral carcinoma, there is no correlation between MIF expression and age, gender, tumor localization, histological grade, tumor stage, or alcohol and tobacco consumption [22]. So, MIF expression does not seem to correlate with these clinical characteristics. However, our data reports an important relationship between MIF secretion and HPV infection, an additional HNSCC risk factor.

HPV infection occurs more often in the oropharyngeal region of the head and neck, and a high proportion of infection are caused by HPV-16 type [6]. The oncoproteins E6 and E7 play a crucial role in the neoplastic transformation of host cells by inactivating p53 and pRb, respectively [23]. In this study, we have demonstrated that, under normoxic conditions, the E6/E7 oncoproteins enhance expression of HIF-1α in HNSCC cells, as it was also reported for human cervical carcinoma cells [24]. Our investigation also showed that HPV infection is conducive to an acidic environment, as evidenced by the increase in lactate production, both in the intracellular compartment and in the culture medium. In addition, we have observed, for the first time, that MIF expression decreased in the tumor cells of HNSCC patients with HPV infection, and that MIF secretion was increased in HPV-positive cell lines, an observation that we confirmed by demonstrating resistance to an inhibitor of MIF (4-IPP) in human cell lines that were infected with HPV, as well as in murine cell lines expressing the E6 and/or E7 oncoproteins. These data were further supported by the increase in the serum MIF in mice receiving the SCCVII E6/E7 cells. In view of these findings, we hypothesized that the acidic environment induced by HPV explains the increase in MIF secretion through the activation of HIF-1α. Consequently, the MIF mRNA level increases, as we have reported in human HPV-positive cell lines, thus leading to elevated protein synthesis and the secretion of MIF.

Other researchers have demonstrated that the E6 and E7 oncoproteins also take part in a perturbation of cellular metabolism termed the Warburg effect, which is a hallmark of cancer cells. Indeed, it was demonstrated that E6 interacts with the transcription factor HIF-1α to induce glycolysis under hypoxia [25]. Moreover, previous studies have shown that the E6 oncoprotein promotes the activity of the mammalian target of rapamycin (mTOR) signaling pathway, thus leading to the accumulation of HIF-1α, pyruvate kinase, lactate dehydrogenase, and pyruvate dehydrogenase kinase 1 [21]. The accumulation of these enzymes induces the Warburg effect by increasing the rate of glycolysis and the production of lactate. It was also reported that the E7 oncoprotein induces the acetylation of the pyruvate kinase M2 isoform (PKM2), thus promoting the dimeric form of PKM2, which leads to the conversion of pyruvate to lactate through lactate dehydrogenase (LDHA) [26].

Furthermore, the high-risk HPV E2 protein, which facilitates the integration of the HPV genome into the host cell genome, could also interact with mitochondrial membranes, thus leading to the production of reactive oxygen species (ROS). This ROS generation correlates with HIF-1α upregulation and lactate production [27]. In contrast, keratinocytes infected with HPV-16 exhibit an increase in monocarboxylate transporter 4 (MCT-4) [28], which is known to participate in lactate export from stromal cells, releasing lactate into the microenvironment and favoring a reverse-Warburg effect for cancer cells. All of these observations established that HPV infection leads to an acidification of the microenvironment. These phenomena may be illustrated by the observations that MIF secretion increased after ROS production, as was demonstrated in clear cell renal cell carcinoma, breast cancer, and lung cancer [29]. Additionally, it is well-known that HIF-1α increases the expression of MIF. Conversely, MIF protects HIF-1α from proteasomal degradation in cancer cells [30–32]. However, the mechanism of MIF secretion remains unknown, and it needs further investigation.

The production of lactate and MIF by cancer cells infected with HPV could partly explain why such cells are poorly immunogenic. Indeed, some studies have demonstrated that HPV-positive tumors contain a low number of tumor-associated immune cells, such as Langerhans cells and cytotoxic T cells, while they recruit high levels of regulatory T lymphocytes [18,33–35]. In addition, lactate production induces the recruitment of immunosuppressive cells such as tumor-associated macrophages (TAMs) and myeloid-derived suppressor cells (MDSCs) [36]. Moreover, it was demonstrated that lactate inhibits the migration of CD4+ T lymphocytes [37]. Concerning MIF, it was observed that the increase in MIF expression induced a reduction in the number of CD3+ T cells in the stromal compartment of laryngeal carcinoma tissues [13]. Furthermore, Dumitru et al. demonstrated that MIF promotes tumor-associated neutrophil recruitment in a CXCR2-dependent manner in vitro; this recruitment enhances the migratory properties of HNSCC tumor cells [38]. Finally, MIF contributes to tumor immune escape by inhibiting CD8+ T lymphocyte and natural killer cell responses through the downregulation of the NKG2D receptor in ovarian cancer cells [39].

In conclusion, we have reported that MIF is more highly secreted in HPV-positive cells than in HPV-negative cell lines, probably by a specific still-unknown mechanism of MIF secretion, and that the E6 and E7 oncoproteins are implicated in this effect. Based on our data and literature, we explain this relationship by the fact that HPV oncoproteins interact with several pathways and metabolic processes, notably, the Warburg effect, thus generating MIF production. Figure 6 summarizes these pathways and our hypothesis. First, E6 activates mTOR, which leads to the accumulation of HIF-1α that induces the expression of several glycolytic enzymes such as PKM2, LDHA, and the lactate transporter MCT4; in addition, HIF-1α induces MIF expression [21,32,40]. Second, the E7 oncoprotein not only promotes the PKM2-mediated generation of lactate, but also induces HIF-1α expression, thus leading to MIF expression [24,26]. Therefore, the increase in MIF secretion as an immune system repressor, and the production of lactate through the Warburg effect, both by HPV oncoproteins, may lead to the development of a pro-tumoral microenvironment.

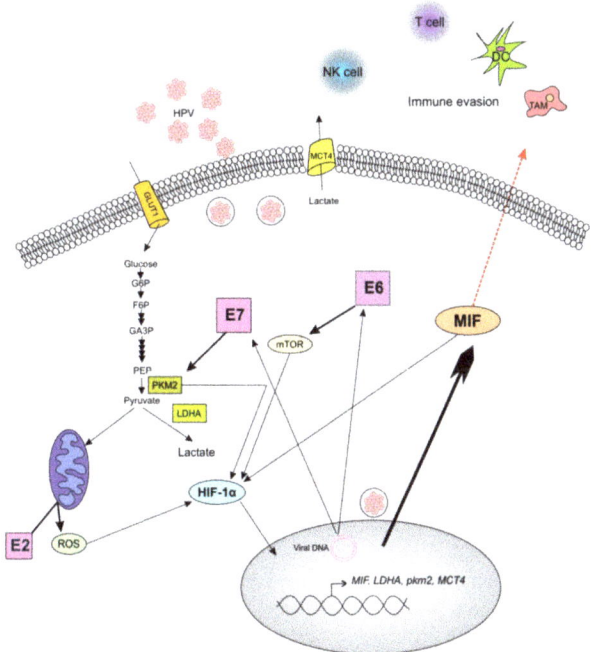

**Figure 6.** Schematic illustration of the role of human papilloma virus (HPV) oncoproteins in the production of macrophage migration inhibitory factor (MIF). The oncoprotein E6 promotes the activation of the mTOR signaling pathway, thus leading to the upregulation of hypoxia inducible factor 1α (HIF-1α), which enhances the production of MIF and increases the production of lactate. The oncoprotein E7 drives the accumulation of the dimeric form of pyruvate kinase M2 (PKM2), thus leading to the conversion of pyruvate to lactate through lactate dehydrogenase (LDHA). Moreover, PKM2 interacts with HIF-1α to amplify the expression of HIF-1α target genes, including MIF and LDHA. Additionally, the HPV E2 protein localizes to the mitochondrial membrane, leading to the increased production of reactive oxygen species (ROS), which increases the stability of HIF-1α. The enrichment of MIF in the extracellular environment could promote the tumor immune escape by the accumulation of pro-tumoral immune cells such as tumor-associated macrophages (TAM), and by the decrease in antitumoral cells such as cytotoxic T cells, Langerhans/dendritic cells (DC), and natural killer (NK) cells. Complete arrows indicate data from the literature, and the red dotted arrow indicates a hypothesis.

## 5. Conclusions

To conclude, we hypothesized that lactate production and HIF-1α expression induces MIF secretion via the HPV E6 and E7 oncoproteins, by the stimulation of enzymes participating in the Warburg effect. This production could lead to development of a pro-tumoral microenvironment.

**Author Contributions:** Study concept and design: N.K., S.S., F.J. Acquisition of data: N.K., J.R.L., G.D. Analysis and interpretation of data: N.K., F.J., R.W., J.-M.C, M.R. and S.S. Drafting and reviewing of the manuscript: N.K., F.J., J.-M.C., R.W., G.B. and S.S.

**Funding:** Nadège Kindt is supported by a PhD grant from the Télévie (grant number 7484615) (Belgian National Fund for Scientific Research, FNRS).

**Acknowledgments:** We thank Grégoire for providing us SCCVII E6, E7, E6/E7 and CT cell lines.

**Conflicts of Interest:** The authors declare no conflict of interests.

## References

1. Global Burden of Disease Cancer Collaboration; Fitzmaurice, C.; Allen, C.; Barber, R.M.; Barregard, L.; Bhutta, Z.A.; Brenner, H.; Dicker, D.J.; Chimed-Orchir, O.; Dandona, R.; et al. Global, Regional, and National Cancer Incidence, Mortality, Years of Life Lost, Years Lived With Disability, and Disability-Adjusted Life-years for 32 Cancer Groups, 1990 to 2015: A Systematic Analysis for the Global Burden of Disease Study. *JAMA Oncol.* **2017**, *3*, 524–548.
2. Elrefaey, S.; Massaro, M.A.; Chiocca, S.; Chiesa, F.; Ansarin, M. HPV in oropharyngeal cancer: The basics to know in clinical practice. *Acta Otorhinolaryngol. Ital.* **2014**, *34*, 299–309. [PubMed]
3. Saraiya, M.; Unger, E.R.; Thompson, T.D.; Lynch, C.F.; Hernandez, B.Y.; Lyu, C.W.; Steinau, M.; Watson, M.; Wilkinson, E.J.; Hopenhayn, C.; et al. US assessment of HPV types in cancers: Implications for current and 9-valent HPV vaccines. *J. Natl. Cancer Inst.* **2015**, *107*, djv086. [CrossRef]
4. Chera, B.S.; Kumar, S.; Shen, C.; Amdur, R.J.; Dagan, R.; Weiss, J.; Grilley-Olson, J.; Zanation, A.; Hackman, T.; Blumberg, J.; et al. Plasma Circulating Tumor HPV DNA for the Surveillance of Cancer Recurrence in HPV-associated Oropharyngeal Cancer. *Int. J. Radiat. Oncol.* **2018**, *102*, 1605–1606. [CrossRef]
5. Gupta, G.P.; Kumar, S.; Marron, D.; Amdur, R.J.; Hayes, D.N.; Weiss, J.; Grilley-Olson, J.; Zanation, A.; Hackman, T.; Zevallos, J.P.; et al. Circulating Tumor HPV16 DNA as a Biomarker of Tumor Genomics and Disease Control in HPV-associated Oropharyngeal Squamous Cell Carcinoma. *Int. J. Radiat. Oncol.* **2018**, *100*, 1310–1311. [CrossRef]
6. Anantharaman, D.; Abedi-Ardekani, B.; Beachler, D.C.; Gheit, T.; Olshan, A.F.; Wisniewski, K.; Wunsch-Filho, V.; Toporcov, T.N.; Tajara, E.H.; Levi, J.E.; et al. Geographic heterogeneity in the prevalence of human papillomavirus in head and neck cancer. *Int. J. Cancer* **2017**, *140*, 1968–1975. [CrossRef] [PubMed]
7. Näsman, A.; Attner, P.; Hammarstedt, L.; Du, J.; Eriksson, M.; Giraud, G.; Ahrlund-Richter, S.; Marklund, L.; Romanitan, M.; Lindquist, D.; et al. Incidence of human papillomavirus (HPV) positive tonsillar carcinoma in Stockholm, Sweden: An epidemic of viral-induced carcinoma? *Int. J. Cancer* **2009**, *125*, 362–366. [CrossRef]
8. Vlantis, A.C. Human Papilloma Virus and Oropharyngeal Carcinoma-Lessons from History. *Chin. J. Dent. Res. Off. J. Sci. Sect. Chin. Stomatol. Assoc. CSA* **2016**, *19*, 9–16.
9. Descamps, G.; Karaca, Y.; Lechien, J.R.; Kindt, N.; Decaestecker, C.; Remmelink, M.; Larsimont, D.; Andry, G.; Hassid, S.; Rodriguez, A.; et al. Classical risk factors, but not HPV status, predict survival after chemoradiotherapy in advanced head and neck cancer patients. *J. Cancer Res. Clin. Oncol.* **2016**, *142*, 2185–2196. [CrossRef] [PubMed]
10. Filleul, O.; Preillon, J.; Crompot, E.; Lechien, J.; Saussez, S. Incidence of head and neck cancers in Belgium: Comparison with world wide and French data. *Bull. Cancer (Paris)* **2011**, *98*, 1173–1183.
11. Bloom, B.R.; Bennett, B. Mechanism of a reaction in vitro associated with delayed-type hypersensitivity. *Science* **1966**, *153*, 80–82. [CrossRef] [PubMed]
12. Kindt, N.; Journe, F.; Laurent, G.; Saussez, S. Involvement of macrophage migration inhibitory factor in cancer and novel therapeutic targets. *Oncol. Lett.* **2016**, *12*, 2247–2253. [CrossRef]
13. Kindt, N.; Preillon, J.; Kaltner, H.; Gabius, H.-J.; Chevalier, D.; Rodriguez, A.; Johnson, B.D.; Megalizzi, V.; Decaestecker, C.; Laurent, G.; et al. Macrophage migration inhibitory factor in head and neck squamous cell carcinoma: Clinical and experimental studies. *J. Cancer Res. Clin. Oncol.* **2013**, *139*, 727–737. [CrossRef] [PubMed]
14. Duray, A.; Descamps, G.; Decaestecker, C.; Sirtaine, N.; Gilles, A.; Khalifé, M.; Chantrain, G.; Depuydt, C.E.; Delvenne, P.; Saussez, S. Human papillomavirus predicts the outcome following concomitant chemoradiotherapy in patients with head and neck squamous cell carcinomas. *Oncol. Rep.* **2013**, *30*, 371–376. [CrossRef] [PubMed]
15. PrimerBank. Available online: https://pga.mgh.harvard.edu/primerbank/ (accessed on 4 October 2018).
16. Sawicka, M.; Pawlikowski, J.; Wilson, S.; Ferdinando, D.; Wu, H.; Adams, P.D.; Gunn, D.A.; Parish, W. The specificity and patterns of staining in human cells and tissues of p16INK4a antibodies demonstrate variant antigen binding. *PLoS ONE* **2013**, *8*, e53313. [CrossRef] [PubMed]
17. Cludts, S.; Decaestecker, C.; Johnson, B.; Lechien, J.; Leroy, X.; Kindt, N.; Kaltner, H.; André, S.; Gabius, H.-J.; Saussez, S. Increased expression of macrophage migration inhibitory factor during progression to hypopharyngeal squamous cell carcinoma. *Anticancer Res.* **2010**, *30*, 3313–3319. [PubMed]

18. Kindt, N.; Descamps, G.; Seminerio, I.; Bellier, J.; Lechien, J.R.; Mat, Q.; Pottier, C.; Delvenne, P.; Journé, F.; Saussez, S. High stromal Foxp3-positive T cell number combined to tumor stage improved prognosis in head and neck squamous cell carcinoma. *Oral Oncol.* **2017**, *67*, 183–191. [CrossRef]
19. Zhou, Q.; Yan, X.; Gershan, J.; Orentas, R.J.; Johnson, B.D. Expression of macrophage migration inhibitory factor by neuroblastoma leads to the inhibition of antitumor T cell reactivity in vivo. *J. Immunol.* **2008**, *181*, 1877–1886. [CrossRef] [PubMed]
20. Fan, R.; Hou, W.-J.; Zhao, Y.-J.; Liu, S.-L.; Qiu, X.-S.; Wang, E.-H.; Wu, G.-P. Overexpression of HPV16 E6/E7 mediated HIF-1α upregulation of GLUT1 expression in lung cancer cells. *Tumour Biol. J. Int. Soc. Oncodev. Biol. Med.* **2016**, *37*, 4655–4663. [CrossRef] [PubMed]
21. Coppock, J.D.; Lee, J.H. mTOR, metabolism, and the immune response in HPV-positive head and neck squamous cell cancer. *World J. Otorhinolaryngol. Head Neck Surg.* **2016**, *2*, 76–83. [CrossRef]
22. Kindt, N.; Lechien, J.; Decaestecker, C.; Rodriguez, A.; Chantrain, G.; Remmelink, M.; Laurent, G.; Gabius, H.-J.; Saussez, S. Expression of macrophage migration-inhibitory factor is correlated with progression in oral cavity carcinomas. *Anticancer Res.* **2012**, *32*, 4499–4505. [PubMed]
23. Howard, J.D.; Chung, C.H. Biology of Human Papillomavirus–Related Oropharyngeal Cancer. *Semin. Radiat. Oncol.* **2012**, *22*, 187–193. [CrossRef]
24. Tang, X.; Zhang, Q.; Nishitani, J.; Brown, J.; Shi, S.; Le, A.D. Overexpression of human papillomavirus type 16 oncoproteins enhances hypoxia-inducible factor 1 alpha protein accumulation and vascular endothelial growth factor expression in human cervical carcinoma cells. *Clin. Cancer Res. Off. J. Am. Assoc. Cancer Res.* **2007**, *13*, 2568–2576. [CrossRef] [PubMed]
25. Guo, Y.; Meng, X.; Ma, J.; Zheng, Y.; Wang, Q.; Wang, Y.; Shang, H. Human papillomavirus 16 E6 contributes HIF-1α induced Warburg effect by attenuating the VHL-HIF-1α interaction. *Int. J. Mol. Sci.* **2014**, *15*, 7974–7986. [CrossRef] [PubMed]
26. Wong, N.; Ojo, D.; Yan, J.; Tang, D. PKM2 contributes to cancer metabolism. *Cancer Lett.* **2015**, *356*, 184–191. [CrossRef] [PubMed]
27. Lai, D.; Tan, C.L.; Gunaratne, J.; Quek, L.S.; Nei, W.; Thierry, F.; Bellanger, S. Localization of HPV-18 E2 at mitochondrial membranes induces ROS release and modulates host cell metabolism. *PLoS ONE* **2013**, *8*, e75625. [CrossRef]
28. Pinheiro, C.; Garcia, E.A.; Morais-Santos, F.; Scapulatempo-Neto, C.; Mafra, A.; Steenbergen, R.D.M.; Boccardo, E.; Villa, L.L.; Baltazar, F.; Longatto-Filho, A. Lactate transporters and vascular factors in HPV-induced squamous cell carcinoma of the uterine cervix. *BMC Cancer* **2014**, *14*, 751. [CrossRef]
29. Gupta, Y.; Pasupuleti, V.; Du, W.; Welford, S.M. Macrophage Migration Inhibitory Factor Secretion Is Induced by Ionizing Radiation and Oxidative Stress in Cancer Cells. *PLoS ONE* **2016**, *11*, e0146482. [CrossRef] [PubMed]
30. Fu, H.; Luo, F.; Yang, L.; Wu, W.; Liu, X. Hypoxia stimulates the expression of macrophage migration inhibitory factor in human vascular smooth muscle cells via HIF-1alpha dependent pathway. *BMC Cell Biol.* **2010**, *11*, 66. [CrossRef] [PubMed]
31. Oda, S.; Oda, T.; Nishi, K.; Takabuchi, S.; Wakamatsu, T.; Tanaka, T.; Adachi, T.; Fukuda, K.; Semenza, G.L.; Hirota, K. Macrophage migration inhibitory factor activates hypoxia-inducible factor in a p53-dependent manner. *PLoS ONE* **2008**, *3*, e2215. [CrossRef]
32. No, Y.R.; Lee, S.-J.; Kumar, A.; Yun, C.C. HIF1α-Induced by Lysophosphatidic Acid Is Stabilized via Interaction with MIF and CSN5. *PLoS ONE* **2015**, *10*, e0137513. [CrossRef] [PubMed]
33. Lechner, A.; Schlößer, H.; Rothschild, S.I.; Thelen, M.; Reuter, S.; Zentis, P.; Shimabukuro-Vornhagen, A.; Theurich, S.; Wennhold, K.; Garcia-Marquez, M.; et al. Characterization of tumor-associated T-lymphocyte subsets and immune checkpoint molecules in head and neck squamous cell carcinoma. *Oncotarget* **2017**, *8*, 44418–44433. [CrossRef] [PubMed]
34. Kindt, N.; Descamps, G.; Seminerio, I.; Bellier, J.; Lechien, J.R.; Pottier, C.; Larsimont, D.; Journé, F.; Delvenne, P.; Saussez, S. Langerhans cell number is a strong and independent prognostic factor for head and neck squamous cell carcinomas. *Oral Oncol.* **2016**, *62*, 1–10. [CrossRef] [PubMed]
35. Nguyen, N.; Bellile, E.; Thomas, D.; McHugh, J.; Rozek, L.; Virani, S.; Peterson, L.; Carey, T.E.; Walline, H.; Moyer, J.; et al. Tumor infiltrating lymphocytes and survival in patients with head and neck squamous cell carcinoma. *Head Neck* **2016**, *38*, 1074–1084. [CrossRef] [PubMed]

36. Ding, J.; Karp, J.E.; Emadi, A. Elevated lactate dehydrogenase (LDH) can be a marker of immune suppression in cancer: Interplay between hematologic and solid neoplastic clones and their microenvironments. *Cancer Biomark. Sect. Dis. Markers* **2017**, *19*, 353–363. [CrossRef] [PubMed]
37. Haas, R.; Smith, J.; Rocher-Ros, V.; Nadkarni, S.; Montero-Melendez, T.; D'Acquisto, F.; Bland, E.J.; Bombardieri, M.; Pitzalis, C.; Perretti, M.; et al. Lactate Regulates Metabolic and Pro-inflammatory Circuits in Control of T Cell Migration and Effector Functions. *PLoS Biol.* **2015**, *13*, e1002202. [CrossRef] [PubMed]
38. Dumitru, C.A.; Gholaman, H.; Trellakis, S.; Bruderek, K.; Dominas, N.; Gu, X.; Bankfalvi, A.; Whiteside, T.L.; Lang, S.; Brandau, S. Tumor-derived macrophage migration inhibitory factor modulates the biology of head and neck cancer cells via neutrophil activation. *Int. J. Cancer* **2011**, *129*, 859–869. [CrossRef]
39. Krockenberger, M.; Dombrowski, Y.; Weidler, C.; Ossadnik, M.; Hönig, A.; Häusler, S.; Voigt, H.; Becker, J.C.; Leng, L.; Steinle, A.; et al. Macrophage migration inhibitory factor contributes to the immune escape of ovarian cancer by down-regulating NKG2D. *J. Immunol.* **2008**, *180*, 7338–7348. [CrossRef]
40. Ullah, M.S.; Davies, A.J.; Halestrap, A.P. The plasma membrane lactate transporter MCT4, but not MCT1, is up-regulated by hypoxia through a HIF-1alpha-dependent mechanism. *J. Biol. Chem.* **2006**, *281*, 9030–9037. [CrossRef]

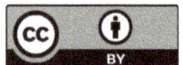

© 2019 by the authors. Licensee MDPI, Basel, Switzerland. This article is an open access article distributed under the terms and conditions of the Creative Commons Attribution (CC BY) license (http://creativecommons.org/licenses/by/4.0/).

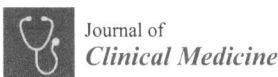 

Article

# Polymorphisms in *ERCC5* rs17655 and *ERCC1* rs735482 Genes Associated with the Survival of Male Patients with Postoperative Oral Squamous Cell Carcinoma Treated with Adjuvant Concurrent Chemoradiotherapy

Thomas Senghore [1,2], Huei-Tzu Chien [3,4], Wen-Chang Wang [5], You-Xin Chen [1], Chi-Kuang Young [6], Shiang-Fu Huang [3,7,*] and Chih-Ching Yeh [1,8,*]

[1] School of Public Health, College of Public Health, Taipei Medical University, Taipei 11031, Taiwan; tsenghore@gmail.com (T.S.); youxin810@gmail.com (Y.-X.C.)
[2] Department of Nursing, School of Medicine and Allied Health Sciences, University of The Gambia, Independence Drive, Banjul, P.O. Box 1646, The Gambia
[3] Department of Public Health, Chang Gung University, Tao-Yuan 33305, Taiwan; kathy.htchien@gmail.com
[4] Department of Nutrition and Health Sciences, Chang Gung University of Science and Technology, Taoyuan 33302, Taiwan
[5] Ph.D. Program for Translational Medicine, College of Medical Science and Technology, Taipei Medical University, Taipei 11031, Taiwan; wangwc@tmu.edu.tw
[6] Department of Otolaryngology, Chang Gung Memorial Hospital, Keelung 20401, Taiwan; riorioroman@gmail.com
[7] Department of Otolaryngology, Head and Neck Surgery, Chang Gung Memorial Hospital, Linkou, Taoyuan 33305, Taiwan
[8] Department of Public Health, College of Public Health, China Medical University, Taichung 40402, Taiwan
* Correspondence: shiangfu.huang@gmail.com (S.-F.H.); ccyeh@tmu.edu.tw (C.-C.Y.); Tel.: +886-3-3281200 (S.-F.H.); +886-2-7361661 (ext. 6534) (C.-C.Y.)

Received: 26 November 2018; Accepted: 25 December 2018; Published: 1 January 2019

**Abstract:** The nucleotide excision repair (NER) pathway plays a major role in the repair of DNA damaged by exogenous agents, such as chemotherapeutic and radiotherapeutic agents. Thus, we investigated the association between key potentially functional single nucleotide polymorphisms (SNPs) in the NER pathway and clinical outcomes in oral squamous cell carcinoma (OSCC) patients treated with concurrent chemoradiotherapy (CCRT). Thirteen SNPs in five key NER genes were genotyped in 319 male OSCC patients using iPLEX MassARRAY. Cox proportional hazards models and Kaplan–Meier survival curves were used to estimate the risk of death or recurrence. Carriers of the *XPC* rs2228000 TT genotype showed a borderline significant increased risk of poor overall survival under the recessive model (hazard ratio (HR) = 1.81, 95% confidence interval (CI) = 0.99–3.29). The CC genotypes of *ERCC5* rs17655 (HR = 1.54, 95% CI = 1.03–2.29) and *ERCC1* rs735482 (HR = 1.65, 95% CI = 1.06–2.58) were associated with an increased risk of worse disease-free survival under the recessive model. In addition, participants carrying both the CC genotypes of *ERCC5* rs17655 and *ERCC1* rs735482 exhibited an enhanced susceptibility for recurrence (HR = 2.60, 95% CI = 1.11–6.09). However, no statistically significant interaction was observed between them. Our findings reveal that the *ERCC5* rs17655 CC and *ERCC1* rs735482 CC genotypes were associated with an increased risk of recurrence in male patients with OSCC treated with CCRT. Therefore, CCRT may not be beneficial, and alternative treatments are required for such patients.

**Keywords:** nucleotide excision repair; genetic polymorphism; oral squamous cell carcinoma; concurrent chemoradiotherapy; prognosis

## 1. Introduction

Oral squamous cell carcinoma (OSCC) is the leading cause of cancer morbidity and mortality, especially among men in Taiwan [1]. Despite new advances in the diagnosis and therapeutic approaches, the 5-year survival remains low [1,2]. While relapse of OSCC remains a major clinical challenge, the incidence of relapse among patients varies, even for those with a similar stage of disease at diagnosis or those who undergo the same treatment [3]. This implies that other factors, such as genetic variations, may play an important role in disease prognosis.

Most patients with OSCC are diagnosed at an advanced stage of the disease [4]. For these patients, the treatment options are limited to mainly systemic therapy, often as concurrent chemoradiotherapy (CCRT) with platinum-based DNA damaging agents as either primary treatment or adjuvant postoperative therapy [5–7]. However, the overall survival (OS) for these patients remains poor because most of them experience recurrence or distance metastases [8–10]. Genetic variations in DNA repair genes affect susceptibility to the efficacy and survival outcome of a certain treatment [11,12]. Increased DNA repair capacity may affect the sensitivity of the tumor cells to chemotherapy and radiotherapy (RT) by allowing cancer cells to repair DNA that has been damaged by these agents. Single nucleotide polymorphism (SNP) in genes involved in the nucleotide excision repair (NER) pathway may modulate DNA repair capacity by influencing gene expression or activity, thereby affecting the anticancer effects of therapeutic agents and treatment response [13,14].

The excision repair cross-complementation genes, including groups 1 (*ERCC1*), 2 (*ERCC2*), and 5 (*ERCC5*) and xeroderma pigmentosium complementation group A (*XPA*) and C (*XPC*) encode proteins that are involved in the NER pathway; and together with other proteins, operate to recognize and repair damaged DNA [15]. The XPC together with XPF initially recognize the DNA lesion that is unwound and remodeled by helicase proteins ERCC3 and ERCC2 that binds to XPA and replication protein A (RPA). The ERCC1 and ERCC5 proteins are involved in the incision of the identified DNA lesion. The difference in treatment response and clinical outcome have been attributed to SNPs in genes that code of the above proteins [13,14]. Therefore, identifying genetic markers in the NER pathway may help develop personalized management strategies, thereby maximizing treatment success and improving survival.

Thus, we conducted a retrospective cohort study to test whether SNPs in genes involved in the NER pathway are associated with prognosis in male patients with OSCC treated with adjuvant CCRT. A total of 13 SNPs in *ERCC5*, *ERCC2*, *ERCC1*, *XPC*, and *XPA* genes, which have been found to affect the risk and/or survival of cancers, were selected in the present study [13,14,16–20]. Their associations with clinical outcomes were evaluated using alternative genetic models, including additive, dominant, and recessive models.

## 2. Material and Methods

### 2.1. Study Population

In total, 360 male participants newly diagnosed with histopathological confirmed advanced OSCC who received surgery plus adjuvant CCRT were recruited from the Head and Neck Surgery Department's Cancer Registry at Chang Gung Memorial Hospital, LinKou, Taiwan, from 1999 to 2016. A total of 41 participants were excluded, including 13 of aboriginal ethnicity, 23 with early-stage oral cancer (TNM stages I and II), and 5 with missing information on clinicopathologic variables (TNM stage, vascular invasion, and extracapsular spread). A final sample of 319 was included for analysis. Information on demographic characteristics (age, education, occupation, and ethnicity), lifestyle habit (cigarette smoking, alcohol drinking, and betel nut chewing), and family cancer history were collected through an interviewer-administered questionnaire. Lifestyle habits were categorized as either never (if the person never engaged in the habit continuously for more than a year) or ever (if the person ever engaged in the habit for more than a year). From the weight and height measurements, body mass index (BMI) was calculated as weight/height$^2$ (kg/m$^2$). Clinical information was also collected before treatment through a detailed medical history, physical examination, completed blood count, routine blood chemistry, computed tomography (CT) or magnetic resonance imaging (MRI) of the head and neck, abdominal ultrasound, and whole body bone scan or positron emission tomography scan. This study was approved by the Chang Gung Memorial Hospital (IRB No. 201800213B0) and Taipei Medical University ethics review committees (IRB No. N201802083). All participants provided written informed consent after a detailed explanation of study objectives.

### 2.2. Sample Preparation and DNA Extraction

For each participant, a pair of tumor and normal adjacent nontumor tissue samples were surgically removed, dissected into small pieces, and immediately stored in liquid nitrogen at −80 °C. The surgically removed samples were then sent for pathological examination and staging as per the seventh edition of the American Joint Committee on Cancer—TNM staging system [21]. Histology diagnosis was defined as squamous cell carcinoma, verrucous carcinoma, cylindric cell carcinoma, adenoid cystic carcinoma, mucoepidermoid carcinoma, and adenocarcinoma. For this study, only those with a diagnosis of squamous cell carcinoma were included. Venous blood samples were also collected and stored in heparinized tubes. Germline DNA was extracted from buffer-coated cells using the standard phenol-chloroform method and prepared for genotyping.

### 2.3. SNP Selection and Genotyping

SNPs in the NER pathway were selected from studies that indicated that SNPs were associated with the risk or prognosis of malignancies in ethnic Chinese [16,18–20]. A total of 13 potentially functional SNPs in *ERCC5* (rs2094258, rs1047768, rs17655, and rs873601), *ERCC2* (rs13181 and rs1799793), *ERCC1* (rs735482, rs3212986, and rs11615), *XPC* (rs2228001 and rs2228000), and *XPA* (rs1800975 and rs10817938) genes were genotyped using the Sequenom iPLEX MassARRAY system (Sequenom, Inc., San Diego, CA, USA). A 10% random sample was reanalyzed, and it showed 100% concordance for all the polymorphisms.

### 2.4. Patient Treatment and Follow-Up

All patients underwent radical tumor excision with clinical stage-based neck dissection after preoperative tumor survey. The primary tumors were resected above 1-cm safety margins (both peripheral and deep margins). Neck dissections were performed according to examination status. If the lesion invaded deeply and crossed the midline, as observed in tongue cancer, bilateral neck dissection was performed. Pathologic parameters included tumor stage, nodal status, extranodal extension (ENE), tumor cell differentiation, perineural invasion, skin invasion, bone invasion, and tumor depth. Postoperative RT was administered to patients with pT4 stage tumor, pathologically close margins (≤4 mm), or pathologically positive lymph nodes. The radiation dose lay between 6000 and 6600 cGy. CCRT with cisplatin-based agents was administered to patients with ENE or pathological multiple lymph node metastases 4 to 8 weeks after the surgical procedure. During the course of RT, 5-fluorouracil was administered orally.

Following commencement of treatment, the participants were monitored during their treatment and after treatment through regular clinical and radiological examinations. Follow-up involved monthly checkups for the first 6 months. This was followed by checkups every 2 months in the second 6 months, then checkups every 3 months within the second year, and checkups every 6 months thereafter. The follow-up included an analysis of medical history, physical examination (including complete oral examination), laboratory examination, X-rays, and CT or MRI. To confirm recurrence, histology of biopsy or imaging studies were conducted. Data for all deaths resulting from OSCC were based on death certificates.

## 2.5. Statistical Analysis

Statistical analysis was performed using SAS (version 9.4 for Windows; SAS institute, Cary, NC, USA). Demographic and clinical characteristics were summarized as mean and standard deviation for continuous variables and frequency and proportions for categorical variables. The distribution of genotypes by clinical characteristics was assessed using Chi-square test. Major clinical outcomes were disease-free survival (DFS) and OS. DFS was measured from the first day of treatment to the time of recurrence, metastasis, or death due to any cause. OS was calculated as the time elapsed (in months) from the date of commencing RT to the date of death. Patients without an event at the date of the last contact were considered as being censored or subject to administrative censoring by the end of the follow-up period. Survival analysis was conducted using the Kaplan–Meier method, and survival curve differences among the genotypes were compared using the log-rank test. Univariate and multivariate Cox proportional hazards models were used to evaluate the effects of demographic, clinical characteristics, and SNPs on survival. Hazard ratios (HRs) and their 95% confidence intervals (CIs) were used to estimate the relative risk of death or recurrence. We evaluated the individual variants in different genetic models, including additive, dominant, and recessive models, on OSCC survival. Sociodemographic and clinical factors significant in the univariate analysis were adjusted in multivariate Cox regression models. Furthermore, multiplicative interactions were evaluated using the likelihood ratio test. Due to the location of multiple SNPs within the same chromosome or gene, linkage disequilibrium (LD) analysis was performed using Haploview (version 4.2). For those SNPs within the same block that were found to be in high LD with each other, further haplotypes analysis was performed using PHASE software (version 2.1) [22]. Statistical significance was set at $p < 0.05$ and was two-sided.

## 3. Results

### 3.1. Demographic and Clinical Characteristics of Study Participants

The demographic and clinical characteristics of the study patients are summarized in Table 1. The mean age was 49.72 ± 9.8. Most participants were under 50 years (51.41%) old, of Taiwanese descent (paternal 72.10% and maternal 74.92%), had normal BMI (49.22%), had smoked cigarettes (according to the "ever" criterion; 85.25%), drank alcohol (69.28%), and chewed betel nut (86.21%). A considerable number of patients exhibited poor clinical characteristics. In total, 55 (17.24%) had poorly differentiated tumors, 197 (61.76%) had primary tumor size in the T3 to T4 range, 217 (67.92%) had N2 to N3 nodal involvement, 177 (55.49%) had perineural invasion, 19 (5.96%) had vascular invasion, 40 (12.54%) had lymphatic invasion, 205 (64.24%) had ENE, and 277 (86.83%) had pathologic TNM stage IV. The genotype frequency distribution analysis showed a statistically significant difference in genotypes of *ERCC1* rs11615 in terms of tumor differentiation ($p = 0.039$), *XPC* rs2228000 in terms of vascular invasion ($p = 0.045$), *ERCC1* rs3212986 and *XPA* rs10817938 in terms of lymphatic invasion ($p = 0.046$ and 0.033, respectively), *XPC* rs2228001 in terms of pathologic TNM stage ($p = 0.039$), and *ERCC5* rs17655 in terms of DFS ($p = 0.049$) (Table S1).

### 3.2. Survival Analysis

The median (range) follow-up duration was 15 months (1–199 months) and 12 months (1–199 months) for OS and DFS, respectively. In the univariate analysis, N2–N3 nodal involvement (HR = 2.41, 95% CI = 1.42–4.10), lymphatic invasion (HR = 2.18, 95% CI = 1.30–3.67), and ENE (HR = 3.91, 95% CI = 2.13–7.19) were significantly associated with OS, whereas primary tumor size in the range of T3 to T4 (HR = 1.72, 95% CI = 1.17–2.53), N2–N3 nodal involvement (HR = 1.63, 95% CI = 1.09–2.44), and ENE (HR = 1.79, 95% CI = 1.20–2.69) were significantly associated with DFS. However, no significant association was observed between demographic and lifestyle factors and survival (Table 2).

**Table 1.** Demographic and clinical characteristics of patients with oral squamous cell carcinoma (OSCC) treated with concurrent chemoradiotherapy (CCRT).

| Variable | n (%) |
|---|---|
| Total | 319 (100) |
| Mean age (SD), years | 49.72 (9.8) |
| Age, years | |
| <50 | 164 (51.41) |
| ≥50 | 155 (48.59) |
| Ethnicity of father | |
| Taiwanese | 230 (72.10) |
| Hakka | 72 (22.57) |
| Mainland Chinese | 17 (5.33) |
| Ethnicity of mother | |
| Taiwanese | 239 (74.92) |
| Hakka | 74 (23.20) |
| Mainland Chinese | 6 (1.88) |
| BMI, kg/m$^2$ | |
| <18.5 | 22 (6.90) |
| 18.5–23.9 | 157 (49.22) |
| ≥24 | 140 (43.89) |
| Cigarette smoking | |
| Never | 47 (14.73) |
| Ever | 272 (85.27) |
| Alcohol drinking | |
| Never | 98 (30.72) |
| Ever | 221 (69.28) |
| Betel nut chewing | |
| Never | 44 (13.79) |
| Ever | 275 (86.21) |
| Tea drinking | |
| Never | 163 (51.10) |
| Ever | 156 (48.90) |
| Coffee drinking | |
| Never | 243 (76.18) |
| Ever | 76 (23.82) |
| Tumor differentiation | |
| Well differentiated | 51 (15.99) |
| Moderate | 210 (65.83) |
| Poor | 55 (17.24) |
| Unclear | 3 (0.94) |
| Primary tumor size | |
| T1–T2 | 122 (38.24) |
| T3–T4 | 197 (61.76) |
| Nodal involvement | |
| N0–N1 | 102 (31.97) |
| N2–N3 | 217 (67.92) |
| Perineural invasion | |
| No | 142 (44.51) |
| Yes | 177 (55.49) |
| Vascular invasion | |
| No | 300 (94.04) |
| Yes | 19 (5.96) |
| Lymphatic invasion | |
| No | 279 (87.46) |
| Yes | 40 (12.54) |
| Extranodal extension | |
| No | 114 (35.74) |
| Yes | 205 (64.26) |
| Pathologic TNM stage | |
| III | 42 (13.17) |
| IV | 277 (86.83) |

OSCC, oral squamous cell carcinoma; SD, standard deviation; BMI, body mass index.

**Table 2.** Univariate association of demographic and clinical factors with survival in patients with OSCC treated with CCRT.

| Variable | Overall Survival | | Disease-Free Survival | |
|---|---|---|---|---|
| | HR (95% CI) | p Value | HR (95% CI) | p Value |
| Age | | | | |
| <50 | 1.00 | | 1.00 | |
| ≥50 | 0.67 (0.44–1.03) | 0.068 | 0.81 (0.57–1.15) | 0.239 |
| Ethnicity of father | | | | |
| Taiwanese | 1.00 | | 1.00 | |
| Hakka | 0.88 (0.51–1.50) | 0.633 | 0.66 (0.40–1.08) | 0.101 |
| Mainland Chinese | 1.27 (0.55–2.93) | 0.577 | 1.72 (0.94–3.14) | 0.079 |
| Ethnicity of mother | | | | |
| Taiwanese | 1.00 | | 1.00 | |
| Hakka | 0.75 (0.43–1.29) | 0.295 | 0.67 (0.42–1.08) | 0.100 |
| Mainland Chinese | 1.80 (0.57–5.72) | 0.320 | 1.60 (0.59–4.37) | 0.355 |
| BMI, kg/m$^2$ | | | | |
| 18.5–23.9 | 1.00 | | 1.00 | |
| <18.5 | 0.85 (0.36–1.98) | 0.705 | 1.49 (0.79–2.84) | 0.223 |
| ≥24 | 0.66 (0.42–1.03) | 0.068 | 0.84 (0.58–1.23) | 0.372 |
| Cigarette smoking | | | | |
| Never | 1.00 | | 1.00 | |
| Ever | 0.89 (0.51–1.57) | 0.675 | 1.02 (0.62–1.68) | 0.938 |
| Alcohol drinking | | | | |
| Never | 1.00 | | 1.00 | |
| Ever | 0.99 (0.64–1.54) | 0.971 | 1.10 (0.75–1.61) | 0.636 |
| Betel nut chewing | | | | |
| Never | 1.00 | | 1.00 | |
| Ever | 1.09 (0.58–2.05) | 0.794 | 1.40 (0.80–2.45) | 0.240 |
| Tea drinking | | | | |
| Never | 1.00 | | 1.00 | |
| Ever | 0.93 (0.61–1.41) | 0.727 | 1.07 (0.75–1.53) | 0.701 |
| Coffee drinking | | | | |
| Never | 1.00 | | 1.00 | |
| Ever | 0.65 (0.37–1.13) | 0.123 | 1.27 (0.85–1.89) | 0.251 |
| Tumor differentiation | | | | |
| Well differentiated | 1.00 | | 1.00 | |
| Moderate | 0.94 (0.55–1.60) | 0.819 | 0.89 (0.56–1.44) | 0.645 |
| Poor | 0.84 (0.40–1.74) | 0.629 | 1.22 (0.68–2.18) | 0.500 |
| Unclear | 2.80 (0.37–1.19) | 0.319 | 1.66 (0.22–2.39) | 0.621 |
| Primary tumor size | | | | |
| T1–T2 | 1.00 | | 1.00 | |
| T3–T4 | 1.29 (0.83–2.01) | 0.258 | 1.72 (1.17–2.53) | 0.006 * |
| Nodal involvement | | | | |
| N0–N1 | 1.00 | | 1.00 | |
| N2–N3 | 2.41 (1.42–4.10) | 0.001 * | 1.63 (1.09–2.44) | 0.018 * |
| Perineural invasion | | | | |
| No | 1.00 | | 1.00 | |
| Yes | 1.29 (0.85–1.98) | 0.238 | 1.27 (0.89–1.83) | 0.189 |
| Vascular invasion | | | | |
| No | 1.00 | | 1.00 | |
| Yes | 1.43 (0.66–3.10) | 0.366 | 0.43 (0.43–2.00) | 0.856 |
| Lymphatic invasion | | | | |
| No | 1.00 | | 1.00 | |
| Yes | 2.18 (1.30–3.67) | 0.003 * | 1.37 (0.82–2.28) | 0.233 |
| Extranodal extension | | | | |
| No | 1.00 | | 1.00 | |
| Yes | 3.91 (2.13–7.19) | <0.001 * | 1.79 (1.20–2.69) | 0.005 * |
| Pathologic TNM stage | | | | |
| III | 1.00 | | 1.00 | |
| IV | 1.64 (0.81–3.29) | 0.168 | 1.66 (0.93–2.96) | 0.087 |

BMI, body mass index; OSCC, oral squamous cell carcinoma; HR, hazard ratio; CI, confidence interval. * $p < 0.05$.

In the univariate Cox proportional hazards models, the *ERCC1* rs735482 CC genotype was marginally significantly associated with poor DFS (HR = 1.53, 95% CI = 0.99–2.38; $p = 0.058$). The *XPA* rs10817938 CC genotype was significantly associated with an increased risk of worse OS (HR = 2.97, 95% CI = 1.20–7.35; $p = 0.019$), and DFS (HR = 2.61, 95% CI = 1.06–6.41; $p = 0.037$), respectively (Table S2).

The results for the multivariate Cox proportional hazards models with covariates adjusted for all selected SPNs are shown in Table 3. Only the *XPC* rs2228000 TT genotype (HR = 1.81, 95% CI = 0.99–3.29, $p$ = 0.053) showed an increased risk of poor OS at borderline significance compared with the CC+CT genotypes. The *ERCC5* rs17655 CC (HR = 1.50, 95% CI = 1.01–2.24; $p$ = 0.045) and *ERCC1* rs735482 CC (HR = 1.61, 95% CI = 1.04–2.51; $p$ = 0.034) genotypes were significantly associated with an increased risk of DFS compared with their counterparts with the GG+GC and AA+AC genotypes, respectively, in the recessive models. The test of LD show that SNPs in *ERCC5* block 1 (rs2094258 and rs1047768; D' = 0.97, $R^2$ = 0.19) and block 2 (rs17655 and rs873601; D' = 0.98, $R^2$ = 0.89), *ERCC1* block (rs3212986 and rs11615; D' = 1.00, $R^2$ = 0.18), *XPC* block (rs2228001 and rs2228000; D' = 1.00, $R^2$ = 0.28), and *XPA* block (rs1800975 and rs10817938; D' = 1.00, $R^2$ = 0.24) were in LD with each other (Figure S1). Of the haplotype constructed from these blocks, only *XPA* GT haplotype (HR = 0.68, 95% CI = 0.47–0.99; $p$ = 0.042) showed statistically significant association with OS (Table S3).

**Table 3.** Multivariate association between nucleotide excision repair (NER) candidate single nucleotide polymorphisms (SNPs) and OSCC survival in patients treated with CCRT.

| SNPs | Overall Survival | | Disease-Free Survival | |
|---|---|---|---|---|
| | HR (95% CI) [a] | $p$ Value | HR (95% CI) [b] | $p$ Value |
| *ERCC5/XPG* | | | | |
| rs2094258 | | | | |
| GG | 1.00 | | 1.00 | |
| GA | 1.14 (0.72–1.79) | 0.574 | 1.07 (0.73–1.57) | 0.726 |
| AA | 0.66 (0.30–1.44) | 0.294 | 1.02 (0.57–1.83) | 0.946 |
| Additive model | 0.91 (0.66–1.25) | 0.559 | 1.03 (0.79–1.34) | 0.839 |
| Dominant model | 1.03 (0.66–1.59) | 0.910 | 1.06 (0.74–1.52) | 0.754 |
| Recessive model | 0.61 (0.29–1.28) | 0.193 | 0.99 (0.57–1.70) | 0.958 |
| rs1047768 | | | | |
| TT | 1.00 | | 1.00 | |
| TC | 1.11 (0.72–1.72) | 0.635 | 0.93 (0.64–1.36) | 0.715 |
| CC | 0.63 (0.25–1.62) | 0.339 | 0.76 (0.39–1.51) | 0.438 |
| Additive model | 0.94 (0.67–1.31) | 0.699 | 0.90 (0.68–1.19) | 0.453 |
| Dominant model | 1.03 (0.67–1.58) | 0.891 | 0.90 (0.63–1.29) | 0.574 |
| Recessive model | 0.60 (0.24–1.49) | 0.272 | 0.79 (0.41–1.53) | 0.482 |
| rs17655 | | | | |
| GG | 1.00 | | 1.00 | |
| GC | 0.95 (0.58–1.54) | 0.829 | 0.86 (0.56–1.31) | 0.482 |
| CC | 0.93 (0.51–1.69) | 0.811 | 1.38 (0.86–2.19) | 0.180 |
| Additive model | 0.96 (0.72–1.30) | 0.803 | 1.16 (0.91–1.49) | 0.238 |
| Dominant model | 0.94 (0.60–1.49) | 0.799 | 1.01 (0.69–1.49) | 0.954 |
| Recessive model | 0.96 (0.58–1.61) | 0.881 | 1.50 (1.01–2.24) | 0.045 * |
| rs873601 | | | | |
| AA | 1.00 | | 1.00 | |
| AG | 0.77 (0.47–1.26) | 0.298 | 0.84 (0.55 1.31) | 0.448 |
| GG | 0.84 (0.47–1.51) | 0.556 | 1.29 (0.80–2.09) | 0.301 |
| Additive model | 0.91 (0.67–1.23) | 0.530 | 1.14 (0.88–1.48) | 0.311 |
| Dominant model | 0.79 (0.50–1.26) | 0.304 | 0.97 (0.65–1.46) | 0.900 |
| Recessive model | 1.00 (0.61–1.64) | 0.988 | 1.44 (0.97–2.14) | 0.070 |
| *ERCC2/XPD* | | | | |
| rs13181 | | | | |
| TT | 1.00 | | 1.00 | |
| TG | 1.03 (0.59–1.81) | 0.909 | 1.00 (0.61–1.64) | 0.997 |
| GG | - | 0.989 | - | 0.984 |
| Additive model | 1.03 (0.59–1.80) | 0.921 | 1.00 (0.61–1.63) | 0.993 |
| Dominant model | 1.03 (0.59–1.81) | 0.915 | 1.00 (0.61–1.64) | 0.998 |
| Recessive model | - | 0.989 | - | 0.984 |
| rs1799793 | | | | |
| GG | 1.00 | | 1.00 | |
| GA | 1.10 (0.58–2.07) | 0.769 | 1.01 (0.58–1.73) | 0.983 |
| AA | - | 0.99 | - | - |
| Additive model | 1.10 (0.58–2.06) | 0.778 | 1.01 (0.58–1.73) | 0.983 |
| Dominant model | 1.10 (0.58–2.07) | 0.773 | 1.01 (0.58–1.73) | 0.983 |
| Recessive model | - | 0.99 | - | - |

Table 3. Cont.

| SNPs | Overall Survival | | Disease-Free Survival | |
|---|---|---|---|---|
| | HR (95% CI) [a] | p Value | HR (95% CI) [b] | p Value |
| ERCC1 | | | | |
| rs735482 | | | | |
| AA | 1.00 | | 1.00 | |
| AC | 0.72 (0.46–1.14) | 0.163 | 0.86 (0.57–1.29) | 0.466 |
| CC | 0.83 (0.44–1.59) | 0.580 | 1.47 (0.89–2.44) | 0.134 |
| Additive model | 0.86 (0.62–1.19) | 0.352 | 1.16 (0.89–1.52) | 0.283 |
| Dominant model | 0.75 (0.48–1.15) | 0.183 | 0.98 (0.67–1.44) | 0.934 |
| Recessive model | 1.01 (0.56–1.83) | 0.975 | 1.61 (1.04–2.51) | 0.034 * |
| rs3212986 | | | | |
| GG | 1.00 | | 1.00 | |
| GT | 1.20 (0.76–1.89) | 0.436 | 0.95 (0.66–1.39) | 0.806 |
| TT | 1.04 (0.48–2.28) | 0.922 | 0.96 (0.50–1.85) | 0.912 |
| Additive model | 1.08 (0.78–1.51) | 0.642 | 0.97 (0.73–1.29) | 0.833 |
| Recessive model | 1.17 (0.75–1.82) | 0.481 | 0.96 (0.67–1.37) | 0.805 |
| Dominant model | 0.94 (0.45–1.97) | 0.870 | 0.99 (0.53–1.85) | 0.967 |
| rs11615 | | | | |
| CC | 1.00 | | 1.00 | |
| CT | 1.23 (0.79–1.91) | 0.351 | 0.85 (0.59–1.23) | 0.388 |
| TT | 0.90 (0.35–2.28) | 0.817 | 0.72 (0.33–1.59) | 0.416 |
| Additive model | 1.08 (0.77–1.51) | 0.661 | 0.85 (0.63–1.14) | 0.282 |
| Dominant model | 1.18 (0.77–1.81) | 0.438 | 0.83 (0.58–1.19) | 0.316 |
| Recessive model | 0.81 (0.33–2.01) | 0.652 | 0.78 (0.36–1.69) | 0.525 |
| XPC | | | | |
| rs2228001 | | | | |
| AA | 1.00 | | 1.00 | |
| AC | 1.07 (0.68–1.69) | 0.766 | 1.21 (0.83–1.78) | 0.329 |
| CC | 0.72 (0.30–1.73) | 0.457 | 0.75 (0.37–1.54) | 0.432 |
| Additive model | 0.94 (0.67–1.32) | 0.716 | 0.99 (0.75–1.31) | 0.941 |
| Dominant model | 1.01 (0.65–1.58) | 0.955 | 1.12 (0.77–1.63) | 0.539 |
| Recessive model | 0.69 (0.30–1.60) | 0.384 | 0.68 (0.34–1.34) | 0.260 |
| rs2228000 | | | | |
| CC | 1.00 | | 1.00 | |
| TC | 1.06 (0.66–1.68) | 0.822 | 0.81 (0.55–1.18) | 0.267 |
| TT | 1.86 (0.97–3.56) | 0.062 | 1.11 (0.59–2.08) | 0.758 |
| Additive model | 1.28 (0.92–1.77) | 0.144 | 0.94 (0.70–1.25) | 0.652 |
| Dominant model | 1.18 (0.76–1.83) | 0.457 | 0.85 (0.59–1.22) | 0.373 |
| Recessive model | 1.81 (0.99–3.29) | 0.053 | 1.23 (0.67–2.26) | 0.501 |
| XPA | | | | |
| rs1800975 | | | | |
| AA | 1.00 | | 1.00 | |
| AG | 0.83 (0.50–1.36) | 0.461 | 0.83 (0.51–1.36) | 0.462 |
| GG | 0.65 (0.35–1.21) | 0.175 | 0.65 (0.35–1.21) | 0.174 |
| Additive model | 0.81 (0.60–1.10) | 0.174 | 0.90 (0.70–1.16) | 0.426 |
| Dominant model | 0.77 (0.48–1.24) | 0.282 | 0.77 (0.48–1.24) | 0.283 |
| Recessive model | 0.74 (0.44–1.25) | 0.260 | 0.73 (0.44–1.25) | 0.258 |
| rs10817938 | | | | |
| TT | 1.00 | | 1.00 | |
| TC | 1.08 (0.68–1.72) | 0.731 | 1.28 (0.87–1.86) | 0.209 |
| CC | 1.68 (0.65–4.33) | 0.286 | 1.88 (0.75–4.74) | 0.180 |
| Additive model | 1.18 (0.82–1.69) | 0.386 | 1.31 (0.95–1.80) | 0.095 |
| Dominant model | 1.15 (0.74–1.77) | 0.543 | 1.32 (0.91–1.90) | 0.139 |
| Recessive model | 1.64 (0.64–4.17) | 0.304 | 1.73 (0.69–4.32) | 0.239 |

OSCC, oral squamous cell carcinoma; SNPs, single nucleotide polymorphisms; HR, hazard ratio; CI, confidence interval. [a] Adjusted for age, BMI, N stage, lymphatic invasion, and extranodal extension. [b] Adjusted for age, T stage, N stage, and extranodal extension. * $p < 0.05$.

We further conducted a combination analysis for the *ERCC5* rs17655 and *ERCC1* rs735482 polymorphisms and DSF in patients with OSCC. The Kaplan–Meier curves showed borderline significant differences in DFS among the four genotypes (log-rank test $p = 0.078$) (Figure 1). The multivariate Cox proportional models indicated that patients with the combination of *ERCC5* rs17655 CC and *ERCC1* rs735482 CC genotypes exhibited a higher risk of disease recurrence than those with the combination of *ERCC5* rs17655 GG+GC and *ERCC1* rs735482 AA+AC genotypes (HR = 2.60, 95% CI = 1.11–6.09; $p = 0.027$) (Table 4). However, this gene-gene interaction was not statistically significant.

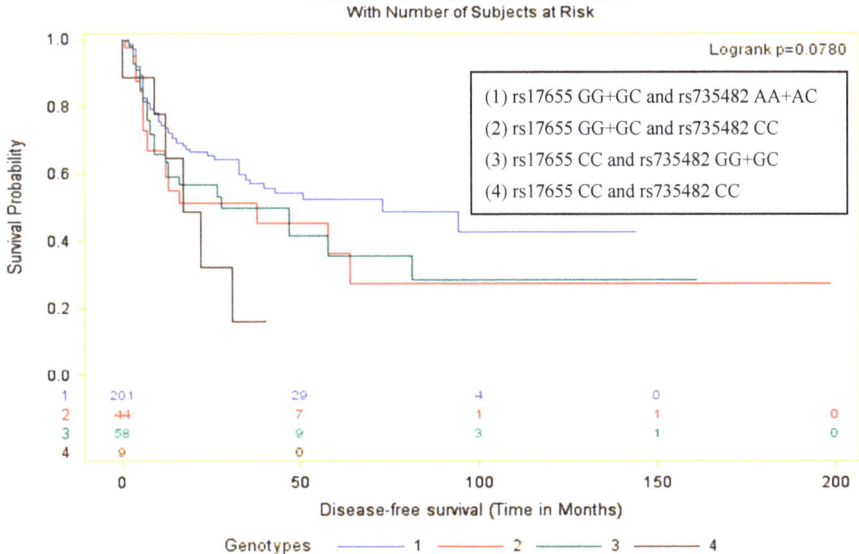

**Figure 1.** Kaplan–Meier survival curve for the combined *ERCC5* rs17655 and *ERCC1* rs735482 polymorphisms and disease-free survival in patients with oral squamous cell carcinoma treated with concurrent chemoradiotherapy. The figure illustrates a borderline significant difference in recurrence among the four groups (log-rank test $p = 0.078$).

**Table 4.** Interaction between the *ERCC5* rs17655 and *ERCC1* rs735482 polymorphisms on the disease-free survival of patients with OSCC treated with CCRT.

| *ERCC5* rs17655 | *ERCC1* rs735482 | No. | Event | HR (95% CI) [a] | *p* Value |
|---|---|---|---|---|---|
| GG+GC | AA+AC | 206 | 71 | 1.00 | |
| GG+GC | CC | 45 | 19 | 1.63 (0.98–2.72) | 0.060 |
| CC | GG+GC | 59 | 29 | 1.52 (0.98–2.37) | 0.062 |
| CC | CC | 9 | 6 | 2.60 (1.11–6.09) | 0.027 * |
| | *p* for interaction | | | | 0.929 |

OSCC, oral squamous cell carcinoma; HR, hazard ratio; CI, confidence interval. [a] Adjusted for age, T stage, N stage, and extranodal extension. * $p < 0.05$.

Table 5 shows the subgroup analysis for the association between significant SNPs and DFS stratified by demographic and clinopathological factors. Results show a significant interaction between *ERCC5* rs17655 polymorphism and perineural invasion on the risk for DFS (interaction $p = 0.008$). The *ERCC5* rs17655 CC genotype individuals with perineural invasion (HR = 2.46, 95% CI = 1.46–4.15; $p < 0.001$) had an increased risk for DFS compared to their counterparts with no perineural invasion. Although a significant interaction between *ERCC1* rs735482 polymorphism and vascular invasion was also observed (interaction $p < 0.001$), the harmful effect of CC genotype on recurrence was not present in any subgroup of vascular invasion.

**Table 5.** Association between the *ERCC5* rs17655 and *ERCC1* rs735482 polymorphisms and the disease-free survival in OSCC patients treated with CCRT stratified by demographic and clinopathological factors.

| Variable | ERCC5 rs17655 HR (95% CI) [a] | p Value | p Interaction | ERCC1 rs735482 HR (95% CI) [a] | p Value | p Interaction |
|---|---|---|---|---|---|---|
| Age | | | 0.486 | | | 0.078 |
| <50 | 1.74 (1.00–3.03) | 0.051 | | 1.04 (0.53–2.06) | 0.911 | |
| ≥50 | 1.24 (0.69–2.23) | 0.473 | | 2.76 (1.47–5.19) | 0.002 * | |
| BMI, kg/m² | | | 0.160 | | | 0.597 |
| 18.5–23.9 | 1.64 (0.95–2.82) | 0.075 | | 1.89 (1.04–3.44) | 0.037 * | |
| <18.5 | 3.06 (0.65–14.49) | 0.159 | | 1.30 (0.05–31.65) | 0.871 | |
| ≥24 | 0.81 (0.37–1.77) | 0.601 | | 1.30 (0.62–2.72) | 0.495 | |
| Cigarette smoking | | | 0.664 | | | 0.975 |
| Never | 1.03 (0.35–2.98) | 0.962 | | 1.99 (0.52–7.58) | 0.316 | |
| Ever | 1.54 (0.99–2.41) | 0.056 | | 1.61 (1.00–2.59) | 0.051 | |
| Alcohol drinking | | | 0.993 | | | 0.676 |
| Never | 1.59 (0.74–3.42) | 0.240 | | 1.43 (0.64–3.22) | 0.387 | |
| Ever | 1.52 (0.94–2.46) | 0.091 | | 1.72 (1.00–2.96) | 0.050 | |
| Betel nut chewing | | | 0.445 | | | 0.968 |
| Never | 2.06 (0.53–8.11) | 0.299 | | 1.64 (0.34–7.86) | 0.536 | |
| Ever | 1.41 (0.92–2.14) | 0.112 | | 1.63 (1.02–2.62) | 0.043 * | |
| Tea drinking | | | 0.331 | | | 0.986 |
| Never | 1.88 (1.05–3.35) | 0.033 * | | 1.60 (0.87–2.94) | 0.134 | |
| Ever | 1.27 (0.73–2.24) | 0.400 | | 1.57 (0.81–3.04) | 0.183 | |
| Coffee drinking | | | 0.073 | | | 0.077 |
| Never | 1.30 (0.82–2.08) | 0.066 | | 2.09 (1.28–3.41) | 0.003 * | |
| Ever | 2.83 (1.27–6.33) | 0.011 * | | 0.72 (0.22–2.42) | 0.601 | |
| Tumor differentiation | | | 0.492 | | | 0.949 |
| Well differentiated | 1.08 (0.43–2.68) | 0.875 | | 3.74 (1.26–11.09) | 0.018 * | |
| Moderate | 1.43 (0.84–2.42) | 0.184 | | 1.06 (0.57–1.98) | 0.858 | |
| Poor | 2.15 (0.88–5.22) | 0.093 | | 3.48 (1.23–9.88) | 0.019 * | |
| Primary tumor size | | | 0.146 | | | 0.394 |
| T1–T2 | 0.96 (0.45–2.03) | 0.905 | | 1.12 (0.49–2.56) | 0.788 | |
| T3–T4 | 1.83 (1.14–2.93) | 0.013 * | | 1.76 (1.04–3.00) | 0.036 * | |
| Nodal involvement | | | 0.328 | | | 0.125 |
| N0–N1 | 2.25 (1.06–4.81) | 0.036 * | | 3.16 (1.47–6.80) | 0.003 * | |
| N2–N3 | 1.32 (0.82–2.13) | 0.252 | | 1.23 (0.69–2.19) | 0.479 | |
| Perineural invasion | | | 0.008 * | | | 0.416 |
| No | 0.77 (0.40–1.49) | 0.429 | | 2.07 (1.06–4.03) | 0.032 * | |
| Yes | 2.46 (1.46–4.15) | <0.001 * | | 1.32 (0.72–2.44) | 0.370 | |
| Vascular invasion | | | 0.410 | | | <0.001 * |
| No | 1.45 (0.96–2.19) | 0.078 | | 1.51 (0.96–2.37) | 0.076 | |
| Yes | 1.27 (0.16–10.34) | 0.826 | | - | | |
| Lymphatic invasion | | | 0.553 | | | 0.449 |
| No | 1.43 (0.92–2.23) | 0.111 | | 1.71 (1.07–2.73) | 0.025 * | |
| Yes | 1.84 (0.64–5.31) | 0.260 | | 0.90 (0.20–4.16) | 0.892 | |
| Extranodal extension | | | 0.253 | | | 0.720 |
| No | 2.35 (1.12–4.94) | 0.024 * | | 2.17 (0.87–5.40) | 0.097 | |
| Yes | 1.31 (0.81–2.13) | 0.277 | | 1.52 (0.90–2.57) | 0.118 | |
| Pathologic TNM stage | | | 0.850 | | | 0.585 |
| III | 1.70 (0.48–6.09) | 0.414 | | 4.82 (0.98–23.58) | 0.053 | |
| IV | 1.51 (0.99–2.31) | 0.055 | | 1.54 (0.96–2.47) | 0.075 | |

OSCC, oral squamous cell carcinoma; HR, hazard ratio; CI, confidence interval; Int, interaction. [a] Adjusted for age, T stage, N stage, and extranodal extension. * $p < 0.05$.

## 4. Discussion

In this study, we investigated the association between potentially functional SNPs in the NER pathway genes and clinical outcomes in male patients with OSCC treated with CCRT. Our findings suggest that the *XPC* rs2228000 TT genotype was marginally significantly associated with increased risk of death, whereas the *ERCC5* rs17655 CC and *ERCC1* rs735482 CC genotypes were significantly associated with the increased risk of relapse.

The NER pathway plays a major role in DNA repair through the removal of bulky DNA lesions formed by ultraviolet (UV) radiation, environmental mutagens, and other chemotherapeutic agents [23,24]. Studies have revealed that variations in DNA-repair capacity are related to cancer risk and prognosis [25,26]. In addition, SNPs in the NER genes modulate susceptibility to efficacy and survival outcome of the treatment in certain types of cancers [11,12]. Therefore, the same phenomena may be exhibited in patients with OSCC, particularly those undergoing CCRT. Such information may be useful in identifying patients who may benefit from alternative therapies to achieve superior survival and improve quality of life.

The *XPC* gene is a key component of the XPC complex, which plays an important role in the early part of the global genome NER. The corresponding protein plays an important function in damage sensing and DNA binding [27]. SNPs in this gene have been found to affect clinical outcomes in various cancer types [18,28,29]. Li and colleagues observed that the *XPC* rs2228000 TT genotypes were associated with shorter OS than the CC+CT genotype individuals in a study of Japanese gastric cancer patients [30]. Another Chinese study demonstrated that patients with the CC genotype of *XPC* rs2228000 have a borderline significant decreased risk of developing gastric cancer compared with those with the CT+TT genotype [31]. This evidence suggests that the T-allele may have a high susceptibility for poor prognosis. Similarly, in our study, the *XPC* rs2228000 TT genotype shows an increased risk of death compared with the CC+CT genotype. Given the importance of the *XPC* gene in the NER pathway, it is possible that variants of *XPC* alter the DNA repair capacity and thereby affect sensitivity to therapeutic agents. However, the association observed in our study was borderline significant and must be interpreted with caution. Furthermore, large studies may be required to confirm these findings.

We also observed that those with the *ERCC5* rs17655 CC and *ERCC1* rs735482 CC genotypes have an increased risk of relapse compared with individuals with the GG+GC and AA+AC genotypes, respectively. Considered a central component in NER, *ERCC5* encodes a specific DNA endonuclease responsible for excision and repair of UV-induced DNA damage [23]. Evidence has linked *ERCC5* polymorphism to chemotherapeutic response and prognosis of tumors [19,20]. The ERCC5 mRNA expression levels were correlated with cytotoxicity of chemotherapy regiments [32]. Additionally, the rs17655 leads to an amino-acid substitution from histidine to aspartic acid, which may lead to differential interacting abilities, thus, influencing the DNA repair efficacy. Song et al. also observed that *ERCC5* rs17655 polymorphism has a moderately increased risk of recurrence in squamous cell carcinoma of the oropharynx [33]. ERCC1 is also a crucial member of the NER pathway that forms a complex with ERCC4, and together with ERCC5, is responsible for DNA incision [34]. Other studies have reported that *ERCC1* affects the clinical outcome and may serve as a potential biomarker for response to cisplatin-based therapy [35,36]. On the basis of these study results, we speculate that the CC genotypes of *ERCC5* rs17655 and *ERCC1* rs735482 may increase the DNA-repair capacity of cancer cells, leading to increased susceptibility to recurrence. Therefore, if these findings are confirmed by other studies, these SNPs may serve as therapeutic biomarkers for clinical outcome in patients with OSCC who undergo CCRT.

Our study has several limitations. First, the hospital-based nature of the patients may have led to selection bias. Secondly, not all SNPs in the entire NER pathway were used. Some rare functional SNPs may have an influence on survival. Finally, the human papilloma virus (HPV) status and inflammatory cytokines expression of patients was not included in the analysis and may limit the interpretation of our findings; hence, HPV and cytokines may affect survival [37,38]. However, a major strength of our study is that all the patients had a similar tumor stage and received the same treatment. This meant that the effect of different treatments was excluded, which might lead to different levels of DNA damage and repair.

## 5. Conclusions

We investigated the association between key potentially functional SNPs in the NER pathway and susceptibility for death or relapse in male patients with advanced OSCC who were treated with adjuvant CCRT. Our findings showed that the CC genotypes of *ERCC5* rs17655 and *ERCC1* rs735482 were associated with an increased risk of recurrence. CCRT may not be beneficial for these patients; therefore, alternative treatments are required. To our knowledge, this is the largest study to investigate the association between NER polymorphisms and survival in patients with OSCC treated with CCRT in ethnic Chinese. Our findings may require further confirmation in studies with a larger sample size or other ethnic populations.

**Supplementary Materials:** The following are available online at http://www.mdpi.com/2077-0383/8/1/33/s1, Figure S1: Linkage disequilibrium (LD) analysis among single nucleotide polymorphisms (SNPs) within the same chromosome or gene, Table S1: Frequency distributions of NER polymorphisms by clinicopathological factors, Table S2: Univariate association between NER candidate SNPs and OSCC survival in CCRT treated patients, Table S3: Haplotype analysis of association between NER candidate SNPs and OSCC survival in patients treated with CCRT.

**Author Contributions:** Conceptualization: S.-F.H. and C.-C.Y.; investigation: H.-T.C. and C.-K.Y.; methodology: T.S., Y.-X.C., W.-C.W., S.-F.H., and C.-C.Y.; resources: H.-T.C., Y.-X.C., and C.-K.Y.; formal analysis: T.S. and Y.-X.C.; validation: T.S., H.-T.C., and Y.-X.C.; writing: (original draft preparation) T.S.; writing (review and editing): T.S., W.-C.W., S.-F.H., and C.-C.Y.; supervision: S.-F.H. and C.-C.Y.; and funding acquisition: S.-F.H. and C.-C.Y.

**Funding:** The research was supported by the Ministry of Science and Technology, Taiwan (MOST 107-2314-B-038-071).

**Acknowledgments:** The authors would like to thank Wallace Academic Editing for the English language review.

**Conflicts of Interest:** The authors declare no conflict of interest.

### References

1. Chiang, C.-J.; Lo, W.-C.; Yang, Y.-W.; You, S.-L.; Chen, C.-J.; Lai, M.-S. Incidence and survival of adult cancer patients in Taiwan, 2002–2012. *J. Formos. Med. Assoc.* **2016**, *115*, 1076–1088. [CrossRef] [PubMed]
2. Amit, M.; Yen, T.C.; Liao, C.T.; Chaturvedi, P.; Agarwal, J.P.; Kowalski, L.P.; Ebrahimi, A.; Clark, J.R.; Kreppel, M.; Zoller, J.; et al. Improvement in survival of patients with oral cavity squamous cell carcinoma: An international collaborative study. *Cancer* **2013**, *119*, 4242–4248. [CrossRef] [PubMed]
3. Leemans, C.R.; Tiwari, R.; Nauta, J.J.; van der Waal, I.; Snow, G.B. Recurrence at the primary site in head and neck cancer and the significance of neck lymph node metastases as a prognostic factor. *Cancer* **1994**, *73*, 187–190. [CrossRef]
4. Markopoulos, A.K. Current Aspects on Oral Squamous Cell Carcinoma. *Open Dent. J.* **2012**, *6*, 126–130. [CrossRef] [PubMed]
5. Adelstein, D.; Gillison, M.L.; Pfister, D.G.; Spencer, S.; Adkins, D.; Brizel, D.M.; Burtness, B.; Busse, P.M.; Caudell, J.J.; Cmelak, A.J.; et al. NCCN Guidelines Insights: Head and Neck Cancers, Version 2.2017. *J. Natl. Compr. Cancer Netw.* **2017**, *15*, 761–770. [CrossRef] [PubMed]
6. Otsuru, M.; Ota, Y.; Aoki, T.; Sasaki, M.; Suzuki, T.; Denda, Y.; Takahashi, M.; Akiba, T.; Kaneko, A. A Study of Adjuvant Chemoradiotherapy with Tri-weekly Cisplatin for Postoperative High-risk Oral Squamous Cell Carcinoma. *Tokai J. Exp. Clin. Med.* **2017**, *42*, 19–24. [PubMed]
7. Ferris, R.L.; Geiger, J.L.; Trivedi, S.; Schmitt, N.C.; Heron, D.E.; Johnson, J.T.; Kim, S.; Duvvuri, U.; Clump, D.A.; Bauman, J.E.; et al. Phase II trial of post-operative radiotherapy with concurrent cisplatin plus panitumumab in patients with high-risk, resected head and neck cancer. *Ann. Oncol.* **2016**, *27*, 2257–2262. [CrossRef]
8. Bernier, J.; Domenge, C.; Ozsahin, M.; Matuszewska, K.; Lefebvre, J.L.; Greiner, R.H.; Giralt, J.; Maingon, P.; Rolland, F.; Bolla, M.; et al. Postoperative irradiation with or without concomitant chemotherapy for locally advanced head and neck cancer. *N. Engl. J. Med.* **2004**, *350*, 1945–1952. [CrossRef]
9. Tanvetyanon, T.; Padhya, T.; McCaffrey, J.; Kish, J.A.; Deconti, R.C.; Trotti, A.; Rao, N.G. Postoperative concurrent chemotherapy and radiotherapy for high-risk cutaneous squamous cell carcinoma of the head and neck. *Head Neck* **2015**, *37*, 840–845. [CrossRef]
10. Leeman, J.E.; Li, J.G.; Pei, X.; Venigalla, P.; Zumsteg, Z.S.; Katsoulakis, E.; Lupovitch, E.; McBride, S.M.; Tsai, C.J.; Boyle, J.O.; et al. Patterns of Treatment Failure and Postrecurrence Outcomes Among Patients With Locally Advanced Head and Neck Squamous Cell Carcinoma After Chemoradiotherapy Using Modern Radiation Techniques. *JAMA Oncol.* **2017**, *3*, 1487–1494. [CrossRef]
11. Jin, H.; Xie, X.; Wang, H.; Hu, J.; Liu, F.; Liu, Z.; Zhou, J.; Zhang, Y.; Xi, X.; Hu, B.; et al. ERCC1 Cys8092Ala and XRCC1 Arg399Gln polymorphisms predict progression-free survival after curative radiotherapy for nasopharyngeal carcinoma. *PLoS ONE* **2014**, *9*, e101256. [CrossRef] [PubMed]

12. Liu, H.; Qi, B.; Guo, X.; Tang, L.Q.; Chen, Q.Y.; Zhang, L.; Guo, L.; Luo, D.H.; Huang, P.Y.; Mo, H.Y.; et al. Genetic variations in radiation and chemotherapy drug action pathways and survival in locoregionally advanced nasopharyngeal carcinoma treated with chemoradiotherapy. *PLoS ONE* **2013**, *8*, e82750. [CrossRef] [PubMed]
13. Lopes-Aguiar, L.; Costa, E.F.D.; Nogueira, G.A.S.; Lima, T.R.P.; Visacri, M.B.; Pincinato, E.C.; Calonga, L.; Mariano, F.V.; de Almeida Milani Altemani, A.M.; Altemani, J.M.C.; et al. XPD c.934G>A polymorphism of nucleotide excision repair pathway in outcome of head and neck squamous cell carcinoma patients treated with cisplatin chemoradiation. *Oncotarget* **2016**, *8*, 16190–16201. [CrossRef] [PubMed]
14. Nanda, S.S.; Gandhi, A.K.; Rastogi, M.; Khurana, R.; Hadi, R.; Sahni, K.; Mishra, S.P.; Srivastava, A.K.; Bhatt, M.L.B.; Parmar, D. Evaluation of XRCC1 Gene Polymorphism as a Biomarker in Head and Neck Cancer Patients Undergoing Chemoradiation Therapy. *Int. J. Radiat. Oncol. Biol. Phys.* **2018**, *101*, 593–601. [CrossRef]
15. Rouillon, C.; White, M.F. The evolution and mechanisms of nucleotide excision repair proteins. *Res. Microbiol.* **2011**, *162*, 19–26. [CrossRef] [PubMed]
16. Gao, C.; Wang, J.; Li, C.; Zhang, W.; Liu, G. A Functional Polymorphism (rs10817938) in the XPA Promoter Region Is Associated with Poor Prognosis of Oral Squamous Cell Carcinoma in a Chinese Han Population. *PLoS ONE* **2016**, *11*, e0160801. [CrossRef] [PubMed]
17. Tan, L.M.; Qiu, C.F.; Zhu, T.; Jin, Y.X.; Li, X.; Yin, J.Y.; Zhang, W.; Zhou, H.H.; Liu, Z.Q. Genetic Polymorphisms and Platinum-based Chemotherapy Treatment Outcomes in Patients with Non-Small Cell Lung Cancer: A Genetic Epidemiology Study Based Meta-analysis. *Sci. Rep.* **2017**, *7*, 5593. [CrossRef]
18. Wang, C.; Nie, H.; Li, Y.; Liu, G.; Wang, X.; Xing, S.; Zhang, L.; Chen, X.; Chen, Y.; Li, Y. The study of the relation of DNA repair pathway genes SNPs and the sensitivity to radiotherapy and chemotherapy of NSCLC. *Sci. Rep.* **2016**, *6*, 26526. [CrossRef]
19. Zhang, R.; Zhou, F.; Cheng, L.; Yu, A.; Zhu, M.; Wang, M.; Zhang, Z.; Xiang, J.; Wei, Q. Genetic variants in nucleotide excision repair pathway predict survival of esophageal squamous cell cancer patients receiving platinum-based chemotherapy. *Mol. Carcinog.* **2018**, *57*, 1553–1565. [CrossRef]
20. Zhou, F.; Zhu, M.; Wang, M.; Qiu, L.; Cheng, L.; Jia, M.; Xiang, J.; Wei, Q. Genetic variants of DNA repair genes predict the survival of patients with esophageal squamous cell cancer receiving platinum-based adjuvant chemotherapy. *J. Transl. Med.* **2016**, *14*, 154. [CrossRef]
21. Amin, M.B.; Greene, F.L.; Edge, S.B.; Compton, C.C.; Gershenwald, J.E.; Brookland, R.K.; Meyer, L.; Gress, D.M.; Byrd, D.R.; Winchester, D.P. The Eighth Edition AJCC Cancer Staging Manual: Continuing to build a bridge from a population-based to a more "personalized" approach to cancer staging. *CA: A Cancer J. Clin.* **2017**, *67*, 93–99. [CrossRef] [PubMed]
22. Stephens, M.; Smith, N.J.; Donnelly, P. A new statistical method for haplotype reconstruction from population data. *Am. J. Hum. Genet.* **2001**, *68*, 978–989. [CrossRef] [PubMed]
23. Schärer, O.D. Nucleotide Excision Repair in Eukaryotes. *Cold Spring Harb. Perspect. Biol.* **2013**, *5*, a012609. [CrossRef] [PubMed]
24. Friedberg, E.C. How nucleotide excision repair protects against cancer. *Nat. Rev. Cancer* **2001**, *1*, 22–33. [CrossRef] [PubMed]
25. Naccarati, A.; Rosa, F.; Vymetalkova, V.; Barone, E.; Jiraskova, K.; Di Gaetano, C.; Novotny, J.; Levy, M.; Vodickova, L.; Gemignani, F.; et al. Double-strand break repair and colorectal cancer: Gene variants within 3′ UTRs and microRNAs binding as modulators of cancer risk and clinical outcome. *Oncotarget* **2016**, *7*, 23156–23169. [CrossRef]
26. Mucha, B.; Pytel, D.; Markiewicz, L.; Cuchra, M.; Szymczak, I.; Przybylowska-Sygut, K.; Dziki, A.; Majsterek, I.; Dziki, L. Nucleotide Excision Repair Capacity and XPC and XPD Gene Polymorphism Modulate Colorectal Cancer Risk. *Clin. Colorectal. Cancer* **2018**, *17*, e435–e441. [CrossRef] [PubMed]
27. Sugasawa, K.; Ng, J.M.; Masutani, C.; Iwai, S.; van der Spek, P.J.; Eker, A.P.; Hanaoka, F.; Bootsma, D.; Hoeijmakers, J.H. Xeroderma pigmentosum group C protein complex is the initiator of global genome nucleotide excision repair. *Mol. Cell* **1998**, *2*, 223–232. [CrossRef]
28. Zheng, Y.; Deng, Z.; Yin, J.; Wang, S.; Lu, D.; Wen, X.; Li, X.; Xiao, D.; Hu, C.; Chen, X.; et al. The association of genetic variations in DNA repair pathways with severe toxicities in NSCLC patients undergoing platinum-based chemotherapy. *Int. J. Cancer* **2017**, *141*, 2336–2347. [CrossRef] [PubMed]

29. Ravegnini, G.; Nannini, M.; Simeon, V.; Musti, M.; Sammarini, G.; Saponara, M.; Gatto, L.; Urbini, M.; Astolfi, A.; Biasco, G.; et al. Polymorphisms in DNA repair genes in gastrointestinal stromal tumours: Susceptibility and correlation with tumour characteristics and clinical outcome. *Tumour Biol.* **2016**, *37*, 13413–13423. [CrossRef]
30. Li, Y.; Liu, Z.; Liu, H.; Wang, L.E.; Onodera, H.; Suzuki, A.; Suzuki, K.; Wadhwa, R.; Elimova, E.; Sudo, K.; et al. Potentially functional variants in the core nucleotide excision repair genes predict survival in Japanese gastric cancer patients. *Carcinogenesis* **2014**, *35*, 2031–2038. [CrossRef]
31. Hua, R.-X.; Zhuo, Z.-J.; Shen, G.-P.; Zhu, J.; Zhang, S.-D.; Xue, W.-Q.; Li, X.-Z.; Zhang, P.-F.; He, J.; Jia, W.-H. Polymorphisms in the XPC gene and gastric cancer susceptibility in a Southern Chinese population. *Onco Targets Ther.* **2016**, *9*, 5513–5519. [CrossRef] [PubMed]
32. Zhao, Y.L.; Yang, L.B.; Geng, X.L.; Zhou, Q.L.; Qin, H.; Yang, L.; Dong, Y.Z.; Zhong, J.J. The association of XPG and MMS19L polymorphisms response to chemotherapy in osteosarcoma. *Pak. J. Med. Sci.* **2013**, *29*, 1225–1229. [CrossRef] [PubMed]
33. Song, X.; Sturgis, E.M.; Jin, L.; Wang, Z.; Wei, Q.; Li, G. Variants in nucleotide excision repair core genes and susceptibility to recurrence of squamous cell carcinoma of the oropharynx. *Int. J. Cancer* **2013**, *133*, 695–704. [CrossRef] [PubMed]
34. Bowden, N.A. Nucleotide excision repair: Why is it not used to predict response to platinum-based chemotherapy? *Cancer Lett.* **2014**, *346*, 163–171. [CrossRef] [PubMed]
35. Arriagada, R.; Bergman, B.; Dunant, A.; Le Chevalier, T.; Pignon, J.P.; Vansteenkiste, J. Cisplatin-based adjuvant chemotherapy in patients with completely resected non-small-cell lung cancer. *N. Engl. J. Med.* **2004**, *350*, 351–360. [CrossRef] [PubMed]
36. Olaussen, K.A.; Dunant, A.; Fouret, P.; Brambilla, E.; Andre, F.; Haddad, V.; Taranchon, E.; Filipits, M.; Pirker, R.; Popper, H.H.; et al. DNA repair by ERCC1 in non-small-cell lung cancer and cisplatin-based adjuvant chemotherapy. *N. Engl. J. Med.* **2006**, *355*, 983–991. [CrossRef] [PubMed]
37. Lafaurie, G.I.; Perdomo, S.J.; Buenahora, M.R.; Amaya, S.; Diaz-Baez, D. Human papilloma virus: An etiological and prognostic factor for oral cancer? *J. Investig. Clin. Dent.* **2018**, *9*, e12313. [CrossRef]
38. Kwon, M.; Kim, J.W.; Roh, J.L.; Park, Y.; Cho, K.J.; Choi, S.H.; Nam, S.Y.; Kim, S.Y.; Lee, B.H. Recurrence and cancer-specific survival according to the expression of IL-4Ralpha and IL-13Ralpha1 in patients with oral cavity cancer. *Eur. J. Cancer (Oxf. Engl.: 1990)* **2015**, *51*, 177–185. [CrossRef]

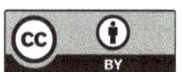

© 2019 by the authors. Licensee MDPI, Basel, Switzerland. This article is an open access article distributed under the terms and conditions of the Creative Commons Attribution (CC BY) license (http://creativecommons.org/licenses/by/4.0/).

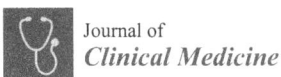 

Article

# Distinct Expression and Clinical Significance of Zinc Finger AN-1-Type Containing 4 in Oral Squamous Cell Carcinomas

Julián Suarez-Canto [1], Faustino Julián Suárez-Sánchez [2], Francisco Domínguez-Iglesias [2], Gonzalo Hernández-Vallejo [3], Juana M. García-Pedrero [4,5,6,*] and Juan C. de Vicente [5,7,8,*]

1. 395 Los Prados Cabueñes, 33394 Gijón, Asturias, Spain; juliansuarezcanto@gmail.com
2. Department of Pathology, Hospital Universitario de Cabueñes, 395 Los Prados Cabueñes, 33394 Gijón, Asturias, Spain; faustinosuarezsanchez@gmail.com (F.J.S.S.); fdoig59@yahoo.es (F.D.I.)
3. School of Dentistry, Complutense University of Madrid, Pza. Ramón y Cajal, s/n, Ciudad Universitaria, 28040 Madrid, Spain; ghervall@odon.ucm.es
4. Department of Otolaryngology, Hospital Universitario Central de Asturias (HUCA), C/Carretera de Rubín, s/n, 33011 Oviedo, Asturias, Spain
5. Instituto de Investigación Sanitaria del Principado de Asturias (ISPA), Instituto Universitario de Oncología del Principado de Asturias (IUOPA), Universidad de Oviedo, C/Carretera de Rubín, s/n, 33011 Oviedo, Asturias, Spain
6. Ciber de Cáncer (CIBERONC), Instituto de Salud Carlos III, Av. Monforte de Lemos, 3-5, 28029 Madrid, Spain
7. Department of Oral and Maxillofacial Surgery, Hospital Universitario Central de Asturias (HUCA), C/Carretera de Rubín, s/n, 33011 Oviedo, Asturias, Spain
8. Department of Surgery, University of Oviedo, Av. Julián Clavería, 6, 33006 Oviedo, Asturias, Spain
* Correspondence: juanagp.finba@gmail.com (J.M.G.-P.); jvicente@uniovi.es (J.C.d.V.); Tel.: +34-985-107937 (J.M.G.-P.); +34-85-103638 (J.C.d.V.)

Received: 27 October 2018; Accepted: 7 December 2018; Published: 10 December 2018

**Abstract:** Zinc finger AN1-type containing 4 (ZFAND4) has emerged as a promising prognostic marker and predictor of metastasis for patients with oral squamous cell carcinoma (OSCC). However, further validation is fundamental before clinical implementation. Hence, this study evaluated the expression pattern of ZFAND4 protein expression by immunohistochemistry using an independent cohort of 125 patients with OSCC, and correlations with the clinicopathologic parameters and disease outcome. Remarkably, ZFAND4 expression, while negligible in normal epithelium, exhibited two distinct expression patterns in tumors that did not overlap. A gross granular staining was characteristic of the undifferentiated cells at the invasive front of tumors, whereas the most differentiated cells located at the center of the tumor nests showed diffuse non-granular staining. ZFAND4 staining was higher in undifferentiated than in differentiated areas of tumors. High ZFAND4 expression in differentiated cells was significantly associated to well-differentiated ($p = 0.04$) and non-recurrent tumors ($p = 0.04$), whereas ZFAND4 expression in undifferentiated cells correlated with tumor location ($p = 0.005$). No correlations between the ZFAND4 expression and patient survival were found. These data question the clinical relevance of ZFAND4 expression as a prognostic biomarker in OSCC, and also reveal distinct ZFAND4 expression patterns depending on the differentiation areas of tumors that should be evaluated separately.

**Keywords:** ZFAND4; ANUBL1; oral squamous cell carcinoma; immunohistochemistry; prognosis

## 1. Introduction

Head and neck squamous cell carcinoma that includes, among others, oral squamous cell carcinoma (OSCC) is the sixth most common cancer in the world, with an annual prevalence of nearly 600,000 new cases worldwide [1,2]. It is generally accepted that OSCC initiates and progresses through a series of multiple genetic alterations caused by chronic exposure to carcinogens, such as alcohol, smoking, and human papilloma virus [3]. Multiple genetic and molecular studies have improved our understanding of the molecular basis of this disease. Indeed, several cellular signaling pathways have been found dysregulated in these tumors through genetic and epigenetic alterations. However, despite major advances in diagnosis and treatment, the survival rate of patients with OSCC has modestly improved over the past 40 years, and it remains at approximately 50% [4].

Sasahira et al. [5] investigated the transcriptional profiles of primary and recurrent OSCC, and found that one of the most upregulated genes identified in recurrent OSCC was zinc finger AN1-type containing 4 (ZFAND4), also known as AN1 and ubiquitin-like homolog (ANUBL1). Although the functional role of ZFAND4 in cancer is still unknown, Kurihara-Shimomura et al. [6] evaluated its prognostic utility in OSCC. They concluded that ZFAND4 could be a useful marker for predicting metastasis and poor prognosis in patients with OSCC. In addition, Tang et al. [7] demonstrated that ZFAND4 expression is upregulated in gastric cancer and positively associated with the grading of this disease.

In the light of these data, ZFAND4 emerges as a promising prognostic biomarker; however, further validation in independent study cohorts is fundamental for implementation to the clinic. Therefore, the objective of this study was to investigate the expression pattern and clinical relevance of ZFAND4 protein expression using an independent cohort of 125 patients with OSCC, and to establish correlations with the clinicopathologic parameters and disease outcome.

## 2. Experimental Section

### 2.1. Patients and Tissue Specimens

A retrospective study was designed. Surgical tissue specimens from 125 patients with OSCC who underwent surgical treatment with curative purposes at the Hospital Universitario Central de Asturias between 1996 and 2007 were retrospectively collected, in accordance to approved institutional review board guidelines. All experimental procedures were conducted in accordance to the Declaration of Helsinki and approved by the Institutional Ethics Committee of the Hospital Universitario Central de Asturias and by the Regional CEIC from Principado de Asturias. Informed consent was obtained from all patients. Clinicopathologic data were collected from medical records. Tissue specimens were obtained from the Biobanco del Principado de Asturias, and representative tissue sections from archival, formalin-fixed paraffin-embedded blocks.

### 2.2. Tissue Microarray Construction

The original archived hematoxylin- and eosin-stained slides were reviewed by an experienced pathologist (FDI) to confirm histological diagnosis. Three representative tissue cores (1 mm diameter) were selected from each tumor block, and transferred to a recipient 'Master' block in a grid-like manner using a manual tissue microarray instrument. In addition, each tissue microarray also contained three cores of normal epithelium as an internal control. A section from each microarray was stained with hematoxylin and eosin, and examined by light microscopy to check the adequacy of tissue sampling.

### 2.3. Immunohistochemistry (IHC)

TMA sections (4 µm) were cut and dried and dried on Flex IHC microscope slides (Dako). The sections were deparaffinized with standard xylene, hydrated through graded alcohols into water, and pretreated by hydrogen peroxide to quench the endogenous peroxidase activity. Antigen retrieval was performed using Envision Flex Target Retrieval solution (Dako), at room temperature on an automatic staining workstation (DakoAutostainer Plus, Dako, Glostrup, Denmark). Staining was carried out at room temperature on an automatic staining workstation (Dako Autostainer Plus) with anti-ZFAND4 antibody (Atlas Antibodies, Stockholm, Sweden) diluted to 0.5 Nµg/mL using the

Dako EnVision detection system (Dako, Glostrup, Denmark). Sections were counterstained with hematoxylin, dehydrated with ethanol, and permanently coverslipped. For negative control purposes, DakoCytomation mouse serum diluted at the same concentration as the primary antibody was used.

Staining was scored blinded to clinical data by two independent observers. ZFAND4 expression was evaluated according to the percentage of stained tumor cells and the staining intensity using the Allred score, as previously described [8]. The proportion of ZFAND4-positive cells was evaluated in both undifferentiated and differentiated areas of the tumors. In all these groups, proportional scores were categorized as: 0, no cells were stained; 1, 1/100 cells were stained; 2, 1/10 cells were stained; 4, 2/3 cells were stained; 5, all cells were stained. Staining intensity was scored as: 0, negative; 1, weak; 2, intermediate; and 3, strong. The total score was calculated by the sum of the proportional and intensity scores, ranging from 0 to 8. Similar to Kurihara-Shimomura et al. [6], the optimal cut-off score for ZFAND4 expression was selected using the receiver operating characteristic (ROC) curve according to the survival status. ZFAND4 staining was independently evaluated in undifferentiated areas of tumors mainly located at the invasive front, and in differentiated areas at the center of the tumor islands.

## 2.4. Statistical Analysis

$\chi^2$ and the Fisher's exact test were used for comparison between categorical variables. Disease-specific survival (DSS) was determined for the date of treatment completion to death for the tumor. For time-to-event analysis, survival curves were plotted using the Kaplan-Meier method. Differences between survival times were analyzed by the log-rank test. Hazard ratios (HR) with their 95% confidence intervals (CI) for clinicopathologic variables were calculated using the univariate Cox proportional hazards model analysis. All tests were two-sided and $p$ values less than 0.05 were considered statistically significant. All statistical analyses were performed using SPSS version 21 (IBM Co., Armonk, NY, USA).

## 3. Results

### 3.1. Patient Characteristics

The cohort of 125 OSCC patients was composed of 82 men and 43 women, ranging from 28 to 91 years, with a median age of 57 years. Forty-one patients (33%) were never-smokers and 56 (45%) never-drinkers. The main clinicopathologic characteristics are summarized in Table 1. Forty-nine cases (39%) showed neck lymph node metastasis, more than 50% were well-differentiated tumors and advanced clinical stages (III or IV), and the most common site was the tongue (41%) followed by the floor of the mouth (30%). Adjuvant radiotherapy was administered to 75 patients (60%), and adjuvant chemotherapy to 14 patients (11.2%). Fifty-four cases (43%) showed loco-regional recurrence, and 19 (15%) suffered from a second primary carcinoma. Over a median follow-up of 61 months (range, 1 to 230 months) 53 deaths occurred.

**Table 1.** Clinical and pathological characteristics of 123 patients with oral squamous cell carcinoma and where zinc finger AN1-type containing 4 (ZFAND4) was valuable.

| Variable | Number (%) |
|---|---|
| Age (year) (mean ± SD; median; range) | 58.6 ± 14.3; 57; 28–91 |
| Gender | |
| Men | 81 (66) |
| Women | 42 (34) |

Table 1. *Cont.*

| Variable | Number (%) |
|---|---|
| Tobacco use | |
| Smoker | 83 (67) |
| Non-smoker | 40 (33) |
| Alcohol use | |
| Drinker | 68 (55) |
| Non-drinker | 55 (45) |
| Location of oral squamous oral cell carcinoma | |
| Tongue | 51 (41) |
| Floor of the mouth | 35 (28) |
| Other sites within te oral cavity | 37 (31) |
| Tumor status | |
| pT1 | 27 (22) |
| pT2 | 53 (43) |
| pT3 | 15 (12) |
| pT4 | 28 (23) |
| Nodal status | |
| pN0 | 74 (60) |
| pN1 | 25 (20) |
| pN2 | 24 (20) |
| Clinical stage | |
| Stage I | 20 (16) |
| Stage II | 31 (25) |
| Stage III | 25 (20) |
| Stage IV | 47 (39) |
| G status | |
| G1 | 78 (63) |
| G2 | 41 (33) |
| G3 | 4 (4) |
| Second primary carcinoma | |
| No | 104 (85) |
| Yes | 19 (15) |
| Local recurrence | |
| No | 69 (56) |
| Yes | 54 (44) |
| Clinical status at the end of the follow-up | |
| Live and without recurrence | 51 (41) |
| Dead of index cancer | 53 (43) |
| Lost or died of other causes (censored) | 19 (16) |

*3.2. Immunohistochemical Analysis of ZFAND4 Expression in OSCC Tissue Specimens*

ZFAND4 staining was not valuable in two (1.6%) of 125 OSCC specimens. While ZFAND4 expression was negligible in normal epithelium, two distinct expression patterns were noted in the tumors that did not overlap in any of the samples (Figure 1). A gross granular staining was characteristic of the undifferentiated cells at the invasive front of tumors, whereas the most differentiated cells located at the center of the tumor nests showed diffuse non-granular staining. The mean percentages of positive ZFAND4 staining were 44.98 (standard deviation –SD-35.38) in undifferentiated cells and 17.18 (SD, 20.61) in differentiated cells. ZFAND4 staining intensity was also evaluated in both undifferentiated and differentiated areas. In undifferentiated cells, there were 13 (11%) negative cases, 37 (30%) weak, 43 (35%) intermediate, and 30 (24%) cases with strong staining. In differentiated cells, 47 (38%) cases were scored negative, 11 (9%) weak, 47 (38%) intermediate, and 18 (15%) had strong staining. Since each tumor was represented by three different tissue cores in the OSCC TMAs, the percentages of stained cells frequently varied in the three tumor areas assessed. Taking this into consideration, the Allred score was determined in two different ways: Either considering the maximum value of ZFAND4 positivity or the mean value of the three tumor cores. Regarding the intensity of immunostaining, the maximum value was always used for all calculations. Finally, the total score was calculated by the sum of the percentages of staining and intensity scores. The resulting indexes ranged between 0 and 8. The receiver operating characteristics (ROC) curve was used to determine the best cut-off score to predict patients' survival, and this value was 4. Accordingly, those cases with an Allred score above 4 were considered as high ZFAND4 expression.

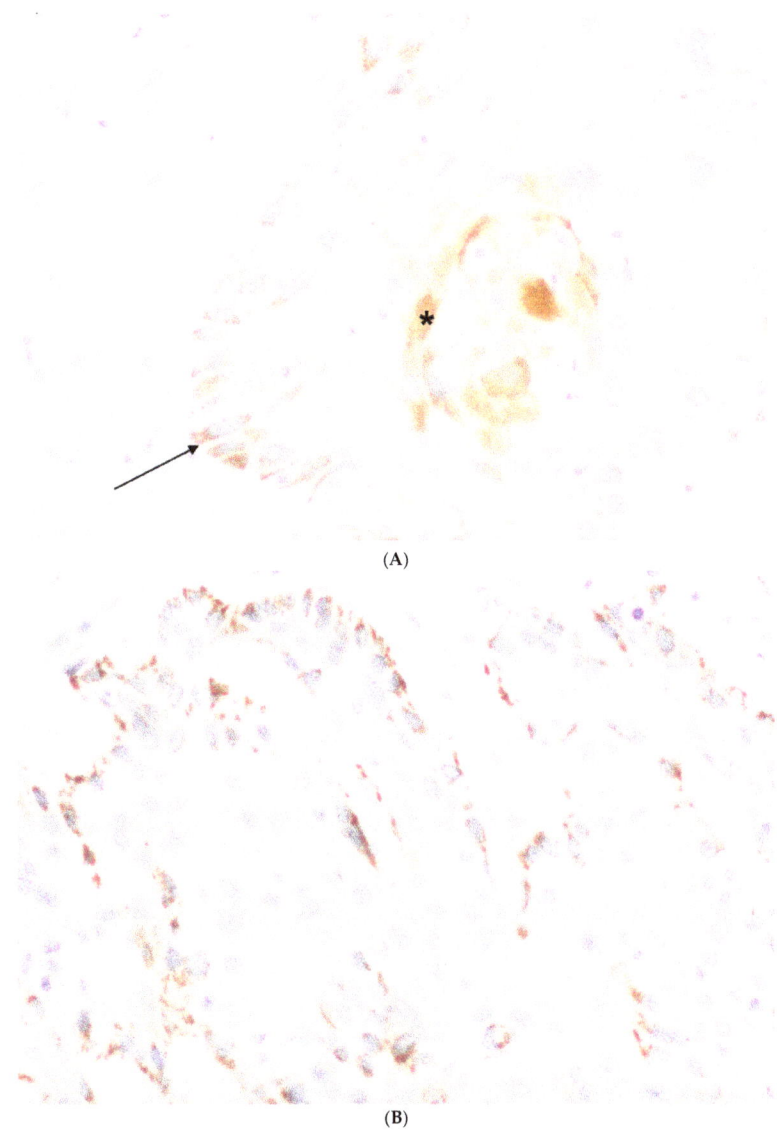

Figure 1. *Cont.*

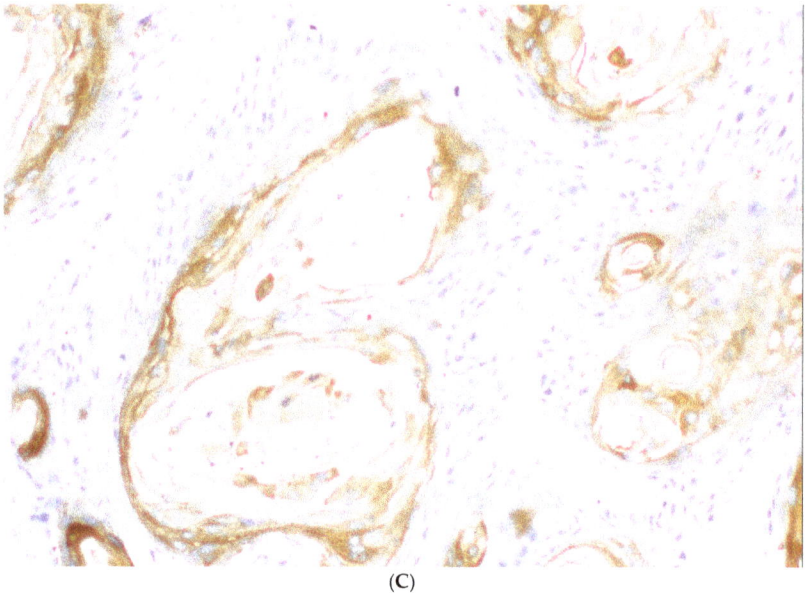

(C)

**Figure 1.** Immunoexpression of ZFAND4 in oral squamous cell carcinoma. (**A**) Staining in undifferentiated areas (arrow) and differentiated areas (*). (**B**) Staining in undifferentiated cells, mainly located in the invasive front of tumor tissue. (**C**) Staining in differentiated cells located at the center of the tumor islands.

### 3.3. Associations of ZFAND4 with Clinicopathologic Characteristics

We next assessed the correlations of high ZFAND4 expression with the clinical data. Table 2 shows the associations of high ZFAND4 expression determined by using the maximum value of the percentage of stained cells to calculate the Allred score. In differentiated areas, high ZFAND4 expression was significantly associated with well-differentiated ($p$ = 0.04) and non-recurrent tumors ($p$ = 0.04), whereas ZFAND4 expression in undifferentiated cells was significantly correlated with tumor location in the tongue ($p$ = 0.005).

On the other hand, when the Allred score was calculated using the mean value of percentage of stained cells (Table 3), ZFAND4 expression in differentiated cells was found to be significantly associated with N status ($p$ = 0.02), being more frequently detected in pN0 and pN1 cases compared to pN2. However, no significant relationship was found between ZFAND4 expression in undifferentiated cells and any clinicopathologic variable.

**Table 2.** Relationships between clinical and pathological variables and high ZFAND4 expression determined by using the maximum value of stained cells to calculate the Allred score.

| Variable | Number of Cases | High ZFAND4 Expression in Undifferentiated Cells (%) | $p$ | High ZFAND4 Expression in Differentiated Cells (%) |
|---|---|---|---|---|
| Gender |  |  |  |  |
| Men | 81 | 50 (62) | 0.98 | 38 (47) |
| Women | 42 | 26 (62) |  | 17 (40) |
| Tobacco use |  |  |  |  |
| Smoker | 83 | 52 (63) | 0.77 | 34 (41) |
| Non-smoker | 40 | 24 (60) |  | 21 (52) |
| Alcohol use |  |  |  |  |
| Drinker | 68 | 42 (62) | 0.99 | 31 (46) |
| Non-drinker | 55 | 34 (62) |  | 24 (44) |

Table 2. Cont.

| Variable | Number of Cases | High ZFAND4 Expression in Undifferentiated Cells (%) | p | High ZFAND4 Expression in Differentiated Cells (%) |
|---|---|---|---|---|
| pT | | | | |
| pT1 | 27 | 19 (70) | | 16 (59) |
| pT2 | 53 | 33 (62) | 0.44 | 25 (47) |
| pT3 | 15 | 10 (67) | | 4 (27) |
| pT4 | 28 | 14 (50) | | 10 (36) |
| pN | | | | |
| pN0 | 74 | 45 (61) | | 34 (46) |
| pN1 | 25 | 17 (68) | 0.75 | 13 (52) |
| pN2 | 24 | 14 (58) | | 8 (33) |
| Clinical stage | | | | |
| Stage I | 20 | 13 (65) | | 9 (45) |
| Stage II | 31 | 20 (64) | 0.69 | 16 (52) |
| Stage III | 25 | 17 (68) | | 11 (44) |
| Stage IV | 47 | 26 (55) | | 19 (40) |
| G status | | | | |
| G1 (Well) | 78 | 52 (67) | 0.14 | 40 (51) |
| G2 + G3 (Moderate + poor) | 45 | 24 (53) | | 15 (33) |
| Tumor location | | | | |
| Tongue | 51 | 39 (76) | 0.005 | 23 (45) |
| Rest | 72 | 37 (51) | | 32 (44) |
| Tumor location | | | | |
| Floor of the mouth | 35 | 20 (57) | 0.5 | 16 (46) |
| Rest | 88 | 56 (64) | | 39 (44) |
| Tumor recurrence | | | | |
| No | 69 | 44 (64) | 0.61 | 36 (52) |
| Yes | 54 | 32 (59) | | 19 (35) |
| Second primary carcinoma | | | | |
| No | 104 | 64 (61) | 0.89 | 48 (46) |
| Yes | 19 | 12 (63) | | 7 (37) |
| Clinical status at the end of the follow-up | | | | |
| Live and without recurrence | 51 | 32 (63) | 0.73 | 26 (51) |
| Dead of index cancer | 53 | 31 (58) | | 20 (38) |
| Lost or died of other causes | 19 | 13 (68) | | 9 (47) |

Table 3. Relationships between clinical and pathological variables and high ZFAND4 expression determined by using the mean value of stained cells to calculate the Allred score.

| Variable | Number of Cases | High ZFAND4 Expression in Undifferentiated Cells (%) | p | High ZFAND4 Expression in Differentiated Cells (%) | p |
|---|---|---|---|---|---|
| Gender | | | | | |
| Men | 81 | 42 (52) | 0.95 | 26 (32) | 0.33 |
| Women | 42 | 22 (52) | | 10 (24) | |
| Tobacco use | | | | | |
| Smoker | 83 | 44 (53) | 0.75 | 23 (28) | 0.58 |
| Non-smoker | 40 | 20 (50) | | 13 (32) | |
| Alcohol use | | | | | |
| Drinker | 68 | 35 (51) | 0.89 | 23 (34) | 0.21 |
| Non-drinker | 55 | 29 (53) | | 13 (24) | |

Table 3. Cont.

| Variable | Number of Cases | High ZFAND4 Expression in Undifferentiated Cells (%) | p | High ZFAND4 Expression in Differentiated Cells (%) | p |
|---|---|---|---|---|---|
| pT | | | | | |
| pT1 | 27 | 16 (59) | | 11 (41) | |
| pT2 | 53 | 27 (51) | 0.29 | 15 (28) | 0.33 |
| pT3 | 15 | 10 (67) | | 2 (13) | |
| pT4 | 28 | 11 (39) | | 8 (29) | |
| pN | | | | | |
| pN0 | 74 | 37 (50) | | 24 (32) | |
| pN1 | 25 | 14 (56) | 0.85 | 10 (40) | 0.02 |
| pN2 | 24 | 13 (54) | | 2 (8) | |
| Clinical stage | | | | | |
| Stage I | 20 | 10 (50) | | 6 (30) | |
| Stage II | 31 | 17 (55) | 0.46 | 11 (35) | 0.81 |
| Stage III | 25 | 16 (64) | | 9 (36) | |
| Stage IV | 47 | 21 (45) | | 10 (21) | |
| G status | | | | | |
| G1 (Well) | 78 | 43 (55) | 0.36 | 27 (35) | 0.08 |
| G2 + G3 (Moderate + poor) | 45 | 21 (47) | | 9 (20) | |
| Tumor location | | | | | |
| Tongue | 51 | 31 (61) | 0.1 | 13 (25) | 0.43 |
| Rest | 72 | 33 (46) | | 23 (32) | |
| Tumor location | | | | | |
| Floor of the mouth | 35 | 19 (54) | 0.75 | 12 (34) | 0.44 |
| Rest | 88 | 45 (51) | | 24 (27) | |
| Tumor recurrence | | | | | |
| No | 69 | 36 (52) | 0.97 | 22 (32) | 0.47 |
| Yes | 54 | 28 (52) | | 14 (26) | |
| Second primary carcinoma | | | | | |
| No | 104 | 52 (50) | 0.29 | 31 (30) | 0.75 |
| Yes | 19 | 12 (63) | | 5 (26) | |
| Clinical status at the end of the follow-up | | | | | |
| Live and without recurrence | 51 | 26 (51) | 0.85 | 17 (33) | 0.59 |
| Dead of index cancer | 53 | 27 (51) | | 15 (28) | |
| Lost or died of other causes | 19 | 11 (58) | | 4 (21) | |

*3.4. ZFAND4 Expression and Patients' Survival*

Over a median follow-up period of 61 months, 27 patients (42.1%) harboring high ZFAND4 expression in undifferentiated cells calculated by using the mean Allred score died due to the index cancer, and 15 patients (41.6%) with high ZFAND4 expression in the differentiated cells. When the maximum Allred score was used, 31 patients (40.7%) with high ZFAND4 expression in the undifferentiated cells, and 20 patients (36.3%) with high ZFAND4 expression in the differentiated cells died due to the index cancer. Kaplan-Meier analysis showed that there were no statistically significant differences in disease-specific survival (DSS) between patients with high versus low ZFAND4 expression in either differentiated or undifferentiated cells (Table 4).

Table 4. Univariate Kaplan-Meier and Cox analysis to assess the association of ZFAND4 expression on disease-specific survival in oral squamous cell carcinoma patients.

| ZFAND4 Expression | Censored Patients (%) | Mean Survival Time (95% CI) | HR (95% CI) | p |
|---|---|---|---|---|
| Undifferentiated cells calculated by using the mean Allred score | | | | |
| Low | 33 (56) | 107.72 (86.32–129.12) | Reference | 0.7 |
| High | 37 (58) | 135.20 (108.87–161.52) | 0.90 (0.52–1.55) | |
| Differentiated cells calculated by using the mean Allred score | | | | |
| Low | 49 (56) | 126.62 (104.38–148.85) | Reference | 0.8 |
| High | 21 (58) | 135.11 (99.60–170.62) | 0.93 (0.51–1.69) | |
| Undifferentiated cells calculated by using the maximum Allred score | | | | |
| Low | 25 (53) | 104.14 (80.46–127.82) | Reference | 0.53 |
| High | 45 (59) | 136.44 (111.81–161.06) | 0.84 (0.48–1.45) | |
| Differentiated cells calculated by using the maximum Allred score | | | | |
| Low | 35 (51) | 105.55 (85.11–126.00) | Reference | 0.25 |
| High | 35 (64) | 144.08 (114.95–173.21) | 0.72 (0.41–1.26) | |

## 4. Discussion

This study aimed to investigate the clinical relevance and prognostic significance of ZFAND4 in OSCC. The prevalence of OSCC is estimated at 264,000 cases and 128,000 deaths annually worldwide [3]. Since the completion of the Human Genome Project in 2003, the subsequent progress in understanding the biology of cancer has led to the development of personalized therapies based on the patient's unique molecular and genetic profile to target defective signaling pathways of tumor cells. It is generally accepted that OSCC arises from multiple genetic alterations, although the molecular basis of carcinogenesis is not fully understood. DNA sequencing technologies coupled with advances in algorithms have enormously contributed to the molecular and functional characterization of mutations, genes, and pathways altered in multiple cancers, including OSCC [9–12]. Furthermore, the majority of tumors showed alterations in multiple targetable genes that are candidates for combination therapy [11]. It is of paramount importance to identify molecular alterations involved in the development of recurrent and metastatic disease, which remains the main cause of morbidity and mortality in OSCC patients.

In a recent paper, Sasahira et al. [5] conducted a cDNA microarray analysis in order to compare the gene expression profile of primary and recurrent OSCC. Ten genes were found to be upregulated in recurrent OSCC compared with the primary tumors. Among these genes, ZFAND4 showed a 100-fold recurrent/primary, thus suggesting a possible role for this gene in tumorigenesis. Tang et al. [7] reported that ZFAND4 expression was consistently highly expressed in gastric cancer compared to normal tissue, and positively associated with increased stage. Functionally, ZFAND4 was found to downregulate the expression of the anti-proliferative miRNAs, miR-148b, miR-375, and miR-182, in SGC-7901 cells, thereby promoting cell proliferation by activation of cyclin-dependent kinase and downregulation of p21 and p53 [7], which supports the notion that ZFAND4 may act as an oncogene in gastric cancer.

In this study, we assumed the same methodology used by Kurihara-Shimomura et al. [6] in order to validate their results in an independent cohort of OSCC patients, and more importantly, the utility of ZFAND4 as a predictor of metastasis and poor prognostic marker. Interestingly, ZFAND4 staining consistently showed distinct expression patterns and distribution in our cohort of 125 OSCC, i.e., granular staining in undifferentiated areas and diffuse staining in differentiated areas of the tumors. These two expression patterns were analyzed separately to evaluate possible correlations with the clinical and follow-up data. Moreover, Allred scores were calculated using both maximum value and mean value of ZFAND4-positive cells for the three tissue cores selected from each tumor.

We found that ZFAND4 staining was higher in undifferentiated than in differentiated areas of tumors. However, ZFAND4 expression in differentiated cells showed the most relevant and significant associations with well-differentiated ($p = 0.04$) and non-recurrent tumors ($p = 0.04$). Nevertheless, ZFAND4 expression did not show a major impact on patient survival. Only a trend was observed between low ZFAND4 expression in differentiated cells and tumor-associated deaths (Table 4). Therefore, the prognostic relevance of ZFAND4 described by Kurihara-Shimomura et al. [6] has not been replicated in our series. Furthermore, Kurihara-Shimomura et al. [6] reported that ZFAND4 is essential for distant metastasis in OSCC, and hypothesized that ZFAND4 could facilitate metastasis to the lymph nodes and distant organs by promoting angiogenesis and/or lymphangiogenesis. In marked contrast, our results only proved a marginal (if any) relationship between ZFAND4 expression and the presence of lymph node metastasis. The limitations of our study are the retrospective design and the use of tissue microarrays to evaluate ZFAND4 immunostaining. Several factors could contribute to the discrepant results between these two studies. On one hand, etiological, clinical, and epidemiological differences in the patient cohorts as well as molecular/biological differences among tumors depending on the geographic areas. Moreover, ZFAND4 expression exhibited a highly heterogeneous pattern within the tumors depending on the differentiation status, which could certainly have a major contribution on the varying results. Particularly since we evaluated separately the clinical significance and correlations of the two distinct ZFAND4 expression patterns in undifferentiated and differentiated areas of tumors, while Kurihara-Shimomura et al. [6] did not distinguish expression patterns within the different tumor areas. Thus, positive ZFAND4 immunostaining was scored in the whole tumor as the diffuse staining in tumor islands, cords, or sheets, irrespective of the cell differentiation status and the grade of keratinization. Since ZFAND4 expression showed two distinct non-overlapping expression patterns depending on the differentiation areas of tumors, each with a clearly distinct clinical significance, evaluation of ZFAND4 expression in the whole tumor could therefore be misleading.

## 5. Conclusions

The herein presented data question the clinical relevance of ZFAND4 expression as a prognostic biomarker in OSCC, and also revealed distinct ZFAND4 expression patterns depending on the differentiation areas of tumors that should be evaluated separately. Further studies are necessary to fully elucidate the pathobiological role of ZFAND4 in OSCC and the potential clinical implications.

**Author Contributions:** Conceptualization, J.C.d.V.; Funding acquisition, J.C.d.V. and J.M.G.-P.; Investigation, J.S.C., F.J.S.S. and F.D.I.; Methodology, J.S.C., F.J.S.S.; Resources, F.D.I., G.H.V. and J.C.d.V.; Writing—original draft, J.C.d.V.; Writing—review & editing, J.M.G.-P.

**Funding:** This study was supported by grants from the Plan Nacional de I + D + I ISCIII PI16/00280 and CIBERONC (CB16/12/00390), the Instituto de Investigación Sanitaria del Principado de Asturias (ISPA), Fundación Bancaria Caja de Ahorros de Asturias-IUOPA and the FEDER Funding Program from the European Union.

**Acknowledgments:** We thank the samples and technical assistance kindly provided by the Principado de Asturias BioBank (PT13/0010/0046), financed jointly by Servicio de Salud del Principado de Asturias, Instituto de Salud Carlos III and Fundación Bancaria Cajastur and integrated in the Spanish National Biobanks Network. This study was supported by grants from the Plan Nacional de I + D + I ISCIII PI16/00280 and CIBERONC (CB16/12/00390), the Instituto de Investigación Sanitaria del Principado de Asturias (ISPA), Fundación Bancaria Caja de Ahorros de Asturias-IUOPA and the FEDER Funding Program from the European Union.

**Conflicts of Interest:** The authors declare no conflict of interest.

## References

1. Rautava, J.; Luukkaa, M.; Heikinheimo, K.; Alin, J.; Grenman, R.; Happonen, R.P. Squamous cell carcinomas arising from different types of oral epithelia differ in their tumor and patient characteristics and survival. *Oral Oncol.* **2007**, *43*, 911–919. [CrossRef] [PubMed]
2. Ferlay, J.; Shin, H.R.; Bray, F.; Forman, D.; Mathers, C.; Parkin, D.M. Estimates of worldwide burden of cancer in 2008: GLOBOCAN 2008. *Int. J. Cancer* **2010**, *127*, 2893–2917. [CrossRef] [PubMed]
3. Sasahira, T.; Kirita, T.; Kuniyasu, H. Update of molecular pathobiology in oral cancer: A review. *Int. J. Clin. Oncol.* **2014**, *19*, 431–436. [CrossRef] [PubMed]
4. Leemans, C.R.; Snijders, P.J.F.; Brakenhoff, R.H. The molecular landscape of head and neck cancer. *Nat. Rev. Cancer* **2018**, *18*, 269–282. [CrossRef] [PubMed]
5. Sasahira, T.; Kurihara, M.; Nishiguchi, Y.; Fujiwara, R.; Kirita, T.; Kuniyasu, H. NEDD 4 binding protein 2-like 1 promotes cancer cell invasion in oral squamous cell carcinoma. *Virchows Arch.* **2016**, *469*, 163–172. [CrossRef] [PubMed]
6. Kurihara-Shimomura, M.; Sasahira, T.; Nakamura, H.; Nakashima, C.; Kuniyasu, H.; Kirita, T. Zinc finger AN1-type containing 4 is a novel marker for predicting metastasis and poor prognosis in oral squamous cell carcinoma. *J. Clin. Pathol.* **2018**, *71*, 436–441. [CrossRef] [PubMed]
7. Tang, L.; Chen, F.; Pang, E.J.; Zhang, Z.Q.; Jin, B.W.; Dong, W.F. MicroRNA-182 inhibits proliferation through targeting oncogenic ANUBL1 in gastric cancer. *Oncol. Rep.* **2015**, *33*, 1707–1716. [CrossRef] [PubMed]
8. Allred, D.C.; Harvey, J.M.; Berardo, M.; Clark, G.M. Prognostic and predictive factors in breast cancer by immunohistochemical analysis. *Mod. Pathol.* **1998**, *11*, 155–168. [PubMed]
9. Kandoth, C.; McLellan, M.D.; Vandin, F.; Ye, K.; Nium, B.; Lu, C.; Xie, M.; Zhang, Q.; McMichael, J.F.; Wyczalkowski, M.A.; et al. Mutational landscape and significance across 12 major cancer types. *Nature* **2013**, *502*, 333–339. [CrossRef] [PubMed]

10. Agrawal, N.; Frederick, M.J.; Pickering, C.R.; Bettegowda, C.; Chang, K.; Li, R.J.; Fakhry, C.; Xie, T.X.; Zhang, J.; Wang, J.; et al. Exome sequencing of head and neck squamous cell carcinoma reveals inactivating mutations in NOTCH1. *Science* **2011**, *333*, 1154–1157. [CrossRef] [PubMed]
11. Pickering, C.R.; Zhang, J.; Yoo, S.Y.; Bengtsson, L.; Moorthy, S.; Neskey, D.M.; Zhao, M.; Ortega Alves, M.V.; Chang, K.; Drummond, J.; et al. Integrative genomic characterization of oral squamous cell carcinoma identifies frequent somatic drivers. *Cancer Discov.* **2013**, *3*, 770–781. [CrossRef] [PubMed]
12. Stransky, N.; Egloff, A.M.; Tward, A.D.; Kostic, A.D.; Cibulskis, K.; Sivachenko, A.; Kryukov, G.V.; Lawrence, M.S.; Sougnez, C.; McKenna, A.; et al. The mutational landscape of head and neck squamous cell carcinoma. *Science* **2011**, *333*, 1157–1160. [CrossRef] [PubMed]

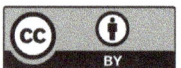

© 2018 by the authors. Licensee MDPI, Basel, Switzerland. This article is an open access article distributed under the terms and conditions of the Creative Commons Attribution (CC BY) license (http://creativecommons.org/licenses/by/4.0/).

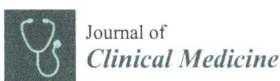 

*Article*

# The Prognostic Significance of Neutrophil-to-Lymphocyte Ratio in Head and Neck Cancer Patients Treated with Radiotherapy

Yeona Cho [1], Jun Won Kim [1], Hong In Yoon [2], Chang Geol Lee [2], Ki Chang Keum [2,*] and Ik Jae Lee [1,*]

1. Department of Radiation Oncology, Gangnam Severance Hospital, Yonsei University College of Medicine, Seoul 06273, Korea; iamyona@yuhs.ac (Y.C.); junwon@yuhs.ac (J.W.K.)
2. Department of Radiation Oncology, Yonsei Cancer Center, Yonsei University College of Medicine, Seoul 03722, Korea; yhi0225@yuhs.ac (H.I.Y.); cglee1023@yuhs.ac (C.G.L.)
* Correspondence: ikjae412@yuhs.ac (I.J.L.); kckeum@yuhs.ac (K.C.K.); Tel.: +82 2-2019-3152 (I.J.L.); +82 2-2227-7823 (K.C.K.); Fax: +82 2-2019-4855 (I.J.L.); +82 2-2228-8112 (K.C.K.)

Received: 12 November 2018; Accepted: 29 November 2018; Published: 3 December 2018

**Abstract:** Background: To investigate the prognostic value of pre-treatment neutrophil/lymphocyte ratio (NLR) in patients treated with definitive radiotherapy (RT) for head and neck cancer. Methods: We retrospectively analyzed 621 patients who received definitive RT for nasopharyngeal, oropharyngeal, hypopharyngeal, and laryngeal cancer. An NLR cut-off value of 2.7 was identified using a receiver operating characteristic curve analysis, with overall survival (OS) as an endpoint. Results: The 5-year progression-free survival (PFS) and OS for all patients were 62.3% and 72.1%, respectively. The patients with a high NLR (68%) had a significantly lower 5-year PFS and OS than their counterparts with a low NLR (32%) (PFS: 39.2% vs. 75.8%, $p < 0.001$; OS: 50.9% vs. 83.8%, $p < 0.001$). In a subgroup analysis according to primary site, a high NLR also correlated with a lower PFS and OS, except in oropharyngeal cancer, where a high NLR only exhibited a trend towards lower survival. In a multivariate analysis, a high NLR remained an independent prognostic factor for PFS and OS. Conclusion: Head and neck cancer tends to be more aggressive in patients with a high NLR, leading to a poorer outcome after RT. The optimal therapeutic approaches for these patients should be reevaluated, given the unfavorable prognosis.

**Keywords:** head and neck cancer; radiotherapy; neutrophil/lymphocyte ratio; survival

## 1. Introduction

Currently, definitive radiotherapy (RT) is one of the main modalities used to treat locally advanced head and neck cancer. However, patients exhibit varying degrees of RT response and may develop recurrences even after a complete response. Although various clinical and molecular predictors of treatment outcomes after definitive RT for head and neck cancer have been investigated, no clear consensus regarding reliable predictive biomarkers has been reached.

Treatment outcomes are known to be affected by both tumor characteristics and host-related factors, including age, sex, and performance status. Recent reports have also described close associations of systemic inflammation with tumorigenesis and treatment outcomes [1,2], and several laboratory markers associated with systemic inflammatory processes, including albumin, hemoglobin, absolute white blood cell (WBC) count or WBC components, and platelet count, have been investigated as prognostic and predictive markers in various types of cancer [3,4]. Inflammation plays a key role in cancer physiology by promoting carcinogenesis, dedifferentiation, and primary tumor growth, and by stimulating tumor cell proliferation by inhibiting apoptosis and increasing mitotic rates [5].

Tumor–host interactions can induce systemic inflammatory responses that affect the numbers of circulating WBCs and the neutrophil/lymphocyte ratio (NLR) in certain types of cancers [6]. Normal NLR values are in the range of 0.78–3.53 in the general population [7]; high NLR values are associated with poor outcomes not only in cancer patients but also in patients with cardiovascular disease [8–10]. To date, some studies of head and neck cancer have suggested an association of high NLR with a poor prognosis. However, data regarding the prognostic significance of a high NLR are limited, especially among patients undergoing definitive RT [11–13]. The antitumor immune response is thought to be part of the ionizing radiation-induced tumor cell death process. Therefore, tumor shrinkage caused by the host immune response may be a direct effect of radiation [14,15]. Accordingly, we postulated that the host immune status, as reflected by the NLR, may predict recurrence after RT in head and neck cancer patients. This study aimed to evaluate the relationships of pretreatment NLR and other hematologic markers with tumor recurrence and survival in patients undergoing definitive RT for head and neck cancer.

## 2. Materials and Methods

### 2.1. Patient Selection and Treatment Protocols

This study was approved by the institutional review board of the Gangnam Severance Hospital (Protocol number: 3-2017-0387). We retrospectively reviewed the medical records of patients who underwent definitive RT with or without concurrent chemotherapy for cancers of the head and neck (including nasopharyngeal, oropharyngeal, hypopharyngeal, and laryngeal cancers) at our institution between 2006 and 2015. Patients who underwent surgery before or after RT, received RT of <30 Gy, had a distant metastasis at the initial diagnosis or previous history of other primary cancer, and whose pre-RT common blood test results were unavailable were excluded. The remaining 621 patients included in the analysis were staged according to the 7th edition of the TNM classification of the American Joint Committee on Cancer (AJCC). Human Papilloma Virus (HPV) infection status was evaluated in oropharyngeal cancer patients. To assess HPV status of each tumor, we used formalin-fixed, paraffin-embedded biopsy tissue to examine p16 expression, which is recognized as a surrogate marker for HPV infection in the oropharynx. Details of this process are described in a previous report of our institution [16].

Patients were treated with definitive RT alone, concurrent chemoradiotherapy (CCRT), or induction chemotherapy followed by CCRT. The choice of treatment was determined by the primary tumor and stage, risk factors, and/or the physicians' discretion. External beam RT comprised either 3D-conformal RT or intensity-modulated RT (IMRT) and was administered 5 days per week in daily fractions of 1.8–2.5 Gy to yield total doses to the primary tumor of 66–75 Gy.

Concurrent chemotherapy regimens included weekly cisplatin (DDP; 40 mg/m$^2$); weekly 5-fluorouracil (5-FU) and cisplatin (FP; 750 mg/m$^2$ and 20 mg/m$^2$, respectively); and 5-FU, taxotere, and cisplatin (TPF; 750 mg/m$^2$, 70 mg/m$^2$, and 75 mg/m$^2$, respectively) every 3 weeks. The anti-epidermal growth factor receptor mAb, cetuximab (Erbitux), was also used. The induction chemotherapy regimen consisted of FP every 3 weeks for 3 cycles or TPF every 3 weeks for 2 cycles.

### 2.2. Hematologic Markers

The patients' blood counts were evaluated prior to performing diagnostic procedures or administering treatments. The WBC count, hemoglobin (Hb) level, absolute neutrophil count (ANC), absolute lymphocyte count (ALC), platelet count, and albumin level were recorded. A diagnosis of anemia was based on a hemoglobin level of <13 g/dL in men and <12 g/dL in women, and hypoalbuminemia was defined as a serum albumin level <3.5 g/dL. Onodera's prognostic nutritional index (PNI) was calculated as $10 \times$ Albumin + $0.005 \times$ ALC.

The NLR was calculated as the neutrophil count divided by the lymphocyte count, and the platelet/lymphocyte ratio (PLR) was calculated as the platelet count divided by the lymphocyte count. The optimum NLR cut-off values were identified via a receiver operating characteristic (ROC) curve analysis, using overall survival (OS) as an end point (Supplement Figure S1), and patients were categorized into high NLR (NLR $\geq$ 2.7) and low (NLR < 2.7) NLR groups.

### 2.3. Outcome Assessment

All patients were followed up for 4–6 weeks after RT, and subsequently at 3-month intervals for the first and second years, 6-month intervals for the third year, and annually for the fourth and fifth years. Progression was defined as regrowth of the primary tumor or the involvement of cervical lymph node(s) (LN) or detection of any new lesion(s) in follow-up imaging studies. Progression-free survival (PFS) was defined as the interval between the date of initial treatment to the detection of first recurrence, death from any cause, or the last follow-up. OS was defined as the interval between the date of initial treatment and death from any cause or the last follow-up.

### 2.4. Statistical Analysis

Categorical data were analyzed using Fisher's exact test or the $\chi^2$ test. Continuous data were compared between groups using the Mann–Whitney U test. The Kaplan–Meier method and log-rank test were used to estimate and compare the PFS and OS rates. Hazard ratios (HRs) were obtained using the cumulative survivor function and are reported with corresponding 95% confidence intervals (CIs). Univariate and multivariate analyses of factors related to OS and PFS were conducted using the Cox proportional hazards model, and multivariate analysis included all variables with $p$ values < 0.05 in the univariate analysis. A $p$ value < 0.05 was considered statistically significant. All analyses were performed using IBM SPSS, version 20.0 (SPSS, Chicago, IL, USA).

## 3. Results

### 3.1. Patient and Treatment Characteristics

Table 1 presents the demographic and treatment characteristics of the 621 included patients, of whom 425 (68.4%) and 196 (31.6%) were stratified into the low and high NLR groups, respectively. Laryngeal cancer was the most frequent type of primary cancer in the low NLR group, whereas nasopharyngeal cancer cases comprised the majority in the high NLR group. Patients with a high NLR tended to have a more advanced clinical T classification and higher frequency of LN metastasis and a significantly higher frequency of systemic chemotherapy (75.2% vs. 48.5%, $p < 0.001$) than those in the low NLR group.

The groups did not differ significantly in terms of the use of IMRT. Of the 16 patients who did not complete the planned course of RT, four (2.0%) and 12 (2.8%) belonged to the high and low NLR groups, respectively ($p = 0.787$). However, more patients in the high NLR group received radiation doses of $\geq$70 Gy (equivalent dose in 2 Gy fractions, $\alpha/\beta = 10$), and the overall duration of RT tended to be longer in this group.

**Table 1.** Patient characteristics.

| Characteristics | | Total N = 621 | (%) | Low NLR Group N = 425 | (%) | High NLR Group N = 196 | (%) | p Value |
|---|---|---|---|---|---|---|---|---|
| Age | Median (Range) | 60 (18–94) | | 60 (18–89) | | 60 (18–94) | | 0.166 |
| Sex | Male | 514 | (82.8) | 365 | (85.9) | 149 | (76.0) | 0.002 |
| | Female | 107 | (17.2) | 60 | (14.1) | 47 | (24.0) | |
| Primary site | Nasopharynx | 192 | (30.9) | 119 | (28.0) | 73 | (37.2) | <0.001 |
| | Oropharynx | 94 | (15.1) | 56 | (13.2) | 38 | (19.4) | |
| | Hypopharynx | 76 | (12.2) | 42 | (9.9) | 34 | (17.3) | |
| | Larynx | 259 | (41.7) | 208 | (48.9) | 51 | (26.0) | |

**Table 1.** *Cont.*

|  |  | Total |  | Low NLR Group |  | High NLR Group |  |  |
|---|---|---|---|---|---|---|---|---|
| Characteristics |  | N = 621 | (%) | N = 425 | (%) | N = 196 | (%) | p Value |
| T classification | T1 | 259 | (41.7) | 206 | (48.5) | 53 | (27.0) | <0.001 |
|  | T2 | 145 | (23.3) | 97 | (22.8) | 48 | (24.5) |  |
|  | T3 | 94 | (15.1) | 52 | (12.2) | 42 | (21.4) |  |
|  | T4 | 123 | (19.8) | 70 | (16.5) | 53 | (27.0) |  |
| N classification | N0 | 294 | (47.3) | 236 | (55.5) | 58 | (29.6) | <0.001 |
|  | N1 | 87 | (14.0) | 56 | (13.2) | 31 | (15.8) |  |
|  | N2 | 219 | (35.3) | 124 | (29.2) | 95 | (48.5) |  |
|  | N3 | 21 | (3.4) | 9 | (2.1) | 12 | (6.1) |  |
| Overall stage | I | 188 | (30.3) | 165 | (38.8) | 23 | (11.7) | <0.001 |
|  | II | 89 | (14.3) | 58 | (13.6) | 31 | (15.8) |  |
|  | III | 118 | (19.0) | 76 | (17.9) | 42 | (21.4) |  |
|  | IVA | 204 | (32.9) | 116 | (27.3) | 88 | (44.9) |  |
|  | IVB | 22 | (3.5) | 10 | (2.4) | 12 | (6.1) |  |
| p16 (in oropharynx) | UE [b] | 56 | (59.6) | 31 | (55.4) | 25 | (65.8) | 0.529 |
|  | negative | 12 | (1.9) | 6 | (10.7) | 6 | (15.8) |  |
|  | positive | 26 | (4.2) | 19 | (33.9) | 7 | (18.4) |  |
| Treatment | RT alone | 270 | (43.5) | 221 | (52.0) | 49 | (25.0) | <0.001 |
|  | CCRT [c] | 234 | (37.7) | 130 | (30.6) | 104 | (53.1) |  |
|  | Induction + CCRT | 117 | (18.8) | 74 | (17.4) | 43 | (21.9) |  |
| RT modality | 3D-CRT [d] | 220 | (35.4) | 156 | (36.7) | 64 | (32.7) | 0.326 |
|  | IMRT [e] | 401 | (64.6) | 269 | (63.3) | 132 | (67.3) |  |
| RT duration | Median | 46 |  | 45 |  | 47 |  | <0.001 |
| (days) | (Range) | (23–99) |  | (23–99) |  | (31–97) |  |  |
| Total dose | <70 | 385 | (61.0) | 277 | (64.6) | 108 | (53.5) | 0.016 |
| (EQD2$_{Gy}$ [a], $\alpha/\beta$ = 10) | ≥70 | 236 | (37.4) | 148 | (34.5) | 88 | (43.6) |  |

Abbreviations: [a] Equivalent dose in 2 Gy fractions, [b] unevaluable, [c] concurrent chemoradiotherapy, [d] 3-dimensional conformal radiotherapy, [e] intensity modulated radiotherapy.

### 3.2. Hematologic Markers

Table 2 presents the values of the measured hematologic markers in all patients. The median baseline WBC count, ANC, and ALC were 6800/µL, 3900/µL, and 1810/µL, respectively, and the WBC and ANC values were significantly higher in the high NLR group. A higher proportion of patients with leukocytosis (WBC count ≥9000/µL) was also observed in the high NLR group (31.7% vs. 7.8% for low NLR, $p < 0.001$). The high NLR group also had higher platelet counts, which expectedly yielded a higher PLR, and was more likely to present with anemia and hypoalbuminemia at the time of diagnosis. Patients with a high NLR also had a significantly lower Onodera's PNI (49.7 vs. 55 for low NLR, $p < 0.001$).

**Table 2.** Hematologic markers.

|  |  | Total |  | low NLR Group |  | High NLR Group |  |  |
|---|---|---|---|---|---|---|---|---|
| Characteristic |  | N = 621 | (%) | N = 425 | (%) | N = 196 | (%) | p Value |
| WBC | Median | 6800 |  | 6300 |  | 7700 |  | <0.001 |
| (cells/µL) | (range) | (2000–21,100) |  | (2000–10,700) |  | (3700–21,100) |  |  |
| ANC [a] | Median | 3900 |  | 3460 |  | 5520 |  | <0.001 |
| (cells/µL) | (range) | (560–18,310) |  | (940–6720) |  | (560–18,300) |  |  |
| ALC [b] | Median | 1810 |  | 2040 |  | 1320 |  | <0.001 |
| (cells/µL) | (range) | (160–3700) |  | (700–3700) |  | (160–2970) |  |  |
| Platelet | Median | 237 |  | 232 |  | 250 |  | <0.001 |
| ($\times 10^3$ cells/µL) | (range) | (14–600) |  | (14–517) |  | (40–600) |  |  |
| PLR [c] | Median | 131 |  | 116 |  | 194 |  | <0.001 |
|  | (range) | (20–1733) |  | 20–269 |  | (26–1733) |  |  |

Table 2. Cont.

| Characteristic | | Total N = 621 | (%) | low NLR Group N = 425 | (%) | High NLR Group N = 196 | (%) | p Value |
|---|---|---|---|---|---|---|---|---|
| Hemoglobin (mg/dL) | Median (range) | 14 (51–15.1) | | 14.1 (5.1–17.4) | | 13.5 (8.3–51.1) | | 0.01 |
| Anemia | No | 497 | (80.0) | 359 | (84.5) | 138 | (70.4) | <0.001 |
| | Yes | 124 | (20.0) | 66 | (15.5) | 58 | (29.6) | |
| Albumin (g/dL) | Median (range) | 4.4 (2.5–5.2) | | 4.4 (2.7–5.2) | | 4.3 (2.5–5.1) | | <0.001 |
| Hypoalbuminemia (<3.3 g/dL) | UE [e] | 69 | (11.1) | 49 | (11.5) | 20 | (10.2) | 0.02 |
| | No | 539 | (86.8) | 371 | (87.3) | 168 | (85.7) | |
| | Yes | 13 | (2.1) | 5 | (1.2) | 8 | (4.1) | |
| Onodera's PNI [d] | Median (range) | 53.1 (27.8–67.6) | | 55 (32.8–67.6) | | 49.7 (27.8–61.7) | | <0.001 |

Abbreviations: [a] Absolute neutrophil count, [b] absolute lymphocyte count, [c] platelet/lymphocyte ratio, [d] prognostic nutritional index, [e] unevaluable.

### 3.3. Survival Analysis

The patients were followed up for a median of 39 (range, 2–130) months. During the follow-up period, 148 patients died and 156 experienced a recurrence. The 5-year PFS and OS rates for all patients were 63.8% and 72.9%, respectively, and both rates were significantly lower in the high NLR group than in the low NLR group (PFS: 39.2% vs. 75.8%, $p < 0.001$; OS: 50.9% vs. 83.8%, $p < 0.001$) (Figure 1). In survival analyses stratified by early- (stage I–II) or advanced-stage disease (stage III–IV), a high NLR remained significantly associated with a poor PFS and OS (Figure 2).

An additional subgroup analysis was performed after stratifying cases by the primary site (nasopharynx, oropharynx, hypopharynx, and larynx). As shown in Figures 3 and 4, patients with nasopharyngeal, hypopharyngeal, and laryngeal cancer and the high NLR group had poorer PFS and OS rates. Among patients with oropharyngeal cancer, however, a high NLR status exhibited only borderline significance in terms of 5-year PFS (42.0% vs. 54.0%, $p = 0.059$) (Figure 3B) and only exhibited a trend with reduced OS (51.5% vs. 65.3%, $p = 0.215$) (Figure 4B).

We also conducted additional analysis according to the treatment scheme. Both PFS and OS were significantly worse in high NLR patients receiving any type of treatment: Patients receiving RT alone, 5-year PFS 84.8% vs. 56.1%, $p < 0.001$ and OS 90.6% vs. 68.6%, $p < 0.001$; patients receiving CCRT, 5-year PFS 66.2% vs. 31.5%, $p < 0.001$ and OS 74.3% vs. 41.7%, $p < 0.001$; patients receiving induction chemotherapy + CCRT, 5-year PFS 68.1% vs. 40.7%, $p < 0.001$ and OS 78.9% vs. 55.2%, $p < 0.001$.

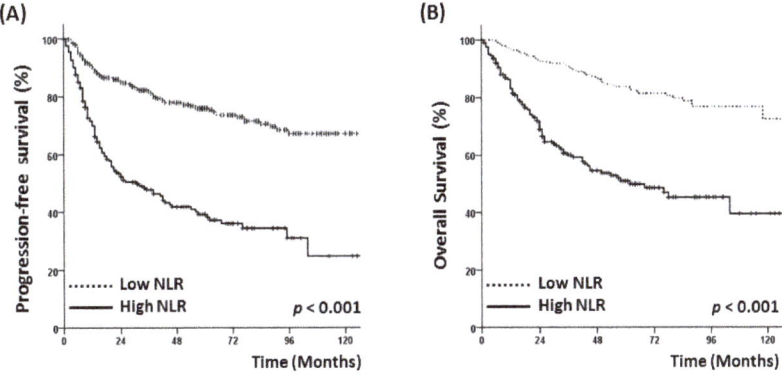

Figure 1. (A) Progression-free survival and (B) overall survival of patients according to neutrophil/lymphocyte ratio (NLR) status.

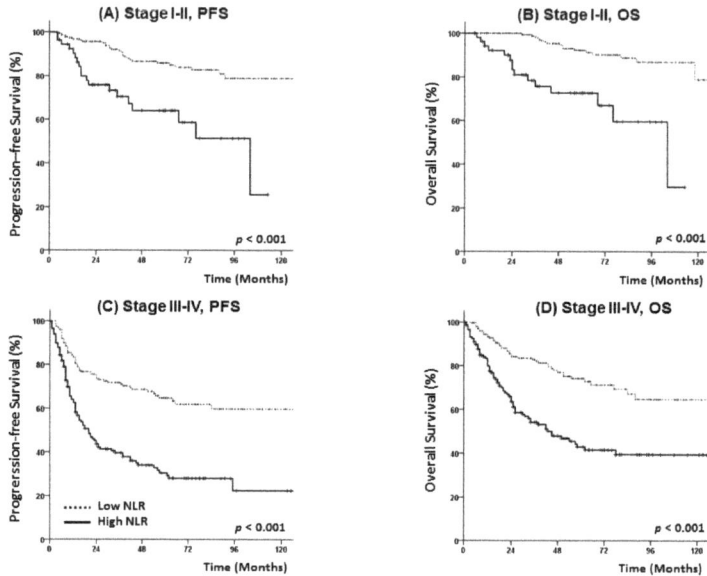

**Figure 2.** Progression-free survival and overall survival of patients with head and neck cancer at (**A**,**B**) stage I–II, and (**C**,**D**) stage III–IV.

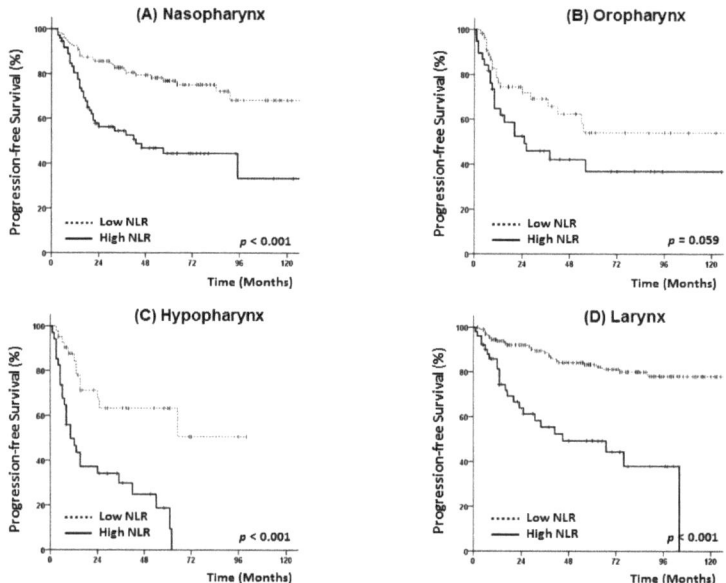

**Figure 3.** Subgroup analysis of progression-free survival according to primary tumor site: Nasopharynx (**A**), oropharynx (**B**), hypopharynx (**C**) and larynx (**D**).

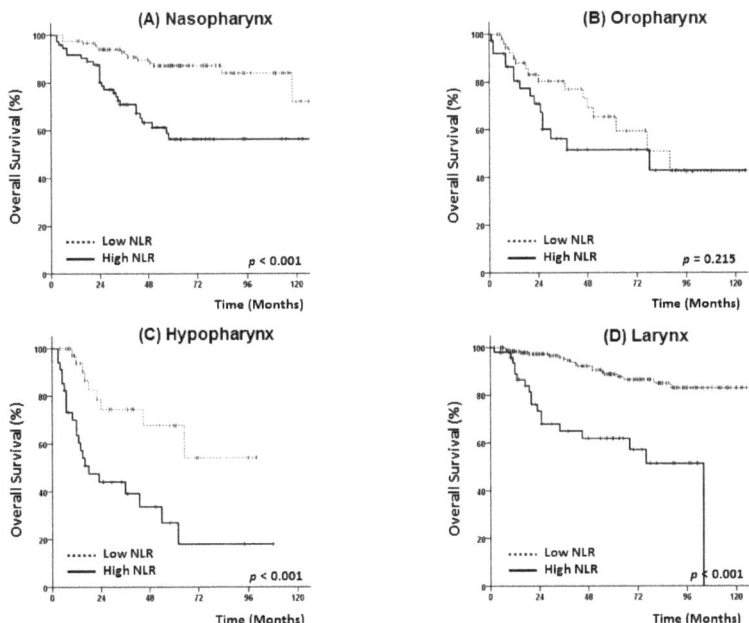

**Figure 4.** Subgroup analysis of overall survival according to primary tumor site: nasopharynx (**A**), oropharynx (**B**), hypopharynx (**C**) and larynx (**D**).

### 3.4. Analysis of Prognostic Factors

The results of univariate and multivariate analyses performed to identify prognostic factors for PFS and OS are shown in Table 3. The multivariate analysis revealed significant associations of a high NLR with poor PFS, an older age, and an advanced T classification. An elevated PLR was also found to be associated with a poor PFS. An older age, advanced T classification, and high NLR were also found to associate significantly with OS, and an elevated PLR exhibited a borderline significant association with a poor OS. Primary hypopharyngeal cancer was associated with both a poor PFS and a poor OS. A low albumin level (<3.3 g/dL) exhibited a negative trend with PFS, but not with OS. LN metastasis, overall stage, leukocytosis (WBC count ≥9000/μL), anemia, and Onodera's PNI were not identified as prognostic factors for PFS or OS.

Table 3. Prognostic factors for progression-free survival and overall survival.

| Variable | | Progression-Free Survival | | | | | | Overall Survival | | | | |
|---|---|---|---|---|---|---|---|---|---|---|---|---|
| | | Univariate Analysis | | | Multivariate Analysis | | | Univariate Analysis | | | Multivariate Analysis | |
| | | HR | 95%CI | p | HR | 95%CI | p | HR | 95%CI | p | HR | 95%CI | p |
| Age | <60 | 1 | | | 1 | | | 1 | | | 1 | | |
| | ≥60 | 1.61 | 1.22–2.12 | 0.001 | 1.54 | 1.08–2.19 | 0.017 | 2.40 | 1.71–3.37 | <0.001 | 2.43 | 1.57–3.75 | <0.001 |
| Sex | Male | 1 | | | | | | 1 | | | | | |
| | Female | 0.97 | 0.68–1.38 | 0.865 | | | | 0.99 | 0.66–1.51 | 0.981 | | | |
| Primary site | Nasopharynx | 1 | | | 1 | | | 1 | | | 1 | | |
| | Oropharynx | 1.78 | 1.21–2.62 | 0.003 | 1.04 | 0.67–1.61 | 0.859 | 2.29 | 1.44–3.62 | <0.001 | 1.19 | 0.68–2.09 | 0.54 |
| | Hypophrynx | 2.46 | 1.66–3.66 | <0.001 | 1.88 | 1.17–3.01 | 0.009 | 3.41 | 2.13–5.44 | <0.001 | 2.01 | 1.13–3.55 | 0.017 |
| | Larynx | 0.63 | 0.44–0.91 | 0.012 | 1.07 | 0.65–1.76 | 0.786 | 0.74 | 0.48–1.15 | 0.181 | 0.97 | 0.49–1.90 | 0.924 |
| T classification | T1, 2 | 1 | | | 1 | | | 1 | | | 1 | | |
| | T3, 4 | 3.05 | 2.32–4.00 | <0.001 | 2.03 | 1.37–3.00 | <0.001 | 3.53 | 2.54–4.90 | <0.001 | 2.39 | 1.48–3.86 | <0.001 |
| N classification | N0 | 1 | | | 1 | | | 1 | | | 1 | | |
| | N1-3 | 2.78 | 2.06–3.77 | <0.001 | 1.37 | 0.81–2.32 | 0.237 | 2.52 | 1.76–3.60 | <0.001 | 1.11 | 0.60–2.04 | 0.749 |
| Overall stage | I-II | 1 | | | 1 | | | 1 | | | 1 | | |
| | III-IVB | 3.48 | 2.52–4.81 | <0.001 | 1.44 | 0.78–2.67 | 0.244 | 3.76 | 2.53–5.60 | <0.001 | 1.58 | 0.71–3.48 | 0.26 |
| Treatment | RT alone | 1 | | | 1 | | | 1 | | | 1 | | |
| | CCRT [e] | 2.83 | 2.06–3.90 | <0.001 | 1.11 | 0.63–1.96 | 0.723 | 2.65 | 1.81–3.88 | <0.001 | 1.02 | 0.53–1.98 | 0.951 |
| | Induction + CCRT | 2.09 | 1.42–3.07 | <0.001 | 0.77 | 0.41–1.46 | 0.425 | 1.98 | 1.25–3.13 | 0.003 | 0.85 | 0.38–1.64 | 0.519 |
| RT modality | 3D CRT [f] | 1 | | | | | | 1 | | | | | |
| | IMRT [g] | 1.26 | 0.95–1.68 | 0.107 | | | | 1.19 | 0.86–1.66 | 0.298 | | | |
| Anemia | No | 1 | | | 1 | | | 1 | | | 1 | | |
| | Yes | 2.25 | 1.69–3.00 | <0.001 | 1.19 | 0.81–1.74 | 0.374 | 0.52 | 0.37–0.72 | <0.001 | 0.96 | 0.63–1.45 | 0.829 |
| WBC (cells/μL) | <9000 | 1 | | | 1 | | | 1 | | | 1 | | |
| | ≥9000 | 1.81 | 1.30–2.52 | <0.001 | 0.93 | 0.61–1.43 | 0.748 | 1.62 | 1.08–2.42 | 0.021 | 0.73 | 0.43–1.23 | 0.233 |
| ANC [a] (cells/μL) | <4000 | 1 | | | 1 | | | 1 | | | 1 | | |
| | ≥4000 | 1.81 | 1.38–2.39 | <0.001 | 0.75 | 0.51–1.10 | 0.142 | 2.02 | 1.45–2.81 | <0.001 | 0.79 | 0.50–1.27 | 0.333 |
| ALC [b] (cells/μL) | <2000 | 1 | | | 1 | | | 1 | | | 1 | | |
| | ≥2000 | 0.61 | 0.45–0.82 | 0.001 | 1.10 | 0.72–1.68 | 0.672 | 0.55 | 0.38–0.79 | 0.001 | 1.10 | 0.64–1.89 | 0.72 |
| Platelet (10³ cells/μL) | <230 | 1 | | | | | | 1 | | | | | |
| | ≥230 | 0.98 | 0.74–1.28 | 0.857 | | | | 1.04 | 0.75–1.44 | 0.825 | | | |
| NLR | <2.7 | 1 | | | 1 | | | 1 | | | 1 | | |
| | ≥2.7 | 3.39 | 2.58–4.46 | <0.001 | 4.10 | 2.66–6.34 | <0.001 | 3.86 | 2.78–5.35 | <0.001 | 4.63 | 2.69–7.94 | <0.001 |
| PLR [c] | <150 | 1 | | | 1 | | | 1 | | | 1 | | |
| | ≥150 | 1.79 | 1.36–2.36 | 0.001 | 1.57 | 1.20–2.06 | 0.03 | 1.96 | 1.42–2.74 | 0.001 | 1.24 | 0.96–2.40 | 0.096 |

Table 3. Cont.

| Variable | | Progression-Free Survival | | | | | | Overall Survival | | | | | |
|---|---|---|---|---|---|---|---|---|---|---|---|---|---|
| | | Univariate Analysis | | | Multivariate Analysis | | | Univariate Analysis | | | Multivariate Analysis | | |
| | | HR | 95%CI | p | HR | 95%CI | p | HR | 95%CI | p | HR | 95%CI | p |
| Hypoalbuminemia | No | 1 | | | 1 | | | 1 | | | 1 | | |
| | Yes | 4.18 | 2.20–7.93 | <0.001 | 1.92 | 0.95–3.85 | 0.068 | 0.44 | 0.3–0.66 | <0.001 | 1.54 | 0.69–3.42 | 0.288 |
| Onodera's PNI [d] | <50 | 1 | | | 1 | | | 1 | | | 1 | | |
| | ≥50 | 0.48 | 0.36–0.65 | <0.001 | 0.80 | 0.53–1.23 | 0.316 | 0.44 | 0.31–0.63 | <0.001 | 0.74 | 0.45–1.24 | 0.259 |

Abbreviations: [a] Absolute neutrophil count, [b] absolute lymphocyte count, [c] platelet/lymphocyte ratio, [d] prognostic nutritional index, [e] concurrent chemoradiotherapy, [f] 3-dimensional conformal radiotherapy, [g] intensity modulated radiotherapy.

*3.5. p16 Status and Hematologic Markers*

We also evaluated the relationship of the p16 status with the levels of various hematologic markers. This status was available for 38 of 94 patients with oropharyngeal cancer (40.4%). In total, 26 patients had p16-positive oropharyngeal cancer and 12 patients had p16-negative oropharyngeal cancer. Patients with a positive p16 status tended to have a lower NLR than those with a negative status (median NLR: 2.1 vs. 2.8, $p = 0.103$). In addition, the WBC count and ANC were lower in p16-positive patients than in their p16-negative counterparts, although these differences were not statistically significant (median WBC: 7100 vs. 8300/µL, $p = 0.073$; median ANC: 4000 vs. 5200/µL, $p = 0.119$) (Supplement Figure S2).

Among the 26 patients with p16-positive oropharyngeal cancer, PFS and OS were not different between the low and high NLR groups (5-year PFS 56.1% vs. 57.1%, $p = 0.781$ and 5-year OS 86.5% vs. 80.0%, $p = 0.646$). In patients with p16-negative oropharyngeal cancer ($n = 12$), PFS was significantly lower in the high NLR group than in the low NLR group (5-year PFS 0% vs. 100%, $p = 0.009$), while OS showed no difference, which may be due to the limited number of cases.

## 4. Discussion

During the past decade, various markers of systemic inflammation have been evaluated with the aims of refining patient stratification to treatment and predictions of survival. Of these markers, the NLR, which is derived from the ANC and ALC of a full blood count, is routinely available. Accordingly, in this study, we evaluated the significance of the pre-treatment NLR in patients who received RT for head and neck cancer and observed significant associations of a high NLR with disease recurrence and OS in the patient sample.

As noted above, we stratified the patients into two groups according to NLR status and found that those with a high NLR had a more advanced clinical stage and therefore more frequently received concurrent chemotherapy with a higher total radiation dose and longer total duration of RT. Despite this more aggressive treatment, however, patients with a high NLR were more likely to experience unfavorable outcomes, and these results remained consistent regardless of disease stage. We further found that adverse hematologic features, such as an elevated WBC, ANC, and platelet count as well as anemia, hypoalbuminemia, and a low Onodera's PNI, were more frequently observed in the high NLR group. These findings suggest that certain types of tumors elicit an enhanced systemic inflammatory response, which may reflect the aggressive nature of the tumor.

We also performed a subgroup analysis according to the primary site of head and neck carcinoma and determined that a high NLR was significantly associated with a poorer PFS and OS among patients with nasopharyngeal, hypopharyngeal, and laryngeal cancers. However, among patients with oropharyngeal cancer, a high NLR was only borderline significant as a prognosticator of PFS and exhibited a trend with OS. Other studies of oropharyngeal cancer have identified NLR as a significant prognostic factor for disease control, and most have used a relatively higher NLR cut-off value ($\geq 5$) [17,18] than those used for other primary sites in the head and neck [19,20]. Additionally, some studies of oropharyngeal cancer have identified the prognostic significance of circulating neutrophil and lymphocyte counts only for recurrence-free survival (RFS), but not for OS [21].

Our above findings may be attributable to the limited number of oropharyngeal cancer patients in our study ($n = 94$) or to the effects of HPV infection. Previous studies suggested that HPV infection might affect the distribution of WBC components and alter inflammatory responses in patients with oropharyngeal cancer [11]. Huang et al. reported that HPV-positive patients had lower levels of circulating neutrophil and monocyte counts when compared to their HPV-negative counterparts, despite similar levels of lymphocyte counts [21]. In the HPV-positive cohort, a high neutrophil or monocyte count was found to correlate with reductions in OS and RFS, whereas in the HPV-negative cohort, the neutrophil and lymphocyte counts were not predictive of either survival parameter. Another study also reported a significantly lower NLR among HPV-positive patients than among their HPV-negative counterparts. Given these findings, we suggest that oropharyngeal cancer may exhibit behaviors or inflammatory responses that are distinct from those of head and neck cancers at other primary sites. Although our study did not reveal significant differences in inflammatory markers among oropharyngeal cancer patients according to p16 status, HPV infection might have altered the WBC distribution and affected disease control and OS.

Some scientists have recommended that more accurate diagnostic tools are needed for risk stratification according to HPV infection. Previous reports have suggested that HPV specific tests such as DNA in situ hybridization and polymerase chain reaction should be used to confirm HPV status, although p16 protein over-expression is very sensitive to the presence of transcriptionally-active HPV, correlates strongly with patient outcomes, is widely available, and is easy to interpret [22]. Gupta et al. also suggested that circulating HPV16 DNA in the plasma may be a clinically useful biomarker [23]. These biomarkers can be measured using a simple blood test, and the level of ctDNA is predictive of an early treatment response. If used in combination with inflammatory markers, this technique will be helpful in predicting a patient's prognosis and determining an appropriate treatment plan.

As noted, NLR is an easily and routinely determined biomarker of systemic inflammation, and in our study population a high NLR correlated strongly and independently with a poorer PFS and OS. Previous studies have also identified a high NLR as an independent prognostic factor for many other types of cancers, including colorectal cancer, renal cell cancer, pancreatic cancer, and head and neck squamous cell carcinoma [2,24–28]. Although the tumorigenic mechanism underlying this relationship with the NLR has not been clearly elucidated, it appears likely that increased levels of several inflammatory cytokines contribute to a microenvironment that promotes carcinogenesis and tumor progression [29]. Several growth factors, including epidermal growth factor, vascular endothelial growth factor, and transforming growth factor-α, also contribute to the creation of microenvironments supportive of angiogenesis and tumor proliferation [30]. Our results are therefore consistent with the concept that a high NLR contributes to poor disease control by suppressing the cytolytic activities of activated effector T cells and the peritumoral infiltration of immuno-suppressive cells such as macrophages [31,32].

We further demonstrated that a higher PLR was associated with PFS in our multivariate analysis. Again, the significance of interactions between platelets and the tumor microenvironment remains somewhat unclear. The platelet count provides an additional index of systemic inflammation elicited by the tumor and degranulation. This inflammation, together with the consequent release of platelet-derived proangiogenic mediators within the tumor microvasculature, may also serve as an important determinant of tumor growth [33–35].

This study had a few limitations. First, the study had a retrospective design and included various primary sites of head and neck cancer. Additionally, patients in the high NLR group tended to have more advanced-stage disease. However, the NLR remained a significant prognostic factor for survival in the multivariate analysis, as well as in an additional analysis according to disease stage. Second, the selection of treatment modalities and regimens was heterogeneous and was determined in accordance with the primary site and physicians' discretion. Third, we did not explore the association of LN metastasis with patient outcomes because of the use of clinical stage and likelihood of upstaging for LNs. Therefore, our findings should be interpreted cautiously. Nevertheless, this is one of the largest studies to evaluate the prognostic significance of systemic inflammation in patients who underwent RT for head and neck cancer, and we have revealed potential differences in the patients' characteristics and outcomes according to their NLR status. In addition, we observed different associations of the NLR status among patients with oropharyngeal cancer versus those with other head and neck cancers, which underscores the need for further studies of the relationship between HPV infection and the NLR.

In conclusion, the results of our large population study validate the suggested association of a high NLR with poorer outcomes after adjusting for potential confounding factors. Although further studies of the biological mechanisms underlying the relationship between inflammation and aggressiveness are needed, our results suggest that a classification system based on pretreatment hematologic markers could identify patients with a high risk of recurrence and poor survival.

**Supplementary Materials:** The following are available online at http://www.mdpi.com/2077-0383/7/12/512/s1, Figure S1: The receiver operating characteristic (ROC) curve analysis for neutrophil/lymphocyte ratio (A) using overall survival OS as an end point. Figure S2. The white blood cell count (A) and neutrophil/lymphocyte ratio (B) in p16 negative and p16 positive patients.

**Author Contributions:** Conceptualization, Y.C., H.I.Y., I.J.L; Data Curation, Y.C., C.G.L., K.C.K.; Formal Analysis, Y.C., J.W.K., H.I.Y.; Resources, C.G.L., K.C.K., I.J.L.; Supervision, K.C.K., I.J.L.; Writing—Original draft, Y.C., J.W.K.; Writing—Review and editing, H.I.Y., C.G.L., K.C.K., I.J.L.

**Funding:** This work was supported by the National Research Foundation of Korea Grant funded by the Korean Government (number NRF-2018R1D1A1B07048234).

**Conflicts of Interest:** The authors declare no conflict of interest.

## References

1. Cho, Y.; Kim, K.H.; Yoon, H.I.; Kim, G.E.; Kim, Y.B. Tumor-related leukocytosis is associated with poor radiation response and clinical outcome in uterine cervical cancer patients. *Ann. Oncol.* **2016**, *27*, 2067–2074. [CrossRef] [PubMed]
2. Kwon, H.C.; Kim, S.H.; Oh, S.Y.; Lee, S.; Lee, J.H.; Choi, H.J.; Park, K.J.; Roh, M.S.; Kim, S.G.; Kim, H.J.; et al. Clinical significance of preoperative neutrophil-lymphocyte versus platelet-lymphocyte ratio in patients with operable colorectal cancer. *Biomarkers* **2012**, *17*, 216–222. [CrossRef]
3. Bhatti, I.; Peacock, O.; Lloyd, G.; Larvin, M.; Hall, R.I. Preoperative hematologic markers as independent predictors of prognosis in resected pancreatic ductal adenocarcinoma: Neutrophil-lymphocyte versus platelet-lymphocyte ratio. *Am. J. Surg.* **2010**, *200*, 197–203. [CrossRef] [PubMed]
4. Lee, S.; Oh, S.Y.; Kim, S.H.; Lee, J.H.; Kim, M.C.; Kim, K.H.; Kim, H.J. Prognostic significance of neutrophil lymphocyte ratio and platelet lymphocyte ratio in advanced gastric cancer patients treated with folfox chemotherapy. *BMC Cancer* **2013**, *13*, 350. [CrossRef] [PubMed]
5. Mantovani, A.; Allavena, P.; Sica, A.; Balkwill, F. Cancer-related inflammation. *Nature* **2008**, *454*, 436–444. [CrossRef] [PubMed]
6. Le Bitoux, M.A.; Stamenkovic, I. Tumor-host interactions: The role of inflammation. *Histochem. Cell Biol.* **2008**, *130*, 1079–1090. [CrossRef] [PubMed]
7. Forget, P.; Khalifa, C.; Defour, J.P.; Latinne, D.; Van Pel, M.C.; De Kock, M. What is the normal value of the neutrophil-to-lymphocyte ratio? *BMC Res. Note* **2017**, *10*, 12. [CrossRef]
8. Wang, J.; Jia, Y.; Wang, N.; Zhang, X.; Tan, B.; Zhang, G.; Cheng, Y. The clinical significance of tumor-infiltrating neutrophils and neutrophil-to-cd8+ lymphocyte ratio in patients with resectable esophageal squamous cell carcinoma. *J. Transl. Med* **2014**, *12*, 7. [CrossRef]
9. Wang, X.; Zhang, G.; Jiang, X.; Zhu, H.; Lu, Z.; Xu, L. Neutrophil to lymphocyte ratio in relation to risk of all-cause mortality and cardiovascular events among patients undergoing angiography or cardiac revascularization: A meta-analysis of observational studies. *Atherosclerosis* **2014**, *234*, 206–213. [CrossRef]
10. Xue, P.; Kanai, M.; Mori, Y.; Nishimura, T.; Uza, N.; Kodama, Y.; Kawaguchi, Y.; Takaori, K.; Matsumoto, S.; Uemoto, S.; et al. Neutrophil-to-lymphocyte ratio for predicting palliative chemotherapy outcomes in advanced pancreatic cancer patients. *Cancer Med.* **2014**, *3*, 406–415. [CrossRef] [PubMed]
11. Rachidi, S.; Wallace, K.; Wrangle, J.M.; Day, T.A.; Alberg, A.J.; Li, Z. Neutrophil-to-lymphocyte ratio and overall survival in all sites of head and neck squamous cell carcinoma. *Head Neck* **2016**, *38*, E1068–E1074. [CrossRef] [PubMed]
12. Kim, D.Y.; Kim, I.S.; Park, S.G.; Kim, H.; Choi, Y.J.; Seol, Y.M. Prognostic value of posttreatment neutrophil-lymphocyte ratio in head and neck squamous cell carcinoma treated by chemoradiotherapy. *Auris Nasus Larynx* **2017**, *44*, 199–204. [CrossRef] [PubMed]
13. Yu, Y.; Wang, H.; Yan, A.; Wang, H.; Li, X.; Liu, J.; Li, W. Pretreatment neutrophil to lymphocyte ratio in determining the prognosis of head and neck cancer: A meta-analysis. *BMC Cancer* **2018**, *18*, 383. [CrossRef]
14. Park, B.; Yee, C.; Lee, K.M. The effect of radiation on the immune response to cancers. *Int. J. Mol. Sci.* **2014**, *15*, 927–943. [CrossRef]
15. Golden, E.B.; Apetoh, L. Radiotherapy and immunogenic cell death. *Semin. Radiat. Oncol.* **2015**, *25*, 11–17. [CrossRef] [PubMed]

16. Lee, J.; Chang, J.S.; Kwon, H.J.; Kim, S.H.; Shin, S.J.; Keum, K.C. Impact of p16 expression in oropharyngeal cancer in the postoperative setting: The necessity of re-evaluating traditional risk stratification. *Jpn. J. Clin. Oncol.* **2016**, *46*, 911–918. [CrossRef] [PubMed]
17. Charles, K.A.; Harris, B.D.; Haddad, C.R.; Clarke, S.J.; Guminski, A.; Stevens, M.; Dodds, T.; Gill, A.J.; Back, M.; Veivers, D.; et al. Systemic inflammation is an independent predictive marker of clinical outcomes in mucosal squamous cell carcinoma of the head and neck in oropharyngeal and non-oropharyngeal patients. *BMC Cancer* **2016**, *16*, 124. [CrossRef] [PubMed]
18. Young, C.A.; Murray, L.J.; Karakaya, E.; Thygesen, H.H.; Sen, M.; Prestwich, R.J. The prognostic role of the neutrophil-to-lymphocyte ratio in oropharyngeal carcinoma treated with chemoradiotherapy. *Clin. Med. Insight Oncol.* **2014**, *8*, 81–86. [CrossRef]
19. Fu, Y.; Liu, W.; OuYang, D.; Yang, A.; Zhang, Q. Preoperative neutrophil-to-lymphocyte ratio predicts long-term survival in patients undergoing total laryngectomy with advanced laryngeal squamous cell carcinoma: A single-center retrospective study. *Medicine* **2016**, *95*, e2689. [CrossRef]
20. Sun, W.; Zhang, L.; Luo, M.; Hu, G.; Mei, Q.; Liu, D.; Long, G.; Hu, G. Pretreatment hematologic markers as prognostic factors in patients with nasopharyngeal carcinoma: Neutrophil-lymphocyte ratio and platelet-lymphocyte ratio. *Head Neck* **2016**, *38*, E1332–E1340. [CrossRef] [PubMed]
21. Huang, S.H.; Waldron, J.N.; Milosevic, M.; Shen, X.; Ringash, J.; Su, J.; Tong, L.; Perez-Ordonez, B.; Weinreb, I.; Bayley, A.J.; et al. Prognostic value of pretreatment circulating neutrophils, monocytes, and lymphocytes in oropharyngeal cancer stratified by human papillomavirus status. *Cancer* **2015**, *121*, 545–555. [CrossRef] [PubMed]
22. Lewis, J.S. P16 immunohistochemistry as a standalone test for risk stratification in oropharyngeal squamous cell carcinoma. *Head Neck Pathol.* **2012**, *6*, S75–S82. [CrossRef] [PubMed]
23. Gupta, G.P.; Kumar, S.; Marron, D.; Amdur, R.J.; Hayes, D.N.; Weiss, J.; Grilley-Olson, J.; Zanation, A.; Hackman, T.; Zevallos, J.P.; et al. Circulating tumor hpv16 DNA as a biomarker of tumor genomics and disease control in hpv-associated oropharyngeal squamous cell carcinoma. *Int. J. Radiat. Oncol. Biol. Phys.* **2018**, *100*, 1310–1311. [CrossRef]
24. Atzpodien, J.; Royston, P.; Wandert, T.; Reitz, M.; Group, D.G.C.R.C.C.-I.T. Metastatic renal carcinoma comprehensive prognostic system. *Br. J. Cancer* **2003**, *88*, 348–353. [CrossRef] [PubMed]
25. Walsh, S.R.; Cook, E.J.; Goulder, F.; Justin, T.A.; Keeling, N.J. Neutrophil-lymphocyte ratio as a prognostic factor in colorectal cancer. *J. Surg. Oncol.* **2005**, *91*, 181–184. [CrossRef] [PubMed]
26. Haram, A.; Boland, M.R.; Kelly, M.E.; Bolger, J.C.; Waldron, R.M.; Kerin, M.J. The prognostic value of neutrophil-to-lymphocyte ratio in colorectal cancer: A systematic review. *J. Surg. Oncol.* **2017**, *115*, 470–479. [CrossRef] [PubMed]
27. Cheng, H.; Long, F.; Jaiswar, M.; Yang, L.; Wang, C.; Zhou, Z. Prognostic role of the neutrophil-to-lymphocyte ratio in pancreatic cancer: A meta-analysis. *Sci. Rep.* **2015**, *5*, 11026. [CrossRef] [PubMed]
28. Rosculet, N.; Zhou, X.C.; Ha, P.; Tang, M.; Levine, M.A.; Neuner, G.; Califano, J. Neutrophil-to-lymphocyte ratio: Prognostic indicator for head and neck squamous cell carcinoma. *Head Neck* **2017**, *39*, 662–667. [CrossRef] [PubMed]
29. Motomura, T.; Shirabe, K.; Mano, Y.; Muto, J.; Toshima, T.; Umemoto, Y.; Fukuhara, T.; Uchiyama, H.; Ikegami, T.; Yoshizumi, T.; et al. Neutrophil-lymphocyte ratio reflects hepatocellular carcinoma recurrence after liver transplantation via inflammatory microenvironment. *J. Hepatol.* **2013**, *58*, 58–64. [CrossRef]
30. Schetter, A.J.; Heegaard, N.H.; Harris, C.C. Inflammation and cancer: Interweaving microrna, free radical, cytokine and p53 pathways. *Carcinogenesis* **2010**, *31*, 37–49. [CrossRef]
31. Mantovani, A.; Schioppa, T.; Porta, C.; Allavena, P.; Sica, A. Role of tumor-associated macrophages in tumor progression and invasion. *Cancer Metastasis Rev.* **2006**, *25*, 315–322. [CrossRef] [PubMed]
32. Templeton, A.J.; McNamara, M.G.; Seruga, B.; Vera-Badillo, F.E.; Aneja, P.; Ocana, A.; Leibowitz-Amit, R.; Sonpavde, G.; Knox, J.J.; Tran, B.; et al. Prognostic role of neutrophil-to-lymphocyte ratio in solid tumors: A systematic review and meta-analysis. *J. Natl Cancer Inst.* **2014**. [CrossRef] [PubMed]
33. Nakahira, M.; Sugasawa, M.; Matsumura, S.; Kuba, K.; Ohba, S.; Hayashi, T.; Minami, K.; Ebihara, Y.; Kogashiwa, Y. Prognostic role of the combination of platelet count and neutrophil-lymphocyte ratio in patients with hypopharyngeal squamous cell carcinoma. *Eur. Arch. Oto-Rhino-Laryngol.* **2016**, *273*, 3863–3867. [CrossRef] [PubMed]

34. Wojtukiewicz, M.Z.; Sierko, E.; Hempel, D.; Tucker, S.C.; Honn, K.V. Platelets and cancer angiogenesis nexus. *Cancer Metastasis Rev.* **2017**, *36*, 249–262. [CrossRef] [PubMed]
35. Sierko, E.; Wojtukiewicz, M.Z. Inhibition of platelet function: Does it offer a chance of better cancer progression control? *Semin. Thrombosis Hemost.* **2007**, *33*, 712–721. [CrossRef] [PubMed]

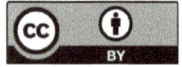

© 2018 by the authors. Licensee MDPI, Basel, Switzerland. This article is an open access article distributed under the terms and conditions of the Creative Commons Attribution (CC BY) license (http://creativecommons.org/licenses/by/4.0/).

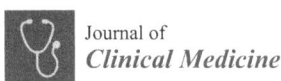 

Article

# Distinctive Expression and Amplification of Genes at 11q13 in Relation to HPV Status with Impact on Survival in Head and Neck Cancer Patients

Francisco Hermida-Prado [1,2,†], Sofía T. Menéndez [1,2,†], Pablo Albornoz-Afanasiev [1,†], Rocío Granda-Diaz [1,2], Saúl Álvarez-Teijeiro [1,2], M. Ángeles Villaronga [1,2], Eva Allonca [1,2], Laura Alonso-Durán [1], Xavier León [3,4], Laia Alemany [5,6], Marisa Mena [2,5], Nagore del-Rio-Ibisate [1,2], Aurora Astudillo [7], René Rodríguez [1,2], Juan P. Rodrigo [1,2,*] and Juana M. García-Pedrero [1,2,*]

1 Department of Otolaryngology, Hospital Universitario Central de Asturias and Instituto de Investigación Sanitaria del Principado de Asturias, Instituto Universitario de Oncología del Principado de Asturias, University of Oviedo, 33011 Oviedo, Spain; franjhermida@gmail.com (F.H.-P.); sofiatirados@gmail.com (S.T.M.); pavlikh@gmail.com (P.A.-A.); rocigd281@gmail.com (R.G.-D.); saul.teijeiro@gmail.com (S.Á.-T.); angelesvillaronga@gmail.com (M.Á.V.); ynkc1@hotmail.com (E.A.); laurita_alonso86@hotmail.com (L.A.-D.); nagoredelrio@gmail.com (N.d.-R.-I.); renerg.finba@gmail.com (R.R.)
2 Centro de Investigación Biomédica en Red Cáncer, CIBERONC, 28029 Madrid, Spain; mmena.iconcologia@gmail.com
3 Otorhinolaryngology Department, Hospital de la Santa Creu i Sant Pau, Universitat Autònoma de Barcelona, 08041 Barcelona, Spain; XLeon@santpau.cat
4 Centro de Investigación Biomédica en Red de Bioingeniería, Biomateriales y Nanomedicina, CIBER-BBN, 28029 Madrid, Spain
5 Cancer Epidemiology Research Program, Catalan Institute of Oncology (ICO), IDIBELL. L'Hospitalet de Llobregat, 08908 Barcelona, Spain; alemanyvilchesico@gmail.com
6 Centro de Investigación Biomédica en Red de Epidemiología y Salud Pública, CIBERESP, Barcelona, Spain
7 Department of Pathology, Hospital Universitario Central de Asturias, Instituto Universitario de Oncología del Principado de Asturias, University of Oviedo, 33011 Oviedo, Spain; astudillo@hca.es
* Correspondence: jprodrigo@uniovi.es (J.P.R.); juanagp.finba@gmail.com (J.M.G.-P.); Tel.: +34-985107937 (J.M.G.-P.)
† These authors contributed equally to this work.

Received: 26 October 2018; Accepted: 29 November 2018; Published: 1 December 2018

**Abstract:** Clear differences have been established between head and neck squamous cell carcinomas (HNSCC) depending on human papillomavirus (HPV) infection status. This study specifically investigated the status of the *CTTN*, *CCND1* and *ANO1* genes mapping at the 11q13 amplicon in relation to the HPV status in HNSCC patients. CTTN, CCND1 and ANO1 protein expression and gene amplification were respectively analyzed by immunohistochemistry and real-time PCR in a homogeneous cohort of 392 surgically treated HNSCC patients. The results were further confirmed using an independent cohort of 279 HNSCC patients from The Cancer Genome Atlas (TCGA). The impact on patient survival was also evaluated. *CTTN*, *CCND1* and *ANO1* gene amplification and protein expression were frequent in HPV-negative tumors, while absent or rare in HPV-positive tumors. Using an independent validation cohort of 279 HNSCC patients, we consistently found that these three genes were frequently co-amplified (28%) and overexpressed (39–46%) in HPV-negative tumors, whereas almost absent in HPV-positive tumors. Remarkably, these alterations (in particular CTTN and ANO1 overexpression) were associated with poor prognosis. Taken together, the distinctive expression and amplification of these genes could cooperatively contribute to the differences in prognosis and clinical outcome between HPV-positive and HPV-negative tumors. These findings could serve as the basis to design more personalized therapeutic strategies for HNSCC patients.

**Keywords:** head and neck squamous cell carcinoma; HPV; 11q13; gene amplification; immunohistochemistry

## 1. Introduction

Head and neck cancer represents a heterogeneous group of tumors that accounts for about 5% of the total annual worldwide cases of cancer, usually associated with poor prognosis [1,2]; however, its incidence and other main features can significantly vary from one region to another. The most prevalent histological type in head and neck cancers is the squamous cell carcinoma (HNSCC), and it is widely accepted that the most important risk factors are tobacco and alcohol consumption [1,3,4]. Interestingly, the incidence of HNSCCs is currently declining in some specific regions, due to a decrease of tobacco and alcohol consumption [4,5]. Nevertheless, there is an increasing incidence of oropharyngeal tumors that are associated with human papillomavirus (HPV) infection in certain developed countries [4,5].

The proportion of HPV-related oropharyngeal tumors can vary considerably among regions; the observed prevalence in Europe varies from an estimated 17% in southern countries to as high as 93% in northern countries like Sweden [5]. More than 90% of HPV-related HNSCC tumors are caused by one specific virus type, the HPV-16, which also leads to HPV-related anogenital tumors [4,5]. On this basis, epidemiological studies have correlated HPV-positive tumors with sexual behaviors, suggesting that the risk increases with the number of sexual partners and is particularly more frequent in men [4,5].

Recent studies have consistently showed that HPV-related (HPV+) and unrelated (HPV−) tumors represent two different entities in terms of clinical, biological, and molecular characteristics. Thus, HPV-positive tumors generally arise in the oropharynx, have a more favorable prognosis, a better response to chemotherapy and radiotherapy, and less genetic alterations when compared to HPV-negative tumors [2,4–6].

One of the most frequent genetic alterations found in HNSCCs is the amplification of the chromosomal region 11q13, which has been associated with tumor aggressive behavior, increased lymph node metastases, and poor outcome [7]. Moreover, the comprehensive molecular analysis of the 11q13 region led to the identification of genes evidenced to be directly related to an improved ability for tumor growth, migration and invasion. Some of the genes mapping to the 11q13 region, are *CTTN* (Cortactin), *CCND1* (Cyclin D1), and the more recently discovered *ANO1* (Anoctamin-1). *CTTN* and *CCND1* are well-established oncogenes, associated with advanced disease stage and poor prognosis [8,9]. On the other hand, the newly characterized *ANO1* encodes a calcium-activated transmembrane chloride channel whose overexpression and amplification have been correlated with increased cell migration and propensity to develop metastases [10,11]. However, data revealing the role and importance of *ANO1* in HNSCC have only recently emerged and, hence, are still limited.

Recent studies have evidenced important differences in the molecular alterations and the impact of the 11q13 chromosomal region in HNSCC, depending on the anatomic site of the tumor and the HPV infection status. These studies suggest that the amplification of 11q13 in HNSCCs is more frequent in HPV-negative than in HPV-positive tumors [12], and this presumably contributes to the better prognosis of the latter. On the basis of the increasing incidence of HPV-related tumors, the current information regarding the clinical differences between HPV-related and unrelated tumors, and the discovery of promising molecular prognosis factors like *ANO1*, we believe it is crucial to study in depth the molecular alterations involved in HNSCC and their relationship with HPV infection, in order to have a better understanding of the pathogenesis of the disease with the ultimate goal of establishing the path for the development of new and more effective treatment strategies. This consideration prompted us to study the status of various genes (*CTTN*, *CCND1* and *ANO1*) mapping at the 11q13 amplicon in relation to HPV infection in two large independent cohorts of HNSCC patients.

## 2. Materials and Methods

### 2.1. Patients and Tissue Specimens

Surgical tissue specimens from 392 patients with HNSCC who underwent resection of their tumors at the Hospital Universitario Central de Asturias and Hospital Sant Pau between 1990 and 2010 were retrospectively collected, in accordance to approved institutional review board guidelines. All experimental protocols were conducted in accordance to the Declaration of Helsinki and approved by the Institutional Ethics Committees of the Hospital Universitario Central de Asturias and Hospital Sant Pau and by the Regional CEIC from Principado de Asturias (approval number: 81/2013 for the project PI13/00259). Informed consent was obtained from all patients. Representative tissue sections were obtained from archival, paraffin-embedded blocks, and the histological diagnoses were confirmed by an experienced pathologist (Aurora Astudillo).

Clinical, sociodemographic, follow-up, and risk factors information was collected from the medical records. The stage of the tumors was determined according to the TNM system of the International Union Against Cancer (7th Edition).

### 2.2. Tissue Microarray (TMA) Construction and DNA Extraction

The original archived hematoxylin- and eosin-stained slides were reviewed by an experienced pathologist (Aurora Astudillo) to confirm the histological diagnoses. Five morphologically representative areas were selected from each individual tumor paraffin block: two for DNA isolation and three for the construction of a TMA. To avoid cross-contamination, two punches of 2 mm diameter were taken first, using a new, sterile punch (Kai Europe GmbH, Solingen, Germany) for every tissue block, and stored in eppendorf tubes (Sigma Aldrich, Saint Louis, MO, USA) at room temperature. Subsequently, three representative tissue cores (1 mm diameter punches) were selected from each tumor block and transferred to a recipient 'Master' block in a grid-like manner using a manual tissue microarray instrument to construct TMA blocks, as described previously [13,14]. In addition, each TMA included three cores of normal epithelium (tonsil) as an internal negative control and three cores of a HPV-positive cervix carcinoma as a positive control. A section from each microarray was stained with hematoxylin and eosin and examined by light microscopy (Leica Microsystems, Wetzlar, Germany) to check the adequacy of tissue sampling.

The protocol for DNA extraction from paraffin-embedded tissue sections has been described elsewhere [13]. Briefly, Formalin-fixed paraffin-embedded (FFPE) tissue samples were subjected to thorough deparaffinization with xylene (Sigma Aldrich, Saint Louis, MO, USA), methanol (Merck, Darmstadt, Germany) washings to remove all traces of the xylene, and a 24 h incubation in 1 mol/L sodium thiocyanate (Sigma Aldrich Inc.) to reduce cross-links. Subsequently, the tissue pellet was digested for 2–3 days in lysis buffer with high doses of proteinase K (final concentration, 2 µg/µL, freshly added twice daily). Finally, DNA extraction was done using the QIAamp DNA Mini Kit (Qiagen GmbH, Hilden, Germany).

### 2.3. HPV Detection

The algorithm used to detect the presence of HPV in these patients has been previously described in detail [13,15]. Briefly, the presence of HPV was assessed by p16-immunohistochemistry in all cases, and those cases showing p16-positive immunostaining (any nuclear and or cytoplasmic staining) were subjected to high-risk HPV DNA detection and genotyping by GP5+/6+-PCR with an enzyme-immuno-assay (EIA) read-out for detection of 14 high-risk HPV types. Subsequent genotyping of EIA-positive cases was performed by bead-based array on the Luminex platform. In addition, in situ hybridization (ISH) with biotinylated HPV DNA probes considered to react with HPV types 16, 18, 31, 33, 35, 39, 45, 51, 52, 56, 58, 59, and 68 (Y1443, DakoCytomation, Glostrup, Denmark) was performed on all carcinomas, using 3 µm tissue sections of the TMAs, according to the manufacturer's instructions.

*2.4. Gene Amplification Analysis*

Gene amplification was evaluated by real-time PCR (Q-PCR) in an ABI PRISM 7500 Sequence detector (Applied Biosystems, Foster City, CA) using Power SYBR Green PCR Master Mix and oligonucleotides designed according to Primer Express software v2.0 (Applied Biosystems, Lincoln Centre Drive Foster City, CA, USA) with the following sequences: for *CCND1* gene, Fw, 5′-GGAAGATCGTCGCCACCTG-3′ and Rv, 5′- GAAACGTGGGTCTGGGCAAC-3′; for *ANO1* gene, Fw, 5′-CAAAGGCAGGTGCTTTGCA-3′ and Rv, 5′-TCTACGGGCCTCTGCTCACT-3′; for *CTTN* gene, Fw, 5′-GATCTCATTTGACCCTGATGACATC-3′ and Rv, 5′-CGTACCGGCCCTTGCA-3′; and for the reference gene *TH* (Tyrosine Hydroxylase, located at 11p15), Fw, 5′-TGAGATTCGGGCCTTCGA-3′ and Rv, 5′-GACACGAAGTAGACTGACTGGTACGT-3′. Dissociation curve analysis of all PCR products showed a single sharp peak, and the correct size of each amplified product was confirmed by agarose gel electrophoresis. The relative gene copy number was calculated using the $2^{-\Delta\Delta C_T}$ method, as we previously described [16,17]. The $\Delta\Delta C_T$ represents the difference between the paired tissue samples ($\Delta C_T$ of tumor $-$ $\Delta C_T$ of normal mucosa), with $\Delta C_T$ being the average $C_T$ for each target gene minus the average $C_T$ for the reference gene (*TH*). Relative copy numbers $\geq$2-fold were considered gene gain, and relative copy numbers $\geq$4-fold were considered positive for gene amplification.

*2.5. Immunohistochemistry*

The formalin-fixed, paraffin-embedded tissues were cut into 3-µm sections and dried on Flex IHC microscope slides (Dako, Glostrup, Denmark). The sections were deparaffinized with standard xylene and hydrated through graded alcohols into water. Antigen retrieval was performed using Envision Flex Target Retrieval solution, high pH (Dako, Glostrup, Denmark). Staining was done at room temperature on an automatic staining workstation (Dako Autostainer Plus) with mouse anti-Cyclin D1 monoclonal antibody DCS-6 (Santa Cruz Biotechnology, Inc. sc-20044) at 1:100 dilution, rabbit polyclonal Anti-TMEM16A antibody (Abcam # ab53212) at 1:500 dilution, or mouse anti-cortactin monoclonal antibody Clone 30 (BD Biosciences Pharmingen, San Jose, CA, USA) at 1:200 dilution, using the Dako EnVision Flex + Visualization System (Dako Autostainer). Counterstaining with hematoxylin was the final step.

The slides were viewed randomly without clinical data by two of the authors, according to the scoring systems previously described [17,18] with a high level of inter-observer concordance (>95%). CCND1 staining was evaluated as the percentage of cells with nuclear staining, scored as 0–2 according to the semiquantitative scale (0–10, 10–50, or >50% positive tumor cells). CCND1 staining scores were classified as negative or positive staining on the basis of values below or above the median value of 10%. Since CTTN and ANO1 staining showed a homogeneous distribution, a semiquantitative scoring system based on staining intensity was applied. Thus, CTTN immunostaining was scored as negative (0), weak (1), moderate (2), and strong protein expression (3). The staining data were dichotomized as negative (scores 0 and 1) versus positive (scores 2 and 3). ANO1 immunostaining was scored as negative (0), weak to moderate (1), and strong protein expression (2). Scores $\geq$1 were considered positive ANO1 expression.

*2.6. Statistical Analysis*

Fisher's exact test was used for comparison between categorical variables, and t Student test for parametric continuous variables. Correlations between protein expression, gene amplification, and HPV status were estimated by Kendall's tau correlation test. All tests were two-sided; $p$ values $\leq$0.05 were considered to be statistically significant.

## 3. Results

### 3.1. Patient Characteristics

A large cohort of 392 homogeneous surgically treated HNSCC patients was selected for study. A flow diagram of the experimental setup is shown in Supplementary Figure S1. All patients had a single primary tumor, microscopically clear surgical margins, and received no treatment prior to surgery. Only 19 patients were women, and the mean age was 60 years (range 30 to 89 years). All but 22 patients were habitual tobacco smokers—202 moderate (1–50 pack-year) and 159 heavy (>50 pack-year)—and 353 were alcohol drinkers. Nineteen tumors were stage I, 25 stage II, 69 stage III, and 279 stage IV. The series included 152 tonsillar, 116 base of tongue, 62 hypopharyngeal, and 62 laryngeal carcinomas. A total of 147 tumors were classified as well-differentiated, 151 as moderately differentiated, and 94 as poorly differentiated. In total, 232 (59%) patients received postoperative radiotherapy.

### 3.2. Distinctive Associations of CCND1, ANO1, and CTTN Protein Expression with HPV Status in HNSCC Patients

We found that 67 cases (17%) showed nuclear and cytoplasmic p16 expression, a surrogate marker for HPV infection (2) (Table 1). HPV DNA was assessed by GP5+/6+-PCR and by in situ hybridization in the 67 p16-positive cases, which resulted in a total of 30 HPV-positive cases (28 oropharyngeal, 1 laryngeal, and 1 hypopharyngeal carcinoma) in our series (all were HPV type 16). Representative images of HPV-positive and HPV-negative cases and also examples of p16 immunostaining are shown in Figure 1. We found a total of 267 (68%) positive cases for CCND1 protein expression, 78 (21%) positive cases for ANO1 expression, and 190 (49%) positive cases for CTTN expression (Table 1). Representative examples of protein staining are shown in Figure 2, and raw data in Supplementary Information. We next investigated the relationship between CCND1, ANO1, and CTTN expression and HPV infection status. The expression of these three proteins was strongly and inversely correlated with HPV infection. Notably, all the HPV-positive cases showed negative ANO1 expression, and 28 HPV-positive cases had also negative CTTN expression (Table 1).

**Table 1.** Analysis of CCND1 (Cyclin D1), ANO1 (Anoctamin-1), and CTTN (Cortactin) protein expression in relation to human papillomavirus (HPV) status and p16 expression in 392 head and neck squamous cell carcinomas (HNSCC) patients.

| Molecular Feature | Number | HPV-Positive | $p$ [#] |
|---|---|---|---|
| **CCND1 protein expression** | | | |
| Negative | 123 | 21 | (−0.239) |
| Positive (scores 1-2) | 267 | 9 | <0.001 |
| **ANO1 protein expression** | | | |
| Negative | 299 | 29 | (−0.147) |
| Positive (scores 1-2) | 78 | 0 | <0.001 |
| **CTTN protein expression** | | | |
| Negative | 199 | 28 | (−0.239) |
| Positive (scores 2-3) | 190 | 2 | <0.001 |
| **p16 protein expression** | | | |
| Negative | 325 | 0 | (0.634) |
| Positive | 67 | 30 | <0.001 |

[#] Kendall's tau correlation coefficient with the associated $p$ value.

### 3.3. Analysis of CCND1, ANO1, and CTTN Gene Amplification in Relation to HPV Status in HNSCC Patients

CCND1, ANO1, and CTTN gene gain and amplification was assessed by real-time PCR in 88 cases selected from the same HNSCC tissue blocks, including 26 HPV-positive cases. We found gene gains and amplifications of *CCND1* in 32 (36%) tumors, *ANO1* in 42 (48%) tumors, and *CTTN* in 26 (30%) tumors (Table 2), with relative gene copy numbers ranging from 2- to 24-fold. Co-amplifications of these three genes were also frequently observed (26 cases, 30%). We also found that tumors harboring gene amplification significantly correlated with higher expression levels of each protein (Figure 3). When analyzing the correlations with HPV infection status, we consistently found that *CCND1*, *ANO1*, and *CTTN* gene amplification inversely correlated with HPV status (Table 2). Thus, amplifications of *CTTN*, *CCND1*, and *ANO1* were frequent in HPV-negative tumors (ranging from 42 to 61%), while absent in HPV-positive tumors.

**Table 2.** Analysis of *CCND1*, *ANO1*, and *CTTN* gene gain and amplification in relation to HPV status in 88 HNSCC patients.

| Copy Number Alteration | No. | HPV-Positive | $p$ [#] |
|---|---|---|---|
| ***CCND1* gene** | | | |
| Negative | 55 | 24 | (−0.430) |
| Gain (≥2 copies) | 6 | 2 | <0.001 |
| Amplification (≥4 copies) | 27 | 0 | |
| ***ANO1* gene** | | | |
| Negative | 45 | 22 | (−0.472) |
| Gain (≥2 copies) | 16 | 4 | <0.001 |
| Amplification (≥4 copies) | 27 | 0 | |
| ***CTTN* gene** | | | |
| Negative | 61 | 26 | (−0.422) |
| Gain (≥2 copies) | 3 | 0 | <0.001 |
| Amplification (≥4 copies) | 24 | 0 | |
| Total Cases | 88 | 26 | |

[#] Kendall's tau correlation coefficient with the associated $p$ value.

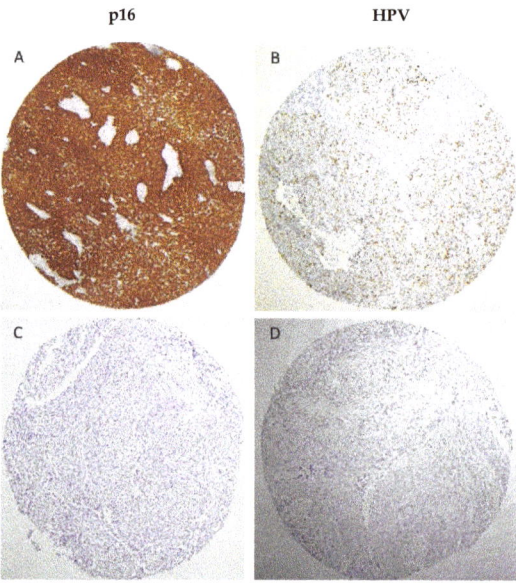

**Figure 1.** Representative images of p16-positive (**A**) and negative (**C**) immunostaining in the HNSCC tissue microarrays (TMAs) and HPV-positive (**B**) and HPV-negative (**D**) cases detected by in situ hybridization. Original magnification ×10.

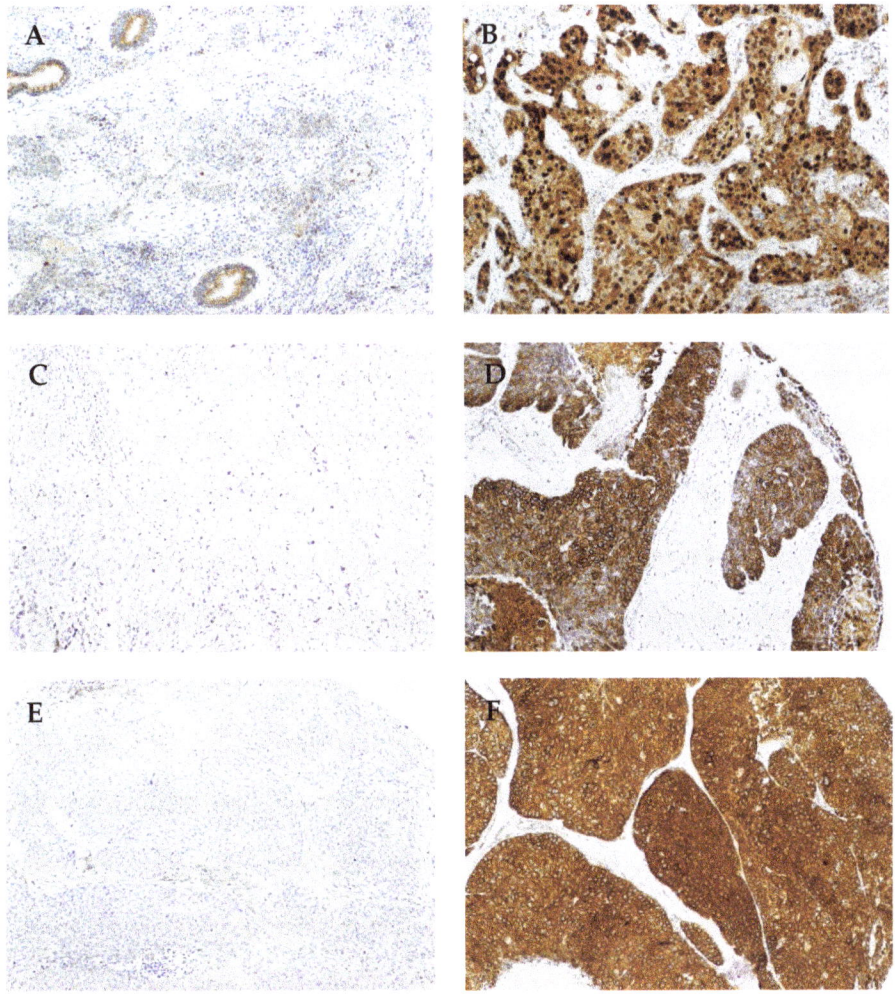

**Figure 2.** Representative examples of negative and strong positive staining for CCND1 (**A**,**B**), ANO1 (**C**,**D**), and CTTN (**E**,**F**). Original magnification ×20.

*3.4. Analysis of CCND1, ANO1, and CTTN mRNA Expression in Relation to HPV Status in 279 HNSCC Patients from the TGCA*

In order to confirm our results, we performed an analysis of the publicly available TCGA data from 279 HNSCC patients [19] using the platform cBioPortal for Cancer Genomics (http://cbioportal.org/) [20]. The clinicopathologic characteristics of this cohort are summarized in Supplementary Table S1 and Figure S2. A total of 36 (13%) patients were positive for HPV infection, most prevalent in the oropharynx (22 cases, 61%), and associated to lower tobacco consumption, lower mutations, improved survival, and a younger age in both men and women. The results also evidenced differential changes in mRNA expression levels of *CTTN*, *CCND1* and *ANO1* depending on HPV infection status. Thus, increased mRNA expression levels of these genes were frequently and significantly observed in HPV-negative tumors (Figure 4A–D), while very rare in HPV-positive patients (Table 3). Similarly, the analysis of copy number alterations of *CTTN*, *CCND1*, and *ANO1* genes also revealed that both amplifications and gains of these three genes were also highly frequent in HPV-negative tumors, whereas almost absent in HPV-positive tumors (Figure 4A,E). Furthermore, the results consistently showed that these three genes were frequently co-amplified (28%) and overexpressed at a higher frequency (39–46%), and, more importantly, these molecular alterations (in particular CTTN and ANO1 overexpression) were associated with a worse clinical outcome in the TCGA cohort of 279 HNSCC patients and also in an extended TCGA cohort which added 251 new HNSCC patients ($n = 530$) (Figure 5).

| CCND1 | | Gene Copy Number | | | Total |
|---|---|---|---|---|---|
| | | No Gain | Gain | Amplification | |
| Protein Score | 0 | 34 | 1 | 1 | 36 |
| | 1 | 16 | 2 | 7 | 25 |
| | 2 | 5 | 3 | 19 | 27 |
| Total | | 55 | 6 | 27 | 88 |

Spearman Coefficient 0.653, $p < 0.001$.

| ANO1 | | Gene Copy Number | | | Total |
|---|---|---|---|---|---|
| | | No Gain | Gain | Amplification | |
| Protein Score | 0 | 40 | 14 | 18 | 72 |
| | 1 | 4 | 2 | 6 | 12 |
| | 2 | 1 | 0 | 3 | 4 |
| Total | | 45 | 16 | 27 | 88 |

Spearman Coefficient 0.237, $p = 0.027$.

| CTTN | | Gene Copy Number | | | Total |
|---|---|---|---|---|---|
| | | No Gain | Gain | Amplification | |
| Protein Score | 0 | 22 | 1 | 0 | 23 |
| | 1 | 32 | 1 | 0 | 33 |
| | 2 | 4 | 1 | 9 | 14 |
| | 3 | 3 | 0 | 15 | 18 |
| Total | | 61 | 3 | 24 | 88 |

Spearman Coefficient 0.711, $p < 0.001$.

**Figure 3.** Crosstab to evaluate the correlations between gene gains and amplification and protein staining scores for CCND1, ANO1, and CTTN.

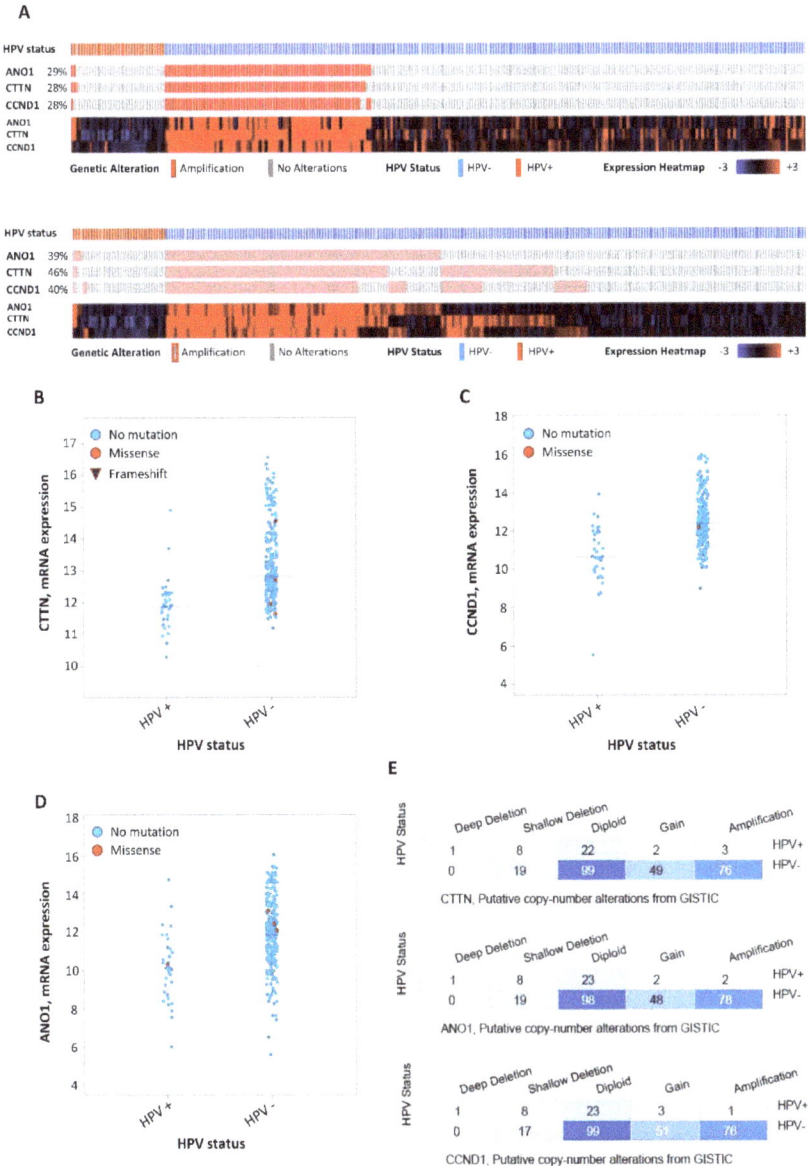

**Figure 4.** Analysis of mRNA expression and copy number alterations of *CTTN*, *CCND1* and *ANO1* in relation to HPV status related to the available HNSCC TCGA data ($n = 279$) obtained from cBioPortal. (**A**) Schematic representation and heat map showing the percentage of cases with *CTTN*, *CCND1*, and *ANO1* gene amplification and mRNA expression in relation to the HPV status. (**B**) CTTN, (**C**) CCND1, and (**D**) ANO1 mRNA expression distributed according to the HPV status. mRNA expression (RNA seq V2 RSEM) values were Log2 transformed (*y*-axis). Whiskers plot (min. to max.) with median values; $p < 0.001$, two-tailed Student *t*-test. (**E**) Copy number alterations of *CTTN*, *CCND1* and *ANO1* according to the HPV status using the GISTIC method.

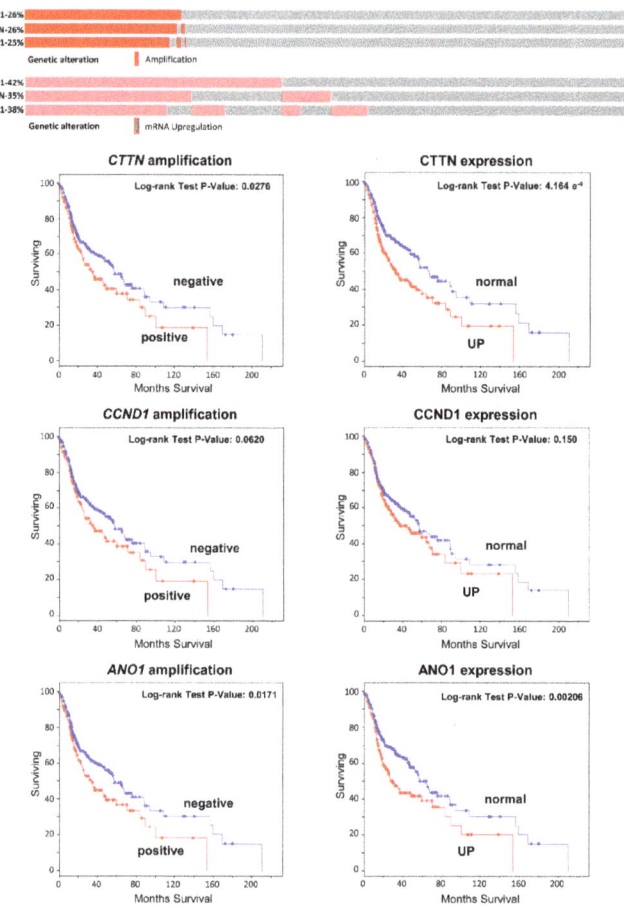

**Figure 5.** Analysis of *CTTN*, *CCND1* and *ANO1* gene amplification and mRNA expression in the TCGA cohort of 530 HNSCC patients using cBioPortal. Schematic representation showing the percentage of cases with amplification or mRNA upregulation of each gene. Kaplan–Meier survival curves categorized by *CTTN*, *CCND1* and *ANO1* gene amplification dichotomized as positive *versus* negative; CTTN, CCND1 and ANO1 mRNA expression (RNA seq V2 RSEM, z-score threshold ±2) dichotomized as normal versus upregulation (UP); *p* values estimated using the Log-rank test.

**Table 3.** Analysis of *CCND1*, *ANO1*, and *CTTN* mRNA expression in relation to HPV status in 279 HNSCC TGCA patients.

| Molecular Feature | No. | HPV-Positive | $p$ [#] |
|---|---|---|---|
| **CCND1 expression** | | | |
| Normal | 206 | 35 | <0.001 |
| UP | 73 | 1 | |
| **ANO1 expression** | | | |
| Normal | 207 | 34 | 0.002 |
| UP | 72 | 2 | |
| **CTTN expression** | | | |
| Normal | 177 | 34 | <0.001 |
| UP | 102 | 2 | |
| Total Cases | 279 | 36 | |

[#] Fisher's exact test.

## 4. Discussion

The incidence of HPV-related HNSCC is currently increasing and gaining importance, while tumors associated to tobacco and alcohol consumption are declining [4,5]. Recent studies have established important differences between HNSCC depending on HPV infection status, including clinical, biological, and molecular features, emphasizing the presence of less genetic alterations, a better response to chemotherapy and radiotherapy, and a more favorable prognosis for HPV-related HNSCC [2,4,5]. These differences could change the way we diagnose, treat, and manage HNSCC. One of the most frequent genetic alterations found in HNSCC is the amplification of the 11q13 locus, which has been associated with increased tumor growth, proliferation, and dissemination [8,9].

Given the importance of the 11q13 locus in HNSCC and to contribute to the molecular characterization of these tumors, we conducted a study on a large unbiased cohort of 392 homogeneous surgically treated HNSCC patients to investigate the role of 11q13 amplification in relation to HPV status. This was accomplished by assessing the specific relationship of the protein expression and amplification of the *CTTN*, *CCND1*, and *ANO1* genes mapping within this locus. Immunohistochemical analysis of CCND1, CTTN, and ANO1 revealed that the expression of these three proteins was strongly and inversely correlated with HPV infection. Noteworthy, all the HPV-positive cases showed negative ANO1 expression, and 28 out of 30 HPV-positive cases had also negative CTTN expression. Likewise, the analysis of gene copy amplification by real-time PCR consistently showed that amplifications of *CTTN*, *CCND1* and *ANO1* were frequently detected in HPV-negative tumors (ranging from 42 to 61%), while absent or rare in HPV-positive tumors (0–15%). Mechanistically, we found that the contribution of gene amplification to protein expression varied widely depending on each gene. Even though tumors harboring amplification also concomitantly expressed high protein levels, positive CCND1 and CTTN expression occurred at a higher frequency than gene amplification, while ANO1 protein expression was less frequent than *ANO1* gene amplification. Additional regulatory mechanisms (transcriptional and post-translational) should contribute to protein expression, as previously reported [18]. A limitation of our study is the use of tissue microarrays to evaluate protein expression, which may constitute a drawback to assess the possible influence of tumor heterogeneity. To minimize this, three different representative tumor areas were selected from each tissue block and analyzed in the TMAs. Of note, the results showed that these proteins presented homogeneous and highly concordant expression patterns in the three tissue punches from each tumor.

These results were further and significantly validated using an independent cohort of 279 TCGA HNSCC patients, thus confirming that the mRNA expression levels of CCND1, CTTN, and ANO1 were significantly increased in a high proportion of HPV-negative tumors, whereas most HPV-positive patients exhibited normal mRNA levels of all these genes. Similar observations were obtained by analyzing the frequencies of copy number alterations. These findings are also consistent with some studies that reported that 11q13 amplifications and gains were less frequent in HPV-related tumors [2,4]. This is also in agreement with the assumption made by Kostareli et al. [6] that, in HPV-positive tumors, a lower amount of genetic alterations is required to achieve the malignant phenotype, because of the inactivation of p53 and pRb proteins by the viral E6 and E7 oncoproteins. To our knowledge, this is the first study to assess specifically the protein expression and copy number alterations of various genes mapping at the 11q13 amplicon in relation to HPV infection status using two large independent cohorts of HNSCC patients. Our study unveils important differences regarding the expression and amplification of the *CCND1*, *CTTN* and *ANO1* genes between HPV-related and unrelated tumors. It is worth mentioning that the two HNSCC cohorts selected for study are representative, sharing multiple of the unique characteristics reported for HPV-positive tumors [13], such as a clear prevalence in the oropharynx, low tobacco and alcohol consumption by the patients, lower tumor stage, basaloid histological pattern, a younger patients' age at diagnosis, lower mutations and CNA, and above all, a better prognosis. A recent study by Dixit et al. [21] provided the first evidence of a link between ANO1 expression and gene amplification and HPV status using a series of 64 pharyngeal tumors and tissue microarrays for IHC evaluation. Therefore, our results further and significantly strength and validate these preliminary findings on ANO1 protein expression using a large independent cohort of 392 HNSCC patients, as well as on ANO1 mRNA levels in the TCGA cohort of 530 HNSCC patients.

Together, these findings suggest that the *CCND1*, *CTTN* and *ANO1* genes within the 11q13 amplicon could play a significant role in HPV-negative tumors but not in HPV-positive tumors. Given that 11q13 amplification has been associated with poor prognosis in HNSCC patients, and, in particular, these three genes have been involved in tumor progression and resistance to radio-, chemotherapy [11,22–26], and EGFR-targeted therapies [27], the herein found distinctive molecular alterations presumably could contribute to the clinical and biological differences between these two different HNSCC subtypes and explain the better prognosis and response to radiotherapy and chemotherapy associated to HPV-positive tumors. In fact, we proved the impact of these molecular alterations on patient survival. In particular, CTTN and ANO1 overexpression, rather than gene amplification, was more frequent and found to associate with a worse clinical outcome in two TCGA cohorts of 279 and 530 HNSCC patients. Nevertheless, given the size of the 11q13 amplicon, it cannot be ruled out that the overexpression of these genes may be secondary and that other genes within the 11q13 amplicon could act as true drivers of HNSCC progression. A recent study has also identified four genes (*ORAOV1*, *CPT1A*, *SHANK2* and *PPFIA1*) as important drivers of 11q13 amplification that showed an impact on prognosis [28]. Therefore, various genes within the 11q13 amplicon could cooperatively contribute to the differences in prognosis and clinical outcome between HPV-positive and HPV-negative tumors. In summary, various studies including ours have provided strong evidence demonstrating that HPV-related and unrelated tumors are two different entities; hence, we consider that the management of HNSCC patients should move toward a more personalized approach.

## 5. Conclusions

*CTTN*, *CCND1* and *ANO1* amplification and overexpression were frequent in HPV-negative tumors and correlated with reduced patient survival, while absent or very rare in HPV-positive tumors. Therefore, these molecular alterations could contribute to the distinct clinical outcomes of these two HNSCC entities and serve as the basis to design more personalized therapeutic strategies for HNSCC patients.

**Supplementary Materials:** The following are available online at http://www.mdpi.com/2077-0383/7/12/501/s1, Figure S1. Schematic representation of the experimental setup designed to analyze CCND1, ANO1 and CTTN protein expression and gene amplification in relation to HPV status in a cohort of 392 HNSCC patients, Figure S2. Clinical and molecular features of the TGCA cohort of 279 HNSCC patients, according to the HPV status. Schematic representation showing the HPV incidence by HNSCC subsites, mutation frequencies, and Kaplan–Meier survival curves ($p = 0.024$, Log-rank test). Raw data of CTTN, CCND1 and ANO1 protein scores in relation to the HPV status for the total cohort of 392 HNSCC patients, Table S1: Clinicopathologic features of the validation cohort of 279 HNSCC patients from the TCGA.

**Author Contributions:** Conceptualization, J.P.R. and J.M.G.-P.; Funding acquisition, X.L., J.P.R. and J.M.G-P; Investigation, F.H.-P., S.T.M., P.A.-A., R.G.-D, M.Á.V., L.A., N.d-R.-I., R.R., J.P.R. and J.M.G-P; Methodology, F.H.-P., S.T.M., E.A., L.A.-D. and A.A.; Resources, X.L., L.A., M.M., A.A. and J.P.R.; Supervision, J.M.G.-P.; Validation, F.H.-P., S.T.M. and S.Á.-T.; Visualization, F.H.-P., P.A.-A. and J.M.G.-P.; Writing—original draft, P.A.-A. and J.M.G.-P.; Writing—review & editing, F.H.-P., S.T.M., X.L., L.A., M.M, R.R. and J.P.R.

**Funding:** This study was supported by grants from the Plan Nacional de I+D+I 2013-2016 ISCIII (PI13/00259), RD12/0036/0015 of Red Temática de Investigación Cooperativa en Cáncer (RTICC), PI16/00280, and CIBERONC (CB16/12/00390 and CB16/12/00401), CIBER-BBN (CB06/01/1031) Spain, Fundación Merck Salud (17-CC-008), the Instituto de Investigación Sanitaria del Principado de Asturias (ISPA), PCTI-Asturias (GRUPIN14-003), Fundación Bancaria Caja de Ahorros de Asturias-IUOPA, and the FEDER Funding Program from the European Union. STM (Sara Borrell Program-CD16/00103) and RR (Miguel Servet II Program-CPII16/00049) were recipients of fellowships from ISCIII.

**Acknowledgments:** We thank the samples and technical assistance kindly provided by the Principado de Asturias BioBank (PT13/0010/0046), financed jointly by Servicio de Salud del Principado de Asturias, Instituto de Salud Carlos III and Fundación Bancaria Cajastur and integrated in the Spanish National Biobanks Network, and IIB Sant Pau. We also thank Aitana Vallina for excellent technical assistance, Pablo Martínez-Camblor for his assistance with statistical analyses.

**Conflicts of Interest:** The authors declare no conflict of interest. Institutional support to L.A. and M.M.: HPV epidemiological studies sponsored by GlaxoSmithKline, Merck and Seegene.

## References

1. Argiris, A.; Karamouzis, M.V.; Raben, D.; Ferris, R.L. Head and neck cancer. *Lancet* **2008**, *371*, 1695–1709. [CrossRef]
2. Klussmann, J.P.; Mooren, J.J.; Lehnen, M.; Claessen, S.M.; Stenner, M.; Huebbers, C.U.; Weissenborn, S.J; Wedemeyer, I.; Preuss, S.F.; Straetmans, J.M.; et al. Genetic signatures of HPV-related and unrelated oropharyngeal carcinoma and their prognostic implications. *Clin. Cancer Res.* **2009**, *15*, 1779–1786. [CrossRef]
3. Haddad, R.I.; Shin, D.M. Recent advances in head and neck cancer. *N. Engl. J. Med.* **2008**, *359*, 1143–1154. [CrossRef]
4. Leemans, C.R.; Snijders, P.J.F.; Brakenhoff, R.H. The molecular landscape of head and neck cancer. *Nat. Rev. Cancer* **2018**, *18*, 269–282. [CrossRef]
5. Marur, S.; Souza, G.D.; Westra, W.H.; Forastiere, A.A. HPV-associated head and neck cancer: A virus-related cancer epidemic. *Lancet Oncol.* **2010**, *11*, 781–789. [CrossRef]
6. Kostareli, E.; Holzinger, D.; Hess, J. New concepts for translational head and neck oncology: Lessons from HPV-related oropharyngeal squamous cell carcinoma. *Font Oncol.* **2012**, *2*, 36. [CrossRef]
7. Wilkerson, P.M.; Reis-Filho, J.S. The 11q13-q14 amplicon: Clinicopathological correlations and potential drivers. *Genes Chromosom. Cancer* **2013**, *52*, 333–355. [CrossRef]
8. Lin, R.J.; Lubpairee, T.; Liu, K.Y.; Anderson, D.W.; Durham, S.; Poh, C.F. Cyclin D1 overexpression is associated with poor prognosis in oropharyngeal cancer. *J. Otolayngol. Head Neck Surg.* **2013**, *42*, 23. [CrossRef]
9. Rodrigo, J.P.; García, L.A.; Ramos, S.; Lazo, P.S.; Suárez, C. EMS1 gene amplification correlates with poor prognosis in squamous cell carcinomas of the head and neck. *Clin. Cancer Res.* **2000**, *6*, 3177–3182.
10. Ayoub, C.; Wasylyk, C.; Li, Y.; Thomas, E.; Marisa, L.; Robé, A.; Roux, M.; Abecassis, J.; de Reyniès, A.; Wasylyk, B. ANO1 amplification and expression in HNSCC with a high propensity for future distant metastasis and its functions in HNSCC cell lines. *Br. J. Cancer* **2010**, *103*, 715–726. [CrossRef]
11. Ruiz, C.; Martins, J.R.; Rudin, F.; Schneider, S.; Dietsche, T.; Fischer, C.A.; Tornillo, L.; Terracciano, L.M.; Schreiber, R.; Bubendorf, L.; et al. Enhanced expression of ANO1 in head and neck squamous cell carcinoma causes cell migration and correlates with poor prognosis. *PLoS ONE* **2012**, *7*, e43265. [CrossRef]
12. Van Kempen, P.M.; Noorlag, R.; Braunius, W.W.; Moelans, C.B.; Rifi, W.; Savola, S.; Koole, R.; Grolman, W.; van Es, R.J.; Willems, S.M. Clinical relevance of copy number profiling in oral and oropharyngeal squamous cell carcinoma. *Cancer Med.* **2015**, *4*, 1525–1535. [CrossRef]
13. Rodrigo, J.P.; Heideman, D.A.; García-Pedrero, J.M.; Fresno, M.F.; Brakenhoff, R.H.; Díaz Molina, J.P.; Snijders, P.J.; Hermsen, M.A. Time trends in the prevalence of HPV in oropharyngeal squamous cell carcinomas in northern Spain (1990-2009). *Int. J. Cancer* **2014**, *134*, 487–492. [CrossRef]
14. Menéndez, S.T.; Rodrigo, J.P.; Alvarez-Teijeiro, S.; Villaronga, M.Á.; Allonca, E.; Vallina, A.; Astudillo, A.; Barros, F.; Suárez, C.; García-Pedrero, J.M. Role of HERG1 potassium channel in both malignant transformation and disease progression in head and neck carcinomas. *Mod. Pathol.* **2012**, *25*, 1069–1078. [CrossRef]
15. Rodrigo, J.P.; Hermsen, M.A.; Fresno, M.F.; Brakenhoff, R.H.; García-Velasco, F.; Snijders, P.J.; Heideman, D.A.; García-Pedrero, J.M. Prevalence of human papillomavirus in laryngeal and hypopharyngeal squamous cell carcinomas in northern Spain. *Cancer Epidemiol.* **2015**, *39*, 37–41. [CrossRef]
16. Rodrigo, J.P.; Álvarez-Alija, G.; Menéndez, S.T.; Mancebo, G.; Allonca, E.; García-Carracedo, D.; Fresno, M.F.; Suárez, C.; García-Pedrero, J.M. Cortactin and focal adhesion kinase as predictors of cancer risk in patients with laryngeal premalignancy. *Cancer Prev. Res.* **2011**, *4*, 1333–1341. [CrossRef]
17. Rodrigo, J.P.; Menéndez, S.T.; Hermida-Prado, F.; Álvarez-Teijeiro, S.; Villaronga, M.Á.; Alonso-Durán, L.; Vallina, A.; Martínez-Camblor, P.; Astudillo, A.; Suárez, C.; et al. Clinical significance of Anoctamin-1 gene at 11q13 in the development and progression of head and neck squamous cell carcinomas. *Sci. Rep.* **2015**, *5*, 15698. [CrossRef]

18. Rodrigo, J.P.; García-Carracedo, D.; García, L.A.; Menéndez, S.; Allonca, E.; González, M.V.; Fresno, M.F.; Suárez, C.; García-Pedrero, J.M. Distinctive clinicopathological associations of amplification of the cortactin gene at 11q13 in head and neck squamous cell carcinomas. *J. Pathol.* **2009**, *217*, 516–523. [CrossRef]
19. Cancer Genome Atlas Network. Comprehensive genomic characterization of head and neck squamous cell carcinomas. *Nature* **2015**, *517*, 576–582. [CrossRef]
20. Cerami, E.; Gao, J.; Dogrusoz, U.; Gross, B.E.; Sumer, S.O.; Aksoy, B.A.; Jacobsen, A.; Byrne, C.J.; Heuer, M.L.; Larsson, E.; et al. The cBio cancer genomics portal: An open platform for exploring multidimensional cancer genomics data. *Cancer Discov.* **2012**, *2*, 401–404. [CrossRef]
21. Dixit, R.; Kemp, C.; Kulich, S.; Seethala, R.; Chiosea, S.; Ling, S.; Ha, P.K.; Duvvuri, U. TMEM16A/ANO1 is differentially expressed in HPV-negative versus HPV-positive head and neck squamous cell carcinoma through promoter methylation. *Sci Rep.* **2015**, *5*, 16657. [CrossRef]
22. Rasamny, J.J.; Allak, A.; Krook, K.A.; Jo, V.Y.; Policarpio-Nicolas, M.L.; Sumner, H.M.; Moskaluk, C.A.; Frierson, H.F., Jr.; Jameson, M.J. Cyclin D1 and FADD as biomarkers in head and neck squamous cell carcinoma. *Otolaryngol. Head Neck Surg.* **2012**, *146*, 923–931. [CrossRef]
23. Feng, Z.; Guo, W.; Zhang, C.; Xu, Q.; Zhang, P.; Sun, J.; Zhu, H.; Wang, Z.; Li, J.; Wang, L.; et al. CCND1 as a predictive biomarker of neoadjuvant chemotherapy in patients with locally advanced head and neck squamous cell carcinoma. *PLoS ONE* **2011**, *6*, e26399. [CrossRef]
24. Kothari, V.; Mulherkar, R. Inhibition of cyclin D1 by shRNA is associated with enhanced sensitivity to conventional therapies for head and neck squamous cell carcinoma. *Anticancer Res.* **2012**, *32*, 121–128.
25. Eke, I.; Deuse, Y.; Hehlgans, S.; Gurtner, K.; Krause, M.; Baumann, M.; Shevchenko, A.; Sandfort, V.; Cordes, N. β$_1$ Integrin/FAK/cortactin signaling is essential for human head and neck cancer resistance to radiotherapy. *J. Clin. Investig.* **2012**, *122*, 1529–1540. [CrossRef]
26. Godse, N.R.; Khan, N.; Yochum, Z.A.; Gomez-Casal, R.; Kemp, C.; Shiwarski, D.J.; Seethala, R.S.; Kulich, S.; Seshadri, M.; Burns, T.F.; et al. TMEM16A/ANO1 Inhibits Apoptosis Via Downregulation of Bim Expression. *Clin. Cancer Res.* **2017**, *23*, 7324–7332. [CrossRef]
27. Bill, A.; Gutierrez, A.; Kulkarni, S.; Kemp, C.; Bonenfant, D.; Voshol, H.; Duvvuri, U.; Gaither, L.A. ANO1/TMEM16A interacts with EGFR and correlates with sensitivity to EGFR-targeting therapy in head and neck cancer. *Oncotarget* **2015**, *6*, 9173–9188. [CrossRef]
28. Barros-Filho, M.C.; Reis-Rosa, L.A.; Hatakeyama, M.; Marchi, F.A.; Chulam, T.; Scapulatempo-Neto, C.; Nicolau, U.R.; Carvalho, A.L.; Pinto, C.A.L.; Drigo, S.A.; et al. Oncogenic drivers in 11q13 associated with prognosis and response to therapy in advanced oropharyngeal carcinomas. *Oral Oncol.* **2018**, *83*, 81–90. [CrossRef]

© 2018 by the authors. Licensee MDPI, Basel, Switzerland. This article is an open access article distributed under the terms and conditions of the Creative Commons Attribution (CC BY) license (http://creativecommons.org/licenses/by/4.0/).

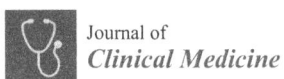 

*Article*

# Nox4 Overexpression as a Poor Prognostic Factor in Patients with Oral Tongue Squamous Cell Carcinoma Receiving Surgical Resection

Yen-Hao Chen [1,2,3], Chih-Yen Chien [4], Fu-Min Fang [5], Tai-Lin Huang [1], Yan-Ye Su [4], Sheng-Dean Luo [4], Chao-Cheng Huang [6,7], Wei-Che Lin [8] and Shau-Hsuan Li [1,*]

[1] Department of Hematology-Oncology, Kaohsiung Chang Gung Memorial Hospital and Chang Gung University College of Medicine, No.123, Dapi Rd., Niaosong Dist., Kaohsiung 833, Taiwan; alex8701125@gmail.com (Y.-H.C.); victor99@cgmh.org.tw (T.-L.H.)
[2] Graduate Institute of Clinical Medical Sciences, College of Medicine, Chang Gung University, Taoyuan 333, Taiwan
[3] School of Medicine, Chung Shan Medical University, Taichung 402, Taiwan
[4] Department of Otolaryngology, Kaohsiung Chang Gung Memorial Hospital and Chang Gung University College of Medicine, No.123, Dapi Rd., Niaosong Dist., Kaohsiung 833, Taiwan; cychien3965@cgmh.org.tw (C.-Y.C.); yanyesu@cgmh.org.tw (Y.-Y.S.); rsd0323@cgmh.org.tw (S.-D.L.)
[5] Department of Radiation Oncology, Kaohsiung Chang Gung Memorial Hospital and Chang Gung University College of Medicine, No.123, Dapi Rd., Niaosong Dist., Kaohsiung 833, Taiwan; fang2569@cgmh.org.tw
[6] Department of Pathology, Kaohsiung Chang Gung Memorial Hospital and Chang Gung University College of Medicine, No.123, Dapi Rd., Niaosong Dist., Kaohsiung 833, Taiwan; huangcc@cgmh.org.tw
[7] Biobank and Tissue Bank, Kaohsiung Chang Gung Memorial Hospital, No.123, Dapi Rd., Niaosong Dist., Kaohsiung 833, Taiwan
[8] Department of Diagnostic Radiology, Kaohsiung Chang Gung Memorial Hospital and Chang Gung University College of Medicine, No.123, Dapi Rd., Niaosong Dist., Kaohsiung 833, Taiwan; alex@cgmh.org.tw
* Correspondence: lee.a0928@msa.hinet.net; Tel.: +886-773-171-23 (ext.8303)

Received: 13 November 2018; Accepted: 27 November 2018; Published: 1 December 2018

**Abstract:** Background: Nox4 has been reported to promote tumor progression of various types of cancer through many different pathways. The current study was designed to evaluate the prognostic significance of Nox4 in patients with oral tongue squamous cell carcinoma (OTSCC) receiving surgical resection. Methods: We retrospectively analyzed the 161 patients with OTSCC treated with surgical resection, including 81 patients with high expression of Nox4 and 80 patients with low expression of Nox4. Two OTSCC cell lines, SAS and SCC4, were used to investigate the proliferation activity. Results: The univariate and multivariable analyses showed that negative nodal metastasis and low expression of Nox4 were significantly associated with superior disease-free survival (DFS) and overall survival (OS). Western blotting analysis indicated that Nox4 was highly expressed in these two OTSCC cell lines and knockdown of Nox4 was successful by transfecting with Nox4 shRNA. In addition, these cell lines were also treated with a Nox4 inhibitor (GKT-137831) and the results showed GKT-137831 could inhibit the proliferation of OTSCC tumor cells in a dose-dependent manner. Conclusion: Our study suggests that Nox4 plays an important role in disease progression of OTSCC and Nox4 overexpression is a poor prognostic factor for patients with OTSCC who received surgical resection.

**Keywords:** Nox4; oral tongue cancer; squamous cell carcinoma; surgery

## 1. Introduction

Head and neck squamous cell carcinoma (HNSCC) is one of the leading cancers worldwide and there are an estimated 500,000 new cases being diagnosed annually [1]. In Taiwan, HNSCC is the sixth most common cancer and fifth leading cause of cancer-related deaths in men [2]. The tongue is the most frequent tumor location for intraoral cancers and tumors most often develop after a long history of tobacco use, alcohol or betel nut consumption and its incidence has increased in recent years. Treatment of oral tongue squamous cell carcinoma (OTSCC) includes a single surgical resection, radiotherapy, chemotherapy, targeted therapy or a combination of these modalities. Despite significant improvements in surgical techniques, chemotherapy, radiotherapy and targeted therapy in the last three decades, the outcome of patients with OTSCC still remains poor [3,4]. Recurrence is the most important prognostic factor and is primarily caused by aggressive local invasion and metastasis, leading to a poor prognosis and a negative quality of life. Thus, OTSCC remains a challenging disease to manage in the field of HNSCC. Therefore, identification of a reliable biomarker to correctly predict the likelihood of a recurrence to potentially reduce mortality in patients with OTSCC is an important research priority.

Nox4 is one of the nicotinamide adenine dinucleotide phosphate (NADPH) oxidases (NOXs) family and is the most frequently expressed isoform in these tumor cells [5]. It generates superoxide or hydrogen peroxide, produces reactive oxygen species (ROS) and been recognized as an important signal molecule in several cancers. Increased generation of ROS has been implicated in the pathogenesis of a variety of tumors [6,7], such as pancreatic cancer, breast cancer, non-small cell lung cancer and colon cancer [8–11]. Some previous studies have identified the biochemical links between Nox4 and cancer through several mechanisms, including angiogenesis, inflammatory cytokines, apoptosis resistance, histone modification, transforming growth factor-β and epidermal growth factor receptor pathway and so forth. [12–17]. Growing evidence confirms that there is a close correlation of Nox4 with cancer development and progression and the inhibition of Nox4 suppresses tumor growth and leads to cancer cell death [18].

However, the role of Nox4 in OTSCC remains unclear thus far. We postulate that Nox4 overexpression accounts for a novel mechanism that contributes to tumor progression and poor clinical outcome in patients with OTSCC. The aim of the present study was to elucidate the prognostic significance of Nox4 on survival in the progression of patients with OTSCC receiving surgical resection. Furthermore, in order to explore the function of Nox4 in cancer ell metabolism of OTSCC, we examined its expression in OTSCC cell lines and we evaluated the effect of Nox4 knockdown on cell proliferation in vitro.

## 2. Experimental Section

### 2.1. Patient Population

We retrospectively reviewed 1256 patients with OTSCC who were treated at Kaohsiung Chang Gung Memorial Hospital between January 2006 and December 2015. Among these 1256 patients with OTSCC, we first excluded those patients with a history of any second primary malignancy, distant metastasis, or who underwent preoperative chemotherapy or radiotherapy. After that, only those patients with OTSCC who received surgical resection as a curative treatment were included. Finally, a total of 161 patients with OTSCC with available paraffin blocks and medical records were identified. The tumor stage of each patient was determined according to the 7th American Joint Committee on Cancer (AJCC) staging system [19].

### 2.2. Immunohistochemistry

Immunohistochemistry staining was achieved using an immunoperoxidase technique and performed on slides (4 μm) of formalin-fixed paraffin-embedded tissue sections using primary antibodies against Nox4 (ab109225, 1:200, Abcam, Cambridge, MA, USA). Briefly, after deparaffinization and rehydration, slides were subjected to a heat-induced epitope retrieval in 10 mM citrate buffer (pH 6.0) in a hot water bath (95 °C) for 20 min. Immunodetection was performed using the LSAB2 kit (Dako, Carpinteria, CA, USA) followed by 3-3′-diaminobenzidine for color development and hematoxylin for counterstaining. For Nox4, incubation without the primary antibody was used as a negative control, while a slide of normal kidney tissue was used as a positive control. The staining assessment was independently carried out by two pathologists (S.L.W. and W.T.H.) without any information about clinicopathologic features or prognosis. Slides were examined at 200× and in each case, at least four sections were examined. We followed the previously published method to score the expression of Nox4 [18]. The percentage of Nox4 positive tumor cells for all neoplastic cells in the section was recorded. Nox4 overexpression was defined as the presence of staining in ≥50% of tumor cells.

### 2.3. Western Blot Analysis

For cell protein extraction, samples were homogenized in RIPA lysis buffer (50 mM Tris-HCl, pH 7.5, 150 mM NaCl, 1% NP-40, 0.5% Na-deoxycholate and 0.1% SDS). The protein concentration in each sample was estimated using a Bio-Rad Protein Assay (Bio-Rad, Hercules, CA, USA). Immunoblotting was performed according to standard procedures. Antibodies used in this study included polyclonal antibodies against Nox4 (ab109225, 1:200, Abcam, Cambridge, MA, USA) and β-actin (Sigma Aldrich, St Louis, MO, USA). The first antibodies were detected by incubation while secondary antibodies were conjugated to horseradish peroxidase (Bio/Can Scientific, Mississauga, ON, Canada) and developed using Western Lighting Reagent. The proteins were explored by X-ray films.

### 2.4. Cell Culture and Transfection

OTSCC cell lines SAS and SCC4 were established and purchased from Bioresource Collection and Research Center in Taiwan. These cell lines were cultured under standard conditions using Dulbecco's modified Eagle's medium (DMEM) with 10% fetal bovine serum, 1X MEM non-essential amino acids, 100 U/mL penicillin, 100 µg/mL streptomycin, 0.25 µg/mL Amphotericin B and 2.0 mmol/L L-glutamine.

To examine the cell proliferative activity of Nox4 in OTSCC, a 3-(4,5-dimethylthiazole-2-yl)-2,5-diphenyltetrazolium bromide (MTT) assay was performed on these cell lines. The procedure was performed as follows: each cell line (7000 cells) was incubated along with a control in a 96-well flat-bottomed plate in triplicate. After incubation for 96 h at 37 °C, 100 µL of MTT (3-(4,5-dimenthylthiazol-2-yl)-2,5-diphenyltetrazolium bromide, 0.5 mg/mL, Sigma, St. Louis, MO, USA) was added to each well and incubation was carried out for another four hours. Then, the supernatant was discarded and the crystal products were eluted with dimethyl sulfoxide (100 µL/well, Sigma). The colorimetric evaluation was tested using a spectrophotometer at 570 nm. The proliferation of each cell line harboring Nox4 overexpression was shown as a percentage of cell growth compared to the control cells.

To confirm the role of Nox4 in the malignant properties of OTSCC cells we transfected Nox4 shRNA into OTSCC cells to generate Nox4 knockdown cells. The above-mentioned OTSCC cell lines were used here. These cells were seeded in a 6 cm dish and allowed to grow to 50%–60% confluence for 24 h. Nox4 shRNA (40 nM) was purchased from RNAi Core of Academia Sinica (Taiwan) and then transfected into OTSCC cells using Hiperfect reagent according to the manufacturer's protocol (Qiagen). To disrupt aggregates formed during lyophilization, shRNA was incubated at 90 °C for one minute and then at 37 °C for 60 min prior to the transfection procedure. The silencing efficiency was evaluated by western blotting 24 to 72 h after shRNA transfection. To examine the cell proliferative activity of Nox4 knockdown in OTSCC, an MTT assay was performed in these cell lines.

To test the role of Nox4 in the progression of OTSCC cells, we treated OTSCC cell lines, with or without a Nox4 inhibitor, with GKT-137831 (Selleck Chemicals, Houston, TX, USA), which is a novel and specific dual Nox1/Nox4 inhibitor. Each cell line (2500 cells) was incubated in 200 µL with GKT-137831 (0, 1, 5, 10, 20, 40, 80 and 100 µM) and control in a 96-well flat-bottomed plate in triplicate.

To examine the cell proliferative activity of Nox4 inhibitor in OTSCC, an MTT assay was performed in these cell lines according to the above-mentioned procedures.

## 2.5. Statistical Analysis

For patient data, the statistical analyses were performed using the SPSS 19 software package (IBM, Armonk, NY, USA). Comparisons between the groups were performed using the chi-square test for categorical variable data. Disease-free survival (DFS) was computed from the time of surgery to the recurrence of cancer or death from any cause without evidence of recurrence. Overall survival (OS) was calculated from the date of diagnosis of the OTSCC to the date of death or last contact. The Kaplan–Meier method was used to estimate DFS and OS and the log-rank test was performed to evaluate the differences between the groups for univariate analysis. In a stepwise forward fashion, significant parameters at the univariate level were entered into a Cox regression model to analyze their relative prognostic importance. For cell line experiments, a $t$-test was used for the statistical analysis. Each experiment was carried out independently at least twice, with three repeats each. For all analyses, a $p$-value $< 0.05$ was considered statistically significant.

## 2.6. Ethics Statement

Study approval was obtained from the Chang Gung Medical Foundation Institutional Review Board (201700414B0) and all the patients provided the written informed consent. All the methods were carried out in accordance with the approved guidelines and the ethical standards of the World Medical Association Declaration of Helsinki.

## 3. Results

### 3.1. Patient Population

A total of 161 patients with OTSCC who received surgical resection were retrospectively examined at Kaohsiung Chang Gung Memorial Hospital. All of the 161 patients with OTSCC had an Eastern Cooperative Oncology Group performance status $\leq 1$. The study group consisted of 148 male patients and 13 female patients with a median age of 53 years (range: 26 to 86 years). A total of 132 patients (82%) had a history of tobacco smoking and alcohol consumption was mentioned in 129 patients (80%). The tumor T status was found to be T1 in 46 patients (29%), T2 in 53 patients (33%), T3 in 13 patients (8%) and T4 in 49 patients (30%). Meanwhile, 93 patients (58%) were diagnosed as having N0 status, 22 patients (14%) as having N1 status, 44 patients (27%) as having N2 status and two patients (1%) as having N3 status. The tumor stage indicated that 36 patients (22%) had stage I, 34 patients (21%) had stage II, 23 patients (14%) had stage III, 62 patients (39%) had stage IVA and six patients (4%) had stage IVB. At the time of analysis, the median period of follow-up was 87.8 months for the 76 living survivors and 62.8 months (range: 2.3–117.6 months) for all 161 patients. The five-year DFS and OS rates were 68.9% and 47.2%, respectively. The clinicopathological parameters of these patients are shown in Table 1.

**Table 1.** Clinicopathological parameters in 161 patients with oral tongue squamous cell carcinoma receiving surgical resection.

| Characteristics | |
| --- | --- |
| Age | 53 years old (26–86) |
| Sex | |
| Male | 148 (92%) |
| Female | 13 (8%) |
| Cigarette smoking | |
| Absent | 29 (18%) |
| Present | 132 (82%) |

Table 1. Cont.

| Characteristics | |
|---|---|
| Alcohol consumption | |
| Absent | 32 (20%) |
| Present | 129 (80%) |
| T status | |
| 1 | 46 (29%) |
| 2 | 53 (33%) |
| 3 | 13 (8%) |
| 4 | 49 (30%) |
| N status | |
| 0 | 93 (58%) |
| 1 | 22 (14%) |
| 2 | 44 (27%) |
| 3 | 2 (1%) |
| Tumor stage | |
| I | 36 (22%) |
| II | 34 (21%) |
| III | 23 (14%) |
| IVA | 62 (39%) |
| IVB | 6 (4%) |
| Nox4 expression | |
| High | 80 (51%) |
| Low | 81 (49%) |

*3.2. Silencing Nox4 Expression Reduces Tumor Cell Proliferation in Vitro*

In the present study, we performed western blotting analyses to determine Nox4 expression phenotype in OTSCC cell lines, SAS and SCC4. After that, these cell lines were stably transfected with Nox4 shRNA and knockdown of Nox4 was shown by western blotting (Figure 1). Furthermore, these cell lines were also treated with GKT-137831, a Nox4 inhibitor. These results showed GKT-137831 could inhibit the proliferation of tumor cells in a dose-dependent manner in SAS and SCC4 cell lines at 24th, 48th and 72nd hour after GKT-137831 treatment (Figure 2).

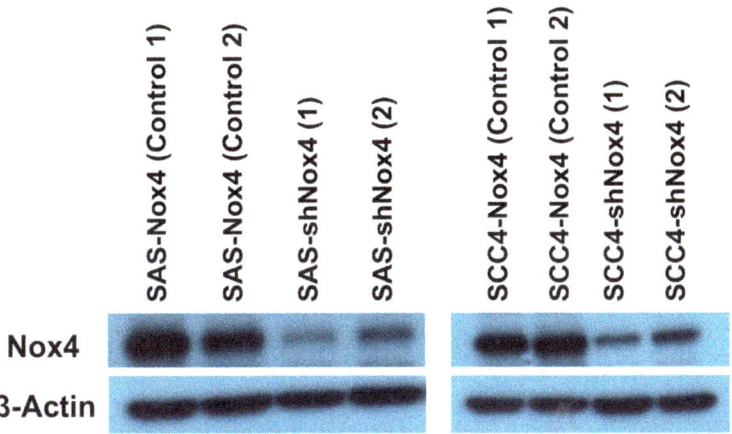

**Figure 1.** Western blotting analysis of Nox4 expression and knockdown of Nox4 in two oral tongue squamous cell carcinoma cell lines, SAS and SCC4.

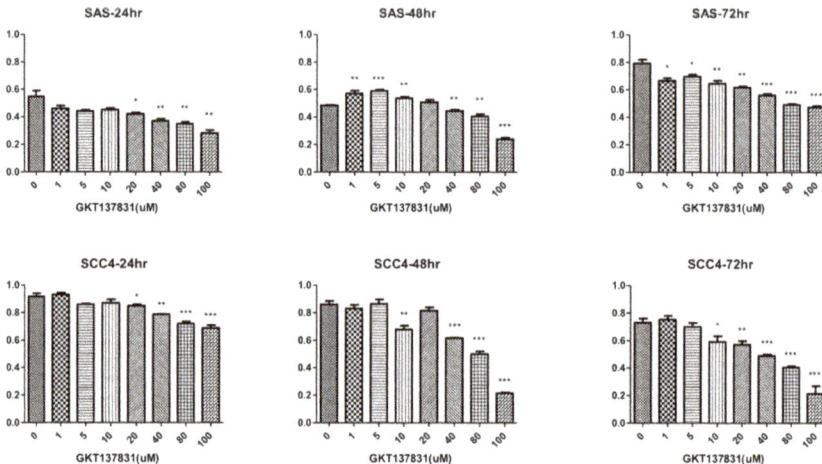

**Figure 2.** Nox4 inhibitor (GKT-137831) displays a growth inhibitory effect in a dose-dependent manner in the two oral tongue squamous cell carcinoma cell lines, SAS and SCC4. Columns, mean; bars, standard deviation. Significant difference in growth inhibition: * $p < 0.05$, ** $p < 0.01$ and *** $p < 0.001$.

### 3.3. Expression of Nox4 and Clinical Outcome

The expression of Nox4 in the immunohistochemical staining is shown in Figure 3. Among the 161 patients, 80 patients (49%) were classified as having a high expression of Nox4 and 81 patients (51%) had a low expression of Nox4. The baseline characteristics did not differ significantly between these two groups, including age, sex, cigarette smoking, alcohol consumption, tumor T status, tumor N status and tumor stage (Table 2).

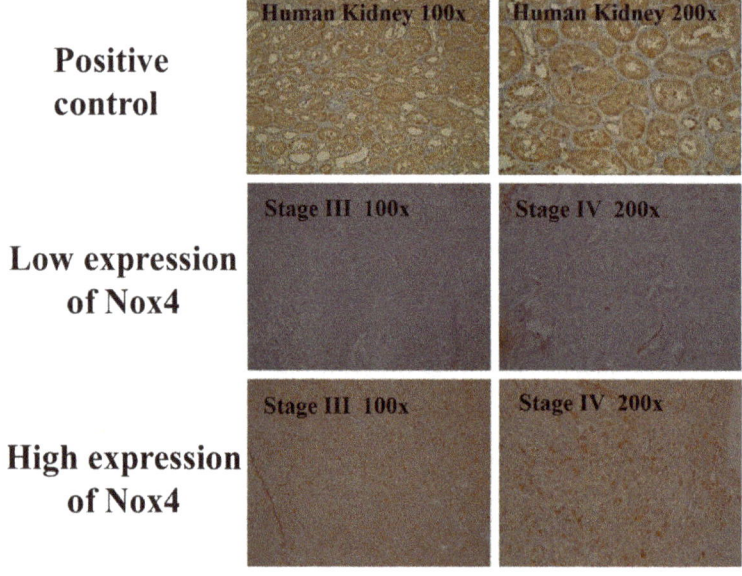

**Figure 3.** Immunohistochemical analysis of Nox4 expression in patients with oral tongue squamous cell carcinoma.

Table 2. Comparison of clinicopathological parameters in 161 patients with oral tongue squamous cell carcinoma receiving surgical resection.

| Characteristics | High expression of Nox4 (N = 80) | Low expression of Nox4 (N = 81) | p-Value |
|---|---|---|---|
| Age | 53 years old (32–86) | 51 years old (26–70) | |
| Sex | | | 0.40 |
| Male | 75 (94%) | 73 (90%) | |
| Female | 5 (6%) | 8 (10%) | |
| Cigarette smoking | | | 0.87 |
| Absent | 14 (17%) | 15 (18%) | |
| Present | 66 (83%) | 66 (82%) | |
| Alcohol consumption | | | 0.97 |
| Absent | 16 (20%) | 16 (20%) | |
| Present | 64 (80%) | 65 (80%) | |
| T status | | | 0.48 |
| 1–2 | 47 (59%) | 52 (64%) | |
| 3–4 | 33 (41%) | 29 (36%) | |
| N status | | | 0.95 |
| 0 | 46 (58%) | 47 (58%) | |
| 1–3 | 34 (42%) | 34 (42%) | |
| Tumor stage | | | 0.95 |
| I–III | 35 (44%) | 35 (43%) | |
| IVA–IVB | 45 (56%) | 46 (57%) | |

With respect to DFS, a univariate analysis found that sex and alcohol consumption were not statistically significant predictors of DFS. The 127 patients who were diagnosed at an age younger than 60 years were found to have superior DFS in comparison with the 34 patients diagnosed at an age older than 60 years (77.5 months versus 10.7 months, $p < 0.001$); meanwhile, 29 patients who never used cigarettes had superior DFS compared to the 132 smokers (not reach versus 40.2 months, $p = 0.047$). Significantly improved DFS was found in the 99 patients who had T1-2 status compared to the 62 patients who had T3-4 status (77.5 months versus 12.1 months, $p = 0.004$) and superior DFS was also found in the 93 patients without nodal metastasis compared to the other 68 patients with positive lymph node metastasis (not reach versus 13.4 months, $p < 0.001$). The 93 patients with stage I–III were found to have superior DFS in comparison with the 68 patients with stage IVA–IVB ($p = 0.025$). The 81 patients with a low expression of Nox4 had better DFS than the other 80 patients with a high expression of Nox4 (77.5 months versus 21.9 months, $p = 0.047$, Figure 4A). In a multivariable analysis, N0 status ($p = 0.009$, hazard ratio (HR): 0.47, 95% confidence interval (CI): 0.27–0.83) and a low expression of Nox4 ($p = 0.0192$, HR: 0.50, 95% CI: 0.28–0.89) were the independent prognostic parameters of better DFS.

With respect to OS, there were no statistically significant differences in parameters of sex and alcohol consumption in a univariate analysis. Significantly better OS was found in the 127 patients aged younger than 60 years than in the 34 patients aged older than 60 years (not reach versus 13.4 months, $p = 0.001$) and superior OS was also found in the 29 patients who never smoked in comparison to the 132 smokers (not reach versus 52.1 months, $p = 0.026$). The 99 patients with T1-2 were found to have better OS compared to the 62 patients with T3-4 (not reach versus 15.5 months, $p = 0.001$); meanwhile, 93 patients without nodal metastasis had superior OS than other 68 patients with positive nodal metastasis (not reach versus 15.5 months, $p < 0.001$). Better OS was found in the 93 patients who were classified as stage I–III compared to the 68 patients classified as having stage IVA–IVB (not reach versus 28.6 months, $p < 0.001$). The 81 patients with a low expression of Nox4 had better OS than the other 80 patients with a high expression of Nox4 (87.9 months versus 33.0 months, $p = 0.032$, Figure 4B).

A multivariable analysis showed that T1-2 status ($p = 0.019$, HR: 0.59, 95% CI: 0.38–0.92), N0 ($p = 0.001$, HR: 0.47, 95% CI: 0.30–0.73) and a low expression of Nox4 ($p = 0.011$, HR: 0.57, 95% CI: 0.37–0.88) were the independent prognostic parameters of superior OS. These univariate and multivariable survival analyses are shown in Table 3.

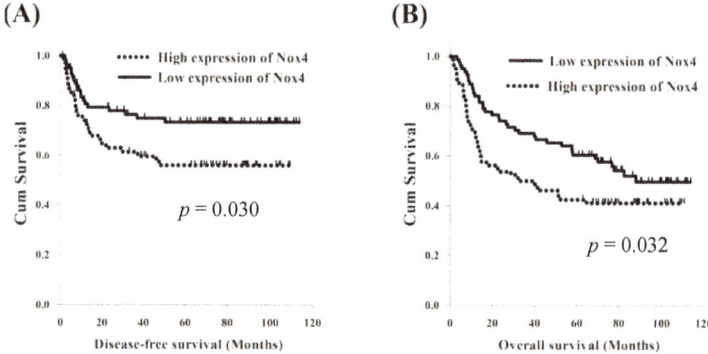

**Figure 4.** Comparison of survival curves for patients with oral tongue squamous cell carcinoma with high and low expression of Nox4. (**A**) Disease-free survival (**B**) Overall survival.

**Table 3.** Univariate and multivariable analysis of disease-free survival and overall survival in 161 patients with oral tongue squamous cell carcinoma receiving surgical resection.

| Characteristics | No. of Patients | Univariate Analysis | | Multivariate Analysis | | Univariate Analysis | | Multivariate Analysis | |
|---|---|---|---|---|---|---|---|---|---|
| | | Median DFS (months) | p-Value | HR (95% CI) | p-Value | Median OS (months) | p-Value | HR (95% CI) | p-Value |
| Age | | | | | | | | | |
| <60 years | 127 (79%) | 77.5 | <0.001 * | | | NR | 0.001 * | | |
| ≥60 years | 34 (21%) | 10.7 | | | | 13.4 | | | |
| Sex | | | | | | | | | |
| Male | 393 (97%) | 46.0 | 0.24 | | | 57.7 | 0.14 | | |
| Female | 11 (3%) | NR | | | | NR | | | |
| Cigarette smoking | | | | | | | | | |
| Absent | 29 (18%) | NR | 0.047 * | | | NR | 0.026 * | | |
| Present | 132 (82%) | 40.2 | | | | 52.1 | | | |
| Alcohol consumption | | | | | | | | | |
| Absent | 32 (20%) | 57.4 | 0.55 | | | NR | 0.42 | | |
| Present | 129 (80%) | 41.2 | | | | 64.5 | | | |
| T status | | | | | | | | | |
| 1 + 2 | 99 (62%) | 77.5 | 0.004 * | | | NR | 0.001 * | 0.59 (0.38–0.92) | 0.019 * |
| 3 + 4 | 62 (38%) | 12.1 | | | | 15.5 | | | |
| N status | | | | | | | | | |
| 0 | 93 (58%) | NR | <0.001 * | 0.47 (0.27–0.83) | 0.009 * | NR | <0.001 * | 0.47 (0.30–0.73) | 0.001 * |
| 1 + 2 + 3 | 68 (42%) | 13.4 | | | | 15.5 | | | |
| Tumor stage | | | | | | | | | |
| I–III | 93 (58%) | NR | 0.025 * | | | NR | <0.001 * | | |
| IVA–IVB | 68 (42%) | NR | | | | 28.6 | | | |
| Nox4 expression | | | | | | | | | |
| High | 80 (49%) | 21.9 | 0.030 * | | | 33.0 | 0.032 * | | |
| Low | 81 (51%) | 77.5 | | 0.50 (0.28–0.89) | 0.018 * | 87.9 | | 0.57 (0.37–0.88) | 0.011 * |

DFS: disease-free survival; OS: overall survival; NR: not reached; HR: hazard ratio; CI: confidence interval * Statistically significant.

## 4. Discussion

Nox4 has been found to promote tumor progression of many types of cancer through various pathways. Nox4 may induce cancer cell progression through promoting tumor angiogenesis. In Nox4 knockout mice with fibrosarcoma, vessel density analysis showed a significant reduction in tumor vascularization, leading to the attenuation of hypoxia-inducible factor 1-alpha, vascular endothelial growth factor, glucose transporter 1 and adrenomedullin [15]. Inflammatory cytokines are one of the critical mediators in inflammation-associated cancer, especially interleukin-6 (IL-6). In non-small cell lung cancer, Nox4 expression is positively correlated with IL-6 expression and exogenous IL-6 treatment significantly enhances Nox4 signaling [16]. The same result was also described in renal cell carcinoma cells [13]. Another possible mechanism for Nox4 inducing cancer progression includes histone modification, transforming growth factor-β and epidermal growth factor receptor (EGFR) pathway and so forth. [12,14,17].

The current study found that Nox4 and lymph node metastasis were both prognostic factors for patients with OTSCC in the univariate and multivariable analyses. Several studies have confirmed that the presence of neck lymph node metastasis is the most reliable prognostic factor of regional or distant treatment failure in patients with OTSCC [20–23]. Recently, growing evidence confirmed the role of Nox4 in the disease progression of various cancer types. Zhang et al. showed that Nox4 was upregulated and promoted tumor cell proliferation in vitro and in vivo and overexpression of Nox4 was closely correlated to tumor stage and contributed to the poor prognosis of patients with non-small cell lung cancer [18]. Lin et al. also demonstrated that Nox4 promoted tumor cell proliferation and apoptosis, migration and invasion and Nox4 overexpression was highly correlated with tumor invasion depth, positive lymph node numbers, distant metastasis and poor prognosis of patients with colorectal cancer [24]. Nox4 also plays a crucial role in regulating gastric cancer cell growth. In a Chinese study, Nox4 expression was correlated with tumor size and poor prognosis in 90 patients with gastric cancer and knockdown of NOX4 expression blocked cell proliferation and the expression of Cyclin D1, BAX and so on in vitro. Nox4 promoted cell proliferation via activation of the GLI1 pathway and overexpression of GLI1 reversed the suppression of tumor cell growth induced by silencing NOX4. Furthermore, overexpression of Nox4 enhanced expression of GLI1 and knockdown of GLI1 expression reduced the effects induced by Nox4 overexpression [25]. A Japanese study, reported by Ito et al., also demonstrated that Nox4 was highly expressed in several oral squamous cell carcinoma cell lines and NOXs knockdown markedly suppressed cell viability and induced apoptosis; in addition, NOXs suppression significantly enhanced the cisplatin-induced cytotoxic effect [26].

In head and neck cancer, an EGFR inhibitor is one of the major therapeutic modalities for HNSCC and is routinely used in clinical practice. Autophagy has been reported to be one of the possible mechanisms of resistance to chemotherapy or EGFR inhibitors and Nox4 plays a critical role in mediating this effect [27]. Chronic inflammation has been confirmed to be strongly associated with tumor invasion, migration and metastasis through increased secretion of pro-inflammatory cytokines, such as IL-2, IL-6, tumor necrosis factor-α and so forth. The antitumor activity of EGFR inhibitors is suppressed by activation of Nox4-mediated pro-inflammatory pathways and knockdown of Nox4 reduced EGFR inhibitor-induced pro-inflammatory cytokine expression [14]. Several studies have highlighted the contribution of the microenvironment to tumor progression and cancer-associated fibroblasts (CAFs) are related to poor prognosis in various cancer types, including head and neck cancer [28–30]. Upregulation of Nox4 expression was strongly correlated with myofibroblastic-CAFs, contributing to decreased cancer-specific survival rates. Suppression of Nox4 was found to revert the myofibroblastic-CAF phenotype, prevent myofibroblastic-CAF accumulation and slower tumor proliferation [31].

The 8th edition of the AJCC staging manual has been introduced into clinical practice in 2018 [32]. There are most significant changes to oral cavity cancer staging, including changes to the T and N staging categories, depth of invasion and extranodal extension (ENE). Several studies have been designed to investigate the importance of the 8th edition of the AJCC staging system. Mascitti et al.

showed that the 8th edition of the AJCC criteria is more suitable for better stratification of patients with OTSCC and the implementation of ENE and lymph node ratio to pathological N classification are indicated to identify patients with poor prognosis [33]. Another study reported by Pollaers et al. revealed that the 8th edition of the AJCC staging system supports better DFS discrimination between overall stages and between T categories in patients with oral cavity squamous cell carcinoma [34]. In our study, although the tumor stage of each OTSCC patient who underwent surgical resection was determined according to the 7th AJCC staging system, the results showed negative nodal metastasis and low expression of Nox4 were significantly associated with superior DFS and OS and the N0 status was not changed whether in the 7th or 8th AJCC staging system.

This study had several limitations. First, it was a retrospective analysis at a single institution with a relatively small sample size. Second, we did not explore the comprehensive mechanisms of Nox4 and downstream pathways, nor investigate how Nox4 overexpression promotes tumor cell proliferation, invasion and metastasis.

However, to the best of our knowledge, this study, at present, covers the largest series of patients with OTSCC who received surgical resection and may thus be useful for understanding the role of Nox4 in the prognosis of OTSCC.

## 5. Conclusions

The results of our study suggest that Nox4 plays an important role in disease progression of OTSCC and Nox4 overexpression is a poor prognostic factor of patients with patients with OTSCC who received surgical resection. Additional studies are warranted in order to clarify the complex mechanism of Nox4 and downstream pathways in patients with OTSCC.

**Author Contributions:** S.-H.L. conceived and designed the experiments. Y.-H.C. wrote the main manuscript text. F.-M.F. and W.-C.L. verified the analytical methods. C.-Y.C., Y.-Y.S. and S.-D.L. contributed to sample preparation. T.-L.H. and C.-C.H. prepared tables and figures. All authors reviewed the manuscript.

**Funding:** This work was supported in part by grant from Chang Gung Memorial Hospital (CMRPG8G0202).

**Acknowledgments:** We thank the Tissue Bank Core Lab at Kaohsiung Chang Gung Memorial Hospital (CLRPG8F1701 and CLRPG8F1602) for their excellent technical support.

**Conflicts of Interest:** The authors declare no conflict of interests.

## Abbreviations

| | |
|---|---|
| HNSCC | Head and neck squamous cell carcinoma |
| OTSCC | Oral tongue squamous cell carcinoma |
| NADPH | Nicotinamide adenine dinucleotide phosphate |
| NOXs | Nicotinamide adenine dinucleotide phosphate oxidases |
| ROS | Reactive oxygen species |
| DMEM | Dulbecco's modified Eagle's medium |
| DFS | Disease-free survival |
| OS | Overall survival |
| IL-6 | Interleukin-6 |
| EGFR | Epidermal growth factor receptor |
| CAFs | Cancer-associated fibroblasts |
| ENE | Extranodal extension |

## References

1. Jemal, A.; Bray, F.; Center, M.M.; Ferlay, J.; Ward, E.; Forman, D. Global cancer statistics. *CA: A Cancer J. Clin.* **2011**, *61*, 69–90. [CrossRef] [PubMed]
2. *Cancer Registry Annual Report 2015*; National Department of Health: Taipei, China, 2015.

3. Camisasca, D.R.; Silami, M.A.; Honorato, J.; Dias, F.L.; de Faria, P.A.; Lourenco Sde, Q. Oral squamous cell carcinoma: Clinicopathological features in patients with and without recurrence. *ORL J. Otorhinolaryngol. Relat. Spec.* **2011**, *73*, 170–176. [CrossRef] [PubMed]
4. Lindenblatt Rde, C.; Martinez, G.L.; Silva, L.E.; Faria, P.S.; Camisasca, D.R.; Lourenco Sde, Q. Oral squamous cell carcinoma grading systems—Analysis of the best survival predictor. *J. Oral. Pathol. Med.* **2012**, *41*, 34–39. [CrossRef] [PubMed]
5. Cheng, G.; Cao, Z.; Xu, X.; van Meir, E.G.; Lambeth, J.D. Homologs of gp91phox: Cloning and tissue expression of Nox3, Nox4, and Nox5. *Gene* **2001**, *269*, 131–140. [CrossRef]
6. Guo, S.; Chen, X. The human Nox4: Gene, structure, physiological function and pathological significance. *J. Drug Target.* **2015**, *23*, 888–896. [CrossRef] [PubMed]
7. Roy, K.; Wu, Y.; Meitzler, J.L.; Juhasz, A.; Liu, H.; Jiang, G.; Lu, J.; Antony, S.; Doroshow, J.H. NADPH oxidases and cancer. *Clin. Sci.* **2015**, *128*, 863–875. [CrossRef] [PubMed]
8. Bauer, K.M.; Watts, T.N.; Buechler, S.; Hummon, A.B. Proteomic and functional investigation of the colon cancer relapse-associated genes NOX4 and ITGA3. *J. Proteome Res.* **2014**, *13*, 4910–4918. [CrossRef] [PubMed]
9. Cheng, G.; Lanza-Jacoby, S. Metformin decreases growth of pancreatic cancer cells by decreasing reactive oxygen species: Role of NOX4. *Biochem. Biophys. Res. Commun.* **2015**, *465*, 41–46. [CrossRef] [PubMed]
10. Choi, J.A.; Jung, Y.S.; Kim, J.Y.; Kim, H.M.; Lim, I.K. Inhibition of breast cancer invasion by TIS21/BTG2/Pc3-Akt1-Sp1-Nox4 pathway targeting actin nucleators, mDia genes. *Oncogene* **2016**, *35*, 83–93. [CrossRef] [PubMed]
11. Vaquero, E.C.; Edderkaoui, M.; Pandol, S.J.; Gukovsky, I.; Gukovskaya, A.S. Reactive oxygen species produced by NAD(P)H oxidase inhibit apoptosis in pancreatic cancer cells. *J. Biol. Chem.* **2004**, *279*, 34643–34654. [CrossRef] [PubMed]
12. Crosas-Molist, E.; Bertran, E.; Sancho, P.; Lopez-Luque, J.; Fernando, J.; Sanchez, A.; Fernandez, M.; Navarro, E.; Fabregat, I. The NADPH oxidase NOX4 inhibits hepatocyte proliferation and liver cancer progression. *Free Radic. Biol. Med.* **2014**, *69*, 338–347. [CrossRef] [PubMed]
13. Fitzgerald, J.P.; Nayak, B.; Shanmugasundaram, K.; Friedrichs, W.; Sudarshan, S.; Eid, A.A.; DeNapoli, T.; Parekh, D.J.; Gorin, Y.; Block, K. Nox4 mediates renal cell carcinoma cell invasion through hypoxia-induced interleukin 6- and 8- production. *PLoS ONE* **2012**, *7*, e30712. [CrossRef] [PubMed]
14. Fletcher, E.V.; Love-Homan, L.; Sobhakumari, A.; Feddersen, C.R.; Koch, A.T.; Goel, A.; Simons, A.L. EGFR inhibition induces proinflammatory cytokines via NOX4 in HNSCC. *Mol. Cancer Res. MCR* **2013**, *11*, 1574–1584. [CrossRef] [PubMed]
15. Helfinger, V.; Henke, N.; Harenkamp, S.; Walter, M.; Epah, J.; Penski, C.; Mittelbronn, M.; Schroder, K. The NADPH Oxidase Nox4 mediates tumour angiogenesis. *Acta Physiol.* **2016**, *216*, 435–446. [CrossRef] [PubMed]
16. Li, J.; Lan, T.; Zhang, C.; Zeng, C.; Hou, J.; Yang, Z.; Zhang, M.; Liu, J.; Liu, B. Reciprocal activation between IL-6/STAT3 and NOX4/Akt signalings promotes proliferation and survival of non-small cell lung cancer cells. *Oncotarget* **2015**, *6*, 1031–1048. [CrossRef] [PubMed]
17. Sanders, Y.Y.; Liu, H.; Liu, G.; Thannickal, V.J. Epigenetic mechanisms regulate NADPH oxidase-4 expression in cellular senescence. *Free Radic. Biol. Med.* **2015**, *79*, 197–205. [CrossRef] [PubMed]
18. Zhang, C.; Lan, T.; Hou, J.; Li, J.; Fang, R.; Yang, Z.; Zhang, M.; Liu, J.; Liu, B. NOX4 promotes non-small cell lung cancer cell proliferation and metastasis through positive feedback regulation of PI3K/Akt signaling. *Oncotarget* **2014**, *5*, 4392–4405. [CrossRef] [PubMed]
19. Edge, S.; Byrd, D.R.; Compton, C.C.; Fritz, A.G.; Greene, F.; Trotti, A. *AJCC Cancer Staging Manual*, 7th ed.; Springer: New York, NY, USA, 2010.
20. Grandi, C.; Alloisio, M.; Moglia, D.; Podrecca, S.; Sala, L.; Salvatori, P.; Molinari, R. Prognostic significance of lymphatic spread in head and neck carcinomas: Therapeutic implications. *Head Neck Surg.* **1985**, *8*, 67–73. [CrossRef] [PubMed]
21. Kalnins, I.K.; Leonard, A.G.; Sako, K.; Razack, M.S.; Shedd, D.P. Correlation between prognosis and degree of lymph node involvement in carcinoma of the oral cavity. *Am. J. Surg.* **1977**, *134*, 450–454. [CrossRef]
22. Schuller, D.E.; McGuirt, W.F.; McCabe, B.F.; Young, D. The prognostic significance of metastatic cervical lymph nodes. *Laryngoscope* **1980**, *90*, 557–570. [CrossRef] [PubMed]
23. Snow, G.B.; Annyas, A.A.; van Slooten, E.A.; Bartelink, H.; Hart, A.A. Prognostic factors of neck node metastasis. *Clin. Otolaryngol. Allied. Sci.* **1982**, *7*, 185–192. [CrossRef] [PubMed]

24. Lin, X.L.; Yang, L.; Fu, S.W.; Lin, W.F.; Gao, Y.J.; Chen, H.Y.; Ge, Z.Z. Overexpression of NOX4 predicts poor prognosis and promotes tumor progression in human colorectal cancer. *Oncotarget* **2017**, *8*, 33586–33600. [CrossRef] [PubMed]
25. Tang, C.T.; Lin, X.L.; Wu, S.; Liang, Q.; Yang, L.; Gao, Y.J.; Ge, Z.Z. NOX4-driven ROS formation regulates proliferation and apoptosis of gastric cancer cells through the GLI1 pathway. *Cell. Signal.* **2018**, *46*, 52–63. [CrossRef] [PubMed]
26. Ito, K.; Ota, A.; Ono, T.; Nakaoka, T.; Wahiduzzaman, M.; Karnan, S.; Konishi, H.; Furuhashi, A.; Hayashi, T.; Yamada, Y.; et al. Inhibition of Nox1 induces apoptosis by attenuating the AKT signaling pathway in oral squamous cell carcinoma cell lines. *Oncol. Rep.* **2016**, *36*, 2991–2998. [CrossRef] [PubMed]
27. Sobhakumari, A.; Schickling, B.M.; Love-Homan, L.; Raeburn, A.; Fletcher, E.V.; Case, A.J.; Domann, F.E.; Miller, F.J., Jr.; Simons, A.L. NOX4 mediates cytoprotective autophagy induced by the EGFR inhibitor erlotinib in head and neck cancer cells. *Toxicol. Appl. Pharmacol.* **2013**, *272*, 736–745. [CrossRef] [PubMed]
28. Erez, N.; Truitt, M.; Olson, P.; Arron, S.T.; Hanahan, D. Cancer-Associated Fibroblasts Are Activated in Incipient Neoplasia to Orchestrate Tumor-Promoting Inflammation in an NF-kappaB-Dependent Manner. *Cancer Cell* **2010**, *17*, 135–147. [CrossRef] [PubMed]
29. Goetz, J.G.; Minguet, S.; Navarro-Lerida, I.; Lazcano, J.J.; Samaniego, R.; Calvo, E.; Tello, M.; Osteso-Ibanez, T.; Pellinen, T.; Echarri, A. Biomechanical remodeling of the microenvironment by stromal caveolin-1 favors tumor invasion and metastasis. *Cell* **2011**, *146*, 148–163. [CrossRef] [PubMed]
30. Marsh, D.; Suchak, K.; Moutasim, K.A.; Vallath, S.; Hopper, C.; Jerjes, W.; Upile, T.; Kalavrezos, N.; Violette, S.M.; Weinreb, P.H. Stromal features are predictive of disease mortality in oral cancer patients. *J. Pathol.* **2011**, *223*, 470–481. [CrossRef] [PubMed]
31. Hanley, C.J.; Mellone, M.; Ford, K.; Thirdborough, S.M.; Mellows, T.; Frampton, S.J.; Smith, D.M.; Harden, E.; Szyndralewiez, C.; Bullock, M. Targeting the Myofibroblastic Cancer-Associated Fibroblast Phenotype through Inhibition of NOX4. *J. Natl. Cancer Inst.* **2018**, *110*, 109–120. [CrossRef] [PubMed]
32. Amin, M.B.; Edge, S.; Greene, F.; Byrd, D.R.; Brookland, R.K.; Washington, M.K.; Gershenwald, J.E.; Compton, C.C.; Hess, K.R.; Sullivan, D.C.; et al. *AJCC Cancer Staging Manual*, 8th ed.; Springer: New York, NY, USA, 2017.
33. Mascitti, M.; Rubini, C.; De Michele, F.; Balercia, P.; Girotto, R.; Troiano, G.; Lo Muzio, L.; Santarelli, A. American Joint Committee on Cancer staging system 7th edition versus 8th edition: Any improvement for patients with squamous cell carcinoma of the tongue? *Oral Surg. Oral Med. Oral Pathol. Oral Radiol.* **2018**, in press. [CrossRef] [PubMed]
34. Pollaers, K.; Hinton-Bayre, A.; Friedland, P.L.; Farah, C.S. AJCC 8th Edition Oral Cavity Squamous Cell Carcinoma Staging—Is It an Improvement on the AJCC 7th Edition? *Oral Oncol.* **2018**, *82*, 23–28. [CrossRef] [PubMed]

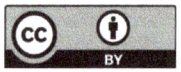

© 2018 by the authors. Licensee MDPI, Basel, Switzerland. This article is an open access article distributed under the terms and conditions of the Creative Commons Attribution (CC BY) license (http://creativecommons.org/licenses/by/4.0/).

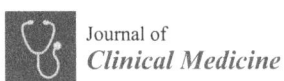

*Article*

# Map1lc3b and Sqstm1 Modulated Autophagy for Tumorigenesis and Prognosis in Certain Subsites of Oral Squamous Cell Carcinoma

Pei-Feng Liu [1,2,†], Hsueh-Wei Chang [3,4,†], Jin-Shiung Cheng [5], Huai-Pao Lee [6,7], Ching-Yu Yen [8,9], Wei-Lun Tsai [5,10], Jiin-Tsuey Cheng [11], Yi-Jing Li [11], Wei-Chieh Huang [12], Cheng-Hsin Lee [1], Luo-Pin Ger [1] and Chih-Wen Shu [13,14,*]

[1] Department of Medical Education and Research, Kaohsiung Veterans General Hospital, Kaohsiung 81362, Taiwan; d908203@gmail.com (P.-F.L.); angioadsc@gmail.com (C.-H.L.); lpger@isca.vghks.gov.tw (L.-P.G.)
[2] Department of Optometry, Shu-Zen Junior College of Medicine and Management, Kaohsiung 82144, Taiwan
[3] Cancer Center, Kaohsiung Medical University Hospital, Kaohsiung Medical University, Kaohsiung 80708, Taiwan; changhw2007@gmail.com
[4] Department of Biomedical Science and Environmental Biology, Kaohsiung Medical University, Kaohsiung 80708, Taiwan
[5] Department of Internal Medicine, Kaohsiung Veterans General Hospital, Kaohsiung 81362, Taiwan; jcheng@vghks.gov.tw (J.-S.C.); tsaiwl@yahoo.com.tw (W.-L.T.)
[6] Department of Pathology and Laboratory Medicine, Kaohsiung Veterans General Hospital, Kaohsiung 81362, Taiwan; hplee0627@vghks.gov.tw
[7] Department of Nursing, Meiho University, Pingtung 91202, Taiwan
[8] Oral and Maxillofacial Surgery Section, Chi Mei Medical Center, Tainan 71004, Taiwan; ycysmc@gmail.com
[9] Department of Dentistry, Taipei Medical University, Taipei 11031, Taiwan
[10] School of Medicine, National Yang-Ming University, Taipei 11221, Taiwan
[11] Department of Biological Science, National Sun Yat-sen University, Kaohsiung 80424, Taiwan; tusya@faculty.nsysu.edu.tw (J.-T.C.); lee720127@yahoo.com.tw (Y.-J.L.)
[12] Graduate Institute of Integrated Medicine, China Medical University, Taichung 40402, Taiwan; jeff20628@gmail.com
[13] School of Medicine for International Students, I-Shou University, Kaohsiung 82445, Taiwan
[14] Institute of Biomedical Sciences, National Sun Yat-sen University, Kaohsiung 80424, Taiwan
* Correspondence: cwshu@isu.edu.tw; Tel.: +886-7-6151100 (ext. 7161); Fax: +886-7-6155910
† These authors contributed equally to this work.

Received: 27 October 2018; Accepted: 22 November 2018; Published: 24 November 2018

**Abstract:** Oral squamous cell carcinoma (OSCC) is one of the most common cancer types worldwide and can be divided into three major subsites: buccal mucosal SCC (BMSCC), tongue SCC (TSCC), and lip SCC (LSCC). The autophagy marker microtubule-associated protein light chain 3B (MAP1LC3B) and adaptor sequestosome 1(SQSTM1) are widely used proteins to evaluate autophagy in tumor tissues. However, the role of MAP1LC3B and SQSTM1 in OSCC is not fully understood, particularly in certain subsites. With a tissue microarray comprised of 498 OSCC patients, including 181 BMSCC, 244 TSCC, and 73 LSCC patients, we found that the expression levels of MAP1LC3B and cytoplasmic SQSTM1 were elevated in the tumor tissues of three subsites compared with those in adjacent normal tissues. MAP1LC3B was associated with a poor prognosis only in TSCC. SQSTM1 was associated with poor differentiation in three subsites, while the association with lymph node invasion was only observed in BMSCC. Interestingly, MAP1LC3B was positively correlated with SQSTM1 in the tumor tissues of BMSCC, whereas it showed no correlation with SQSTM1 in adjacent normal tissue. The coexpression of higher MAP1LC3B and SQSTM1 demonstrated a significantly worse disease-specific survival (DSS) and disease-free survival (DFS) in patients with BMSCC and LSCC, but not TSCC. The knockdown of MAP1LC3B and SQSTM1 reduced autophagy, cell proliferation, invasion and tumorspheres of BMSCC cells. Additionally, silencing both

MAP1LC3B and SQSTM1 enhanced the cytotoxic effects of paclitaxel in the tumorspheres of BMSCC cells. Taken together, MAP1LC3B and SQSTM1 might modulate autophagy to facilitate tumorigenesis and chemoresistance in OSCC, particularly in BMSCC.

**Keywords:** MAP1LC3B; SQSTM1; autophagy; subsites; tumorigenesis; prognosis; oral cancer

## 1. Introduction

Oral squamous cell carcinoma (OSCC), a type of head and neck cancer, is one of the most common malignant tumors worldwide [1,2]. Oral cancer mainly originates from the epithelium of the oral cavity, of which the tongue, buccal mucosa, and lip are the top three most common subsites [3]. Oral cancer is a multistep process modulated by environmental and endogenous factors, such as alcohol and tobacco and betel chewing. Other factors include poor oral hygiene and chronic infections caused by viruses or bacteria. Although the standard treatment is effective for patients diagnosed at the early stage, the morbidity rate for patients with advanced-stage disease has not decreased much in the past few decades [4], requiring more precise biomarkers for either an early diagnosis or therapeutic targets for a better outcome.

Autophagy is a clearance pathway that involves more than 38 autophagy-related (ATG) proteins to recruit impaired proteins and organelles for bulk degradation for new synthesis [5]. Autophagy plays a crucial role in physiological homeostasis, and its dysfunction may cause various diseases, such as cancer, neurodegeneration disease and infection. However, the role of autophagy in tumor progression is a "double-edged sword", with opposite functions in tumor imitation and malignancy. Autophagy exhibits suppressive effects on chronic inflammation and ROS production, thereby inhibiting carcinogenesis in the early phase [6,7] and facilitates cancer cell growth and survival under microenvironmental stress conditions [8]. Autophagy can support tumor cell survival through suppressing the p53 response and maintaining mitochondrial metabolism to prevent metabolic stress and mitigate the accumulation of toxic substances [9–11]. Regarding the clinical association of autophagy markers, microtubule-associated light chain 3B (MAP1LC3B), an essential protein for autophagosome elongation, is associated with poor survival in various cancer types; however, some studies have indicated that cancer patients with high MAP1LC3B expression have a better outcome [12], particularly in K-Ras-mutated colorectal cancer cells. Additionally, SQSTM1 contains an MAP1LC3B-interacting (LIR) domain and a ubiquitin-associated (UBA) domain, which serve as an autophagy adaptor to recruit ubiquitinated proteins to the autophagosome for selective autophagy [13,14]. High levels of cytoplasmic SQSTM1 have also been found to be associated with poor survival in several cancer types [12]. However, little is known about the detailed clinical relevance and functions of MAP1LC3B and SQSTM1 in certain subsites of OSCC. In this study, we compared the MAP1LC3B and SQSTM1 protein levels in tumor tissues and adjacent normal tissues in three major subsites of OSCC, including BMSCC, TSCC and LSCC. Our results show that both MAP1LC3B and cytoplasmic SQSTM1 were elevated in tumor tissues in three subsites of OSCC compared with that in adjacent normal tissues. Moreover, SQSTM1 was associated with poor survival in patients with BMSCC, but not in those with TSCC and LSCC. The SQSTM1 protein level was also found to be positively correlated with MAP1LC3B in the tumor tissues of BMSCC but not in adjacent normal tissues. In contrast to the single expression of MAP1LC3B or SQSTM1, high coexpression of MAP1LC3B and SQSTM1 showed a worse DSS and DFS in BMSCC. Silencing MAP1LC3B and SQSTM1 diminished autophagy, cell proliferation, invasion, tumorsphere formation and paclitaxel resistance in BMSCC cell lines, supporting our findings in clinical samples. Our results suggest that MAP1LC3B and SQSTM1 could serve as biomarkers or therapeutic targets for BMSCC.

## 2. Experimental Procedure

### 2.1. Tissue Specimens and Tissue Microarray (TMA) Construction

In total, 498 margin-free (margin-size $\geq 0.2$ cm) paraffin-embedded materials of primary BMSCC ($n = 181$), TSCC ($n = 244$), and LSCC ($n = 73$) were established previously [3]. The data of sex, age, cell differentiation, pathological stage, tumor TNM classification, tumor subsites, and tumor recurrence time were also collected. Pathologic TNM classification was determined according to the guidelines of the 2002 American Joint Committee on Cancer (AJCC) system. The Institutional Review Board at Kaohsiung Veterans General Hospital (KVGH) approved this study to comply with the Declaration of Helsinki (IRB number: VGHKS 11-CT12-13). All information was obtained from the archives of the KVGH pathology department between 1993 and 2006.

The TMA block contained 144 cores, including 48 trios consisting of 2 cores from the tumor tissue and 1 core from the adjacent normal tissue. After construction, TMA blocks were cut in 4-μm paraffin sections using standard techniques [3].

### 2.2. Immunohistochemistry (IHC)

TMA blocks were cut into 4-μm paraffin sections for immunostaining processes as previously reported [15]. Antigen retrieval was performed by a pressure boiler at 125 °C for 10 min in Tris-EDTA (10 mM, pH 9.0) for MAP1LC3B and sodium citrate (10 mM, pH 6.0) for SQSTM1. After blocking with 3% hydrogen peroxide in methanol, the slides were incubated with antibody against MAP1LC3B (dilution 1:100; 5F10; NanoTools, Munich, Germany) and SQSTM1 (dilution 1:1000; BML-PW9860; Enzo Life Sciences, Farmingdale, NY, USA) in a cold room overnight. The color was developed at room temperature, and the sections were counterstained with hematoxylin.

### 2.3. Immunohistochemistry Analysis and Score

All the slides were independently reviewed by an oral cancer pathologist and a senior pathology technician. Subsequently, 5%–20% of core samples were randomly selected for re-evaluation. If disagreement occurred (intensity score discrepancy >1 or percentage level >20%), the slide was re-evaluated to obtain a consensus diagnosis by a senior pathologist until all the discrepancies was resolved. During the evaluation, none of them were aware of the clinical outcomes of the patients. The scores for cytoplasmic staining were based on the staining intensity (0, no signal; 1, mild; 2, moderate; and 3, strong) and percentage of positive staining (0, <5%; 1, 5%–25%; 2, 26%–50%; 3, 51%–75%; and 4, >75%). In our preliminary test, the intensity score of staining for LC3 and cytoplasmic SQSTM1 was measured and standardized (0, no expression; 1, weak expression; 2, moderate expression; and 3, strong expression; Figure 1) in OSCC. The final score, ranging from 0 to 7, was used to analyze the association of MAP1LC3B and SQSTM1 with clinicopathological features. For survival analysis, the expression levels were dichotomized as low expression and high expression with the cutoff based on the receiver operating characteristic (ROC) curve. The cutoff values were determined for MAP1LC3B and SQSTM1 in BMSCC, TSCC, LSCC and OSCC.

### 2.4. Cell Culture and Transient Transfection

The buccal mucosal squamous cell lines TW2.6 and OC3 or OC3-I5 (gift of Dr. Lu-Hai Wang) [16] were cultured in DMEM/F12 (Gibco, Life Technologies, CA, USA) with 10% FBS, 100 μg/mL of streptomycin, 100 U/mL of penicillin, and 1% L-glutamine at 37 °C with 5% $CO_2$:95% air. The cells were cultured in Corning tissue culture-treated plastic dishes (Corning, Inc., Corning, NY, USA). BMSCC cells were seeded with RNAiMAX (13778150; Life Technologies, CA, USA) in the presence of 5 nM scrambled siRNA or siRNA against human MAP1LC3B (L-012846-00-0005; Dharmacon, IL, USA) or SQSTM1 (L-010230-00-0005; Dharmacon, IL, USA) for 48 h. The knockdown efficiency was determined with immunoblotting using anti-MAP1LC3B or SQSTM1 antibody as previously reported [17].

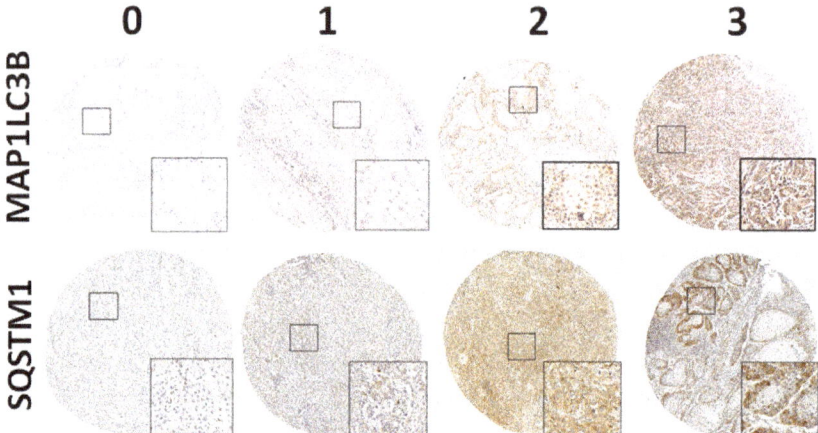

**Figure 1.** Protein levels of MAP1LC3B puncta and SQSTM1 in OSCC. The MAP1LC3B puncta and cytoplasmic SQSTM1 were stained by immunohistochemistry and categorized into four different levels as follows: 0 = negative staining; 1 = weak; 2 = moderate; 3 = strong.

*2.5. Analysis of Cell Viability*

The cell viability assay was performed using the CellTiter-Glo luminescent cell viability assay kit (Promega, Madison, WI, USA). Briefly, 5–7 × $10^5$ cells/mL were cultured in sterile 96-well plates for 24–48 h, and then 100 µL of CellTiter-Glo reagent was added to lyse the cells for 10 min. The luminescence signal was measured using a Fluoroskan Ascent FL reader (Thermo Fisher Scientific, Waltham, CA, USA). For tumorsphere formation, the cells (OC3: 5 × $10^3$ cells/well, TW2.6: 5 × $10^3$ cells/well) were seeded into Nano Culture Plates (NCPs) (MBL Corporation, Nagoya, Japan) in the presence of siRNA for 7 days to form spheroid cells that might induce stem cell-like properties. The tumorspheres were then treated with or without the anticancer drug paclitaxel (Selleckchem, Houston, TX, USA) for two days. The sphere viability was measured using the CellTiter Glo 3D system (Promega, Madison, WI, USA).

*2.6. Invasion Assay*

For the wound-healing assay, Transwell invasion assays were performed using 8-µm pore inserts (Greiner Bio-One, Stroud, UK). The cells were knocked down with siRNA for 48 h and then were seeded into the top chamber of Transwell plates coated with 0.5% Matrigel in 300 µL of DMEM containing 1% FBS. To the bottom wells were added with complete medium to stimulate invasion. After seeding for 24 h, the cells were fixed and stained with 0.1% crystal violet. The cells that had invaded through the Matrigel and had reached to the reverse side were pictured under a microscope at a magnification of 200× and were quantified with ImageJ. Each assay was performed in triplicate.

*2.7. Statistical Analysis*

The Kruskal–Wallis one-way ANOVA test was used to evaluate the differential protein expression in TAN tissues and tumor tissues in various OSCC types. The protein expression levels between TAN tissues and tumor tissues were analyzed by the Wilcoxon signed-rank test. Student's t test, Mann–Whitney U test, Kruskal–Wallis one-way ANOVA test and one-way ANOVA test were used to evaluate the correlation between each protein expression level and clinicopathologic parameters. The Kaplan–Meier method was used to analyze cumulative survival curves, and survival curve analysis was performed using the log-rank test. The Cox proportional hazards model was used to evaluate the impact of the protein expression on survival using factors significant in univariate analysis as covariates. The association between cell differentiation and the relative protein expression levels in tumor tissues compared with that in paired TAN tissues of individual OSCC patients with different AJCC pathological stages was determined by Fisher's exact test. A two-sided value of $p < 0.05$ was considered statistically significant.

## 3. Results

*3.1. Association of the MAP1LC3B and SQSTM1 Protein Levels with Tumorigenesis and Clinicopathological Outcomes*

MAP1LC3B can be divided into two major forms: cytosolic MAP1LC3B-I and autophagosome membrane-bound MAP1LC3B-II (MAP1LC3B puncta), which indicates autophagy. We initially checked for MAP1LC3B puncta with IHC staining in tissues. Representative photomicrographs of MAP1LC3B and SQSTM1 for negative (0), weak (1+), moderate (2+), and strong (3+) expression in tumor tissue are shown in Figure 1. However, we found that only a few slides contained MAP1LC3B puncta in most of the OSCC TMA. Thus, we scored the total MAP1LC3B expression levels in all tissues and found that the MAP1LC3B levels were increased in tumor tissues compared with those in adjacent normal tissues in three major subsites of OSCC, including BMSCC ($3.31 \pm 1.44$ vs. $2.30 \pm 1.06$, $p < 0.001$), TSCC ($1.48 \pm 1.02$ vs. $0.59 \pm 0.94$, $p < 0.001$) and LSCC ($3.14 \pm 1.43$ vs. $2.32 \pm 0.71$, $p < 0.001$) (Table 1). Although SQSTM1 was found in both the nucleus and cytoplasm of cells, SQSTM1 interacts with MAP1LC3B to recruit damaged proteins to the autophagosome for degradation in the lysosome via selective autophagy, suggesting SQSTM1 functions as an autophagy adaptor in nonnuclear regions. Herein, we scored the cytoplasmic SQSTM1 level of tissues to analyze its correlation with tumorigenesis and clinicopathological outcomes at three subsites of OSCC. Similar to the results of MAP1LC3B, cytoplasmic SQSTM1 was elevated in three subsites of OSCC (BMSCC: $2.89 \pm 1.11$ vs. $1.89 \pm 1.00$, $p < 0.001$; TSCC: $2.78 \pm 1.08$ vs. $1.88 \pm 0.77$, $p < 0.001$; and LSCC: $3.22 \pm 1.25$ vs. $2.03 \pm 0.64$, $p < 0.001$) (Table 1). Regarding the expression levels of MAP1LC3B and cytoplasmic SQSTM1 and clinicopathological outcomes, including cell differentiation, pathological stage, sex and age, the MAP1LC3B expression levels in BMSCC and LSCC were significantly higher than those in TSCC ($p < 0.001$, Table 2). A high MAP1LC3B protein level was associated with poor differentiation in only TSCC ($p = 0.042$, Table 2) but not in BMSCC and LSCC. On the other hand, SQSTM1 protein levels were associated with poor differentiation in BMSCC ($p = 0.015$), TSCC ($p = 0.042$) and LSCC ($p = 0.003$, Table 3). High SQSTM1 expression was correlated with lymph node invasion in BMSCC ($3.22 \pm 1.29$ vs. $2.74 \pm 1.02$, $p = 0.033$, Table 3) but not in TSCC and LSCC.

**Table 1.** Comparisons of MAP1LC3B and SQSTM1 expression between tumor tissues and corresponding tumor adjacent normal tissues at three subsites of oral SCC.

| Variables | No. | Tumor adjacent normal | | Tumor | | Z | p-value * |
|---|---|---|---|---|---|---|---|
| | | Mean ± SD | Median | Mean ± SD | Median | | |
| BMSCC | | | | | | | |
| MAP1LC3B | 135 | 2.01 ± 1.08 | 2.00 | 3.31 ± 1.44 | 3.00 | 7.787 | **<0.001** |
| SQSTM1 | 132 | 1.89 ± 1.00 | 2.00 | 2.89 ± 1.11 | 2.00 | 6.821 | **<0.001** |
| TSCC | | | | | | | |
| MAP1LC3B | 174 | 0.59 ± 0.94 | 0.00 | 1.48 ± 1.02 | 2.00 | 7.710 | **<0.001** |
| SQSTM1 | 192 | 1.88 ± 0.77 | 2.00 | 2.78 ± 1.08 | 2.00 | 7.939 | **<0.001** |
| LSCC | | | | | | | |
| MAP1LC3B | 59 | 2.32 ± 0.71 | 2.00 | 3.14 ± 1.43 | 3.00 | 4.084 | **<0.001** |
| SQSTM1 | 59 | 2.03 ± 0.64 | 2.00 | 3.22 ± 1.25 | 3.00 | 5.049 | **<0.001** |
| OSCC | | | | | | | |
| MAP1LC3B | 368 | 1.39 ± 1.23 | 2.00 | 2.42 ± 1.54 | 2.00 | 11.717 | **<0.001** |
| SQSTM1 | 383 | 1.91 ± 0.84 | 2.00 | 2.89 ± 1.13 | 2.00 | 11.620 | **<0.001** |

Abbreviations: SCC, squamous cell carcinoma; SD, standard deviation. * $p$-values were estimated by the Wilcoxon signed-rank test. Bold values denote statistically significant.

Table 2. Expression of MAP1LC3B and clinicopathologic outcomes in patients with OSCC and three primary subsites.

| Variable | BMSCC (n = 181) | | | | TSCC (n = 244) | | | | LSCC (n = 73) | | | | OSCC (n = 498) | | | |
|---|---|---|---|---|---|---|---|---|---|---|---|---|---|---|---|---|
| | % | Mean ± SD | Median | p-value | % | Mean ± SD | Median | p-value | % | Mean ± SD | Median | p-value | % | Mean ± SD | Median | p-value |
| Sex | | | | | | | | | | | | | | | | |
| Female | 2.2 | 2.50 ± 0.58 | 2.50 | 0.240 * | 11.9 | 1.69 ± 1.34 | 2.00 | 0.311 * | 9.6 | 3.71 ± 0.95 | 4.00 | 0.246 * | 8.0 | 2.13 ± 1.44 | 2.00 | 0.256 * |
| Male | 97.8 | 3.34 ± 1.42 | 3.00 | | 88.1 | 1.47 ± 1.03 | 2.00 | | 90.4 | 3.00 ± 1.58 | 3.00 | | 92.0 | 2.41 ± 1.56 | 2.00 | |
| Age, year | | | | | | | | | | | | | | | | |
| ≤50 | 44.2 | 3.39 ± 1.31 | 3.00 | 0.570 * | 51.6 | 1.52 ± 1.04 | 2.00 | 0.812 * | 21.9 | 2.69 ± 1.62 | 2.00 | 0.266 * | 44.6 | 2.27 ± 1.48 | 2.00 | 0.131 * |
| >50 | 55.8 | 3.27 ± 1.49 | 3.00 | | 48.4 | 1.48 ± 1.11 | 2.00 | | 78.1 | 3.18 ± 1.51 | 3.00 | | 55.4 | 2.49 ± 1.60 | 2.00 | |
| Subsite | | | | | | | | | | | | | | | | |
| Buccal | 100.0 | 3.32 ± 1.41 | 3.00 | - | - | - | - | - | - | - | - | - | 36.3 | 3.32 ± 1.41 [a] | 3.00 | <0.001 † |
| Tongue | - | - | - | | 100.0 | 1.50 ± 1.07 | 2.00 | | - | - | - | | 49.0 | 1.50 ± 1.07 [ab] | 2.00 | |
| Lip | - | - | - | | - | - | - | | 100.0 | 3.07 ± 1.54 | 3.00 | | 14.7 | 3.07 ± 1.54 [b] | 3.00 | |
| Cell differentiation | | | | | | | | | | | | | | | | |
| Well | 26.0 | 3.04 ± 1.38 | 3.00 | 0.213 ‡ | 10.7 | 1.08 ± 1.06 [c] | 1.00 | 0.042 ‡ | 46.6 | 3.00 ± 0.98 | 3.00 | 0.726 † | 21.5 | 2.55 ± 1.45 | 2.00 | 0.209 ‡ |
| Moderate | 69.1 | 3.39 ± 1.40 | 3.00 | | 82.4 | 1.52 ± 1.06 | 2.00 | | 47.9 | 3.06 ± 1.80 | 3.00 | | 72.5 | 2.32 ± 1.55 | 2.00 | |
| Poor | 5.0 | 3.78 ± 1.56 | 3.00 | | 7.0 | 1.88 ± 1.05 [c] | 2.00 | | 5.5 | 3.75 ± 2.99 | 4.00 | | 6.0 | 2.70 ± 1.76 | 2.00 | |
| AJCC pathological stage | | | | | | | | | | | | | | | | |
| I, II | 61.3 | 3.30 ± 1.33 | 3.00 | 0.782 * | 68.9 | 1.45 ± 1.05 | 2.00 | 0.246 * | 79.5 | 3.21 ± 1.48 | 3.00 | 0.132 * | 67.7 | 2.36 ± 1.53 | 2.00 | 0.498 * |
| III, IV | 38.7 | 3.36 ± 1.53 | 3.00 | | 31.1 | 1.62 ± 1.12 | 2.00 | | 20.5 | 2.53 ± 1.68 | 2.00 | | 32.3 | 2.46 ± 1.59 | 2.00 | |
| T classification | | | | | | | | | | | | | | | | |
| T1, T2 | 75.7 | 3.25 ± 1.38 | 3.00 | 0.224 * | 79.5 | 1.47 ± 1.04 | 2.00 | 0.460 * | 82.2 | 3.17 ± 1.47 | 3.00 | 0.245 * | 78.5 | 2.36 ± 1.52 | 2.00 | 0.321 * |
| T3, T4 | 24.3 | 3.55 ± 1.50 | 4.00 | | 20.5 | 1.60 ± 1.18 | 2.00 | | 17.8 | 2.62 ± 1.80 | 3.00 | | 21.5 | 2.52 ± 1.66 | 2.00 | |
| N classification | | | | | | | | | | | | | | | | |
| N0 | 75.1 | 3.26 ± 1.36 | 3.00 | 0.296 * | 79.9 | 1.45 ± 1.07 | 2.00 | 0.157 * | 94.5 | 3.12 ± 1.57 | 3.00 | 0.277 * | 80.3 | 2.35 ± 1.54 | 2.00 | 0.256 * |
| N1, N2 | 24.9 | 3.51 ± 1.55 | 3.00 | | 20.1 | 1.69 ± 1.08 | 2.00 | | 5.5 | 2.25 ± 0.50 | 2.00 | | 19.7 | 2.55 ± 1.57 | 2.00 | |

Abbreviations: SCC, squamous cell carcinoma; AJCC, American Joint Committee on Cancer. * p values were estimated by student's t-test. † p values were estimated by Kruskal–Wallis one-way ANOVA test. ‡ p values were estimated by one-way ANOVA test. [a] $p < 0.001$; [b] $p < 0.001$; [c] $p = 0.054$. Bold values denote statistically significant.

Table 3. Expression of SQSTM1 and clinicopathologic outcomes in patients with OSCC and three primary subsites.

| Variable | BMSCC (n = 181) | | | | TSCC (n = 244) | | | | LSCC (n = 73) | | | | OSCC (n = 498) | | | |
|---|---|---|---|---|---|---|---|---|---|---|---|---|---|---|---|---|
| | % | Mean ± SD | Median | p-value | % | Mean ± SD | Median | p-value | % | Mean ± SD | Median | p-value | % | Mean ± SD | Median | p-value |
| Sex | | | | | | | | | | | | | | | | |
| Female | 2.2 | 3.50 ± 1.73 | 3.50 | 0.246 * | 11.9 | 3.03 ± 1.27 | 3.00 | 0.155 * | 9.6 | 3.29 ± 1.11 | 3.00 | 0.622 * | 8.0 | 3.13 ± 1.26 | 3.00 | 0.099 * |
| Male | 97.8 | 2.85 ± 1.09 | 2.00 | | 88.1 | 2.73 ± 1.05 | 2.00 | | 90.4 | 3.03 ± 1.31 | 3.00 | | 92.0 | 2.82 ± 1.11 | 2.00 | |
| Age, year | | | | | | | | | | | | | | | | |
| ≤50 | 44.2 | 2.80 ± 1.10 | 2.00 | 0.506 * | 51.6 | 2.68 ± 1.06 | 2.00 | 0.211 * | 21.9 | 3.00 ± 1.10 | 3.00 | 0.849 * | 44.6 | 2.75 ± 1.07 | 2.00 | 0.089 * |
| >50 | 55.8 | 2.91 ± 1.12 | 3.00 | | 48.4 | 2.86 ± 1.10 | 2.00 | | 78.1 | 3.07 ± 1.35 | 3.00 | | 55.4 | 2.92 ± 1.16 | 3.00 | |
| Subsite | | | | | | | | | | | | | | | | |
| Buccal | 100.0 | 2.86 ± 1.11 | 2.00 | - | - | - | - | - | - | - | - | - | 36.3 | 2.86 ± 1.11 | 2.00 | 0.152 † |
| Tongue | - | - | - | | 100.0 | 2.77 ± 1.08 | 2.00 | | - | - | - | | 49.0 | 2.77 ± 1.08 | 2.00 | |
| Lip | - | - | - | | - | - | - | | 100 | 3.05 ± 1.29 | 3.00 | | 14.7 | 3.05 ± 1.29 | 3.00 | |
| Cell differentiation | | | | | | | | | | | | | | | | |
| Well | 26.0 | 2.53 ± 0.97 ᵃ | 2.00 | 0.015 † | 10.7 | 2.58 ± 0.95 ᵇ | 2.00 | 0.040 ‡ | 46.6 | 2.53 ± 1.02 ᵈ | 2.00 | 0.003 † | 21.5 | 2.54 ± 0.97 ᵉᶠ | 2.00 | 0.001 ‡ |
| Moderate | 69.1 | 2.94 ± 1.11 | 3.00 | | 82.4 | 2.72 ± 1.02 ᶜ | 2.00 | | 47.9 | 3.46 ± 1.24 ᵈ | 3.00 | | 72.5 | 2.87 ± 1.09 ᵉᵍ | 2.00 | |
| Poor | 5.0 | 3.56 ± 1.33 ᵃ | 4.00 | | 7.0 | 3.59 ± 1.58 ᵇᶜ | 4.00 | | 5.5 | 4.00 ± 2.16 | 3.50 | | 6.0 | 3.63 ± 1.54 ᶠᵍ | 4.00 | |
| AJCC pathological stage | | | | | | | | | | | | | | | | |
| I, II | 61.3 | 2.79 ± 1.05 | 2.00 | 0.293 * | 68.9 | 2.74 ± 1.01 | 2.00 | 0.935 § | 79.5 | 2.97 ± 1.34 | 3.00 | 0.248 * | 67.7 | 2.80 ± 1.09 | 2.00 | 0.415 § |
| III, IV | 38.7 | 2.97 ± 1.19 | 2.00 | | 31.1 | 2.82 ± 1.23 | 2.00 | | 20.5 | 3.40 ± 1.06 | 4.00 | | 32.3 | 2.94 ± 1.20 | 2.00 | |
| T classification | | | | | | | | | | | | | | | | |
| T1, T2 | 75.7 | 2.88 ± 1.11 | 2.00 | 0.765 * | 79.5 | 2.80 ± 1.07 | 2.00 | 0.355 * | 82.2 | 2.97 ± 1.33 | 3.00 | 0.212 * | 78.5 | 2.85 ± 1.13 | 2.00 | 0.754 * |
| T3, T4 | 24.3 | 2.82 ± 1.11 | 2.00 | | 20.5 | 2.64 ± 1.12 | 2.00 | | 17.8 | 3.46 ± 1.05 | 4.00 | | 21.5 | 2.81 ± 1.13 | 2.00 | |
| N classification | | | | | | | | | | | | | | | | |
| N0 | 75.1 | 2.74 ± 1.02 | 2.00 | 0.033 § | 79.9 | 2.75 ± 1.04 | 2.00 | 0.718 * | 94.5 | 3.07 ± 1.31 | 3.00 | 0.630 * | 80.3 | 2.81 ± 1.09 | 2.00 | 0.285 § |
| N1, N2 | 24.9 | 3.22 ± 1.29 | 3.00 | | 20.1 | 2.82 ± 1.24 | 2.00 | | 5.5 | 2.75 ± 0.96 | 2.50 | | 19.7 | 3.00 ± 1.26 | 2.00 | |

Abbreviations: SCC, squamous cell carcinoma; AJCC, American Joint Committee on Cancer. * p values were estimated by student's t-test. † p values were estimated by one-way ANOVA test. ‡ p values were estimated by Kruskal–Wallis one-way ANOVA test. § p values was estimated by Mann–Whitney U test. ᵃ p = 0.001; ᵇ p = 0.031; ᶜ p = 0.016; ᵈ p = 0.008; ᵉ p = 0.019; ᶠ p < 0.001; ᵍ p = 0.005. Bold values denote statistically significant.

## 3.2. Expression Levels of MAP1LC3B and SQSTM1 and Disease-Specific Survival (DSS) of OSCC Patients

We further determined whether MAP1LC3B expression was correlated with SQSTM1 in tumor tissues and adjacent normal tissues in three subsites of OSCC. Interestingly, Pearson's correlation analysis showed that MAP1LC3B was positively correlated with SQSTM1 in the tumor tissues of BMSCC but showed no correlation in adjacent normal tissues (Table 4). Nevertheless, opposite effects were observed in TSCC, whereas MAP1LC3B was correlated with SQSTM1 expression in both tumor and adjacent normal tissues in LSCC (Table 4), suggesting these molecules might be differentially regulated at diverse subsites of OSCC. Moreover, to determine whether MAP1LC3B and SQSTM1 could be used as prognostic factors in the different subsites of OSCC, we further investigated the relationship of MAP1LC3B and SQSTM1 expression with DSS. Kaplan–Meier curve analysis showed that higher MAP1LC3B (Figure 2) expression was associated with a poor DSS in LSCC ($p = 0.008$), whereas high SQSTM1 (Figure 3) expression was associated with a poor DSS in BMSCC ($p = 0.005$). After adjustment for cell differentiation (moderate + poor vs. well) and AJCC pathological stage (stage III + IV vs. stage I + II) following Cox's regression analysis, both MAP1LC3B (AHR: 1.59, 95% CI: 1.00–2.52, $p = 0.05$, Table 5) and SQSTM1 (AHR: 1.92, 95% CI: 1.19–3.09, $p = 0.008$, Table 4) were correlated with unfavorable DSS in BMSCC. High MAP1LC3B expression showed a worse DSS in LSCC (AHR: 19.93, 95% CI: 1.61–246.87, $p = 0.02$, Table 4). Additionally, BMSCC and LSCC with high coexpression of MAP1LC3B and SQSTM1 had a shorter DSS than those with low coexpression of MAP1LC3B and SQSTM1 (BMSCC: $p = 0.019$, LSCC: $p = 0.012$, Figure 3). After adjusting for cell differentiation and AJCC pathological stage, the results also showed that BMSCC (AHR: 2.38, 95% CI: 1.27–4.46, $p = 0.007$, Table 5) and LSCC (AHR: 20.72, 95% CI: 1.72–250.12, $p = 0.017$, Table 5) patients with high coexpression of MAP1LC3B and SQSTM1 had higher hazard of death.

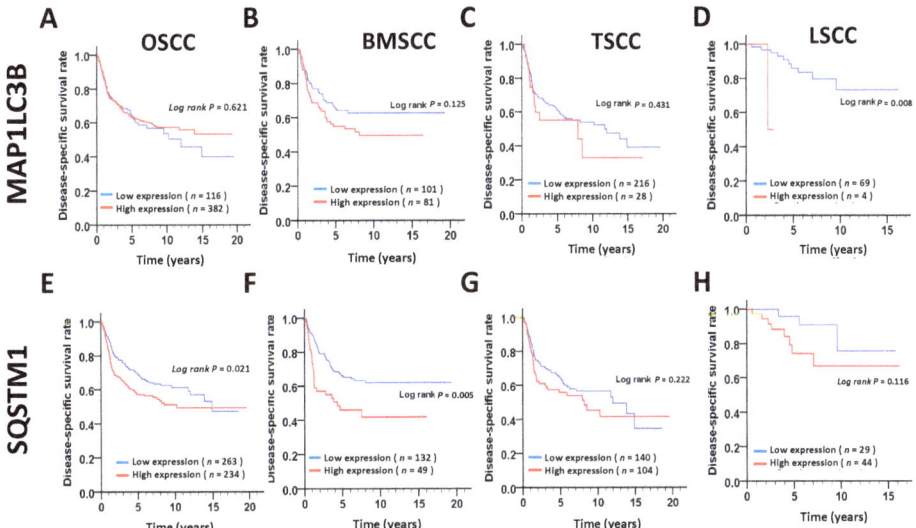

**Figure 2.** DSS survival curves for MAP1LC3B and SQSTM1 expression in patients with different subsites of OSCC. DSS survival curves of MAP1LC3 (**A–D**) and SQSTM1 (**E–H**) are shown for OSCC (**A,E**) and three main subsites, BMSCC (**B,F**), TSCC (**C,G**) and LSCC (**D,H**). The cutoff values for high or low expression of MAP1LC3B and SQSTM1 in tumor tissues were based on the receiver operating characteristic (ROC) curve.

Table 4. Correlation coefficients (*r*) between MAP1LC3B and SQSTM1 in OSCC.

|  | Adjacent Normal MAP1LC3B | Tumor MAP1LC3B |
|---|---|---|
| BMSCC SQSTM1 | (*n* = 114) *r* = −0.053 *p* = 0.578 | (*n* = 181) *r* = 0.155 *p* = 0.038 |
| TSCC SQSTM1 | (*n* = 166) *r* = 0.162 *p* = 0.037 | (*n* = 244) *r* = 0.095 *p* = 0.140 |
| LSCC SQSTM1 | (*n* = 55) *r* = 0.266 *p* = 0.049 | (*n* = 73) *r* = 0.504 *p* < 0.001 |
| OSCC SQSTM1 | (*n* = 365) 0.068 *p* = 0.218 | (*n* = 498) 0.181 *p* < 0.001 |

The correlation coefficient and *p*-value were estimated by the Spearman's rank correlation coefficient.

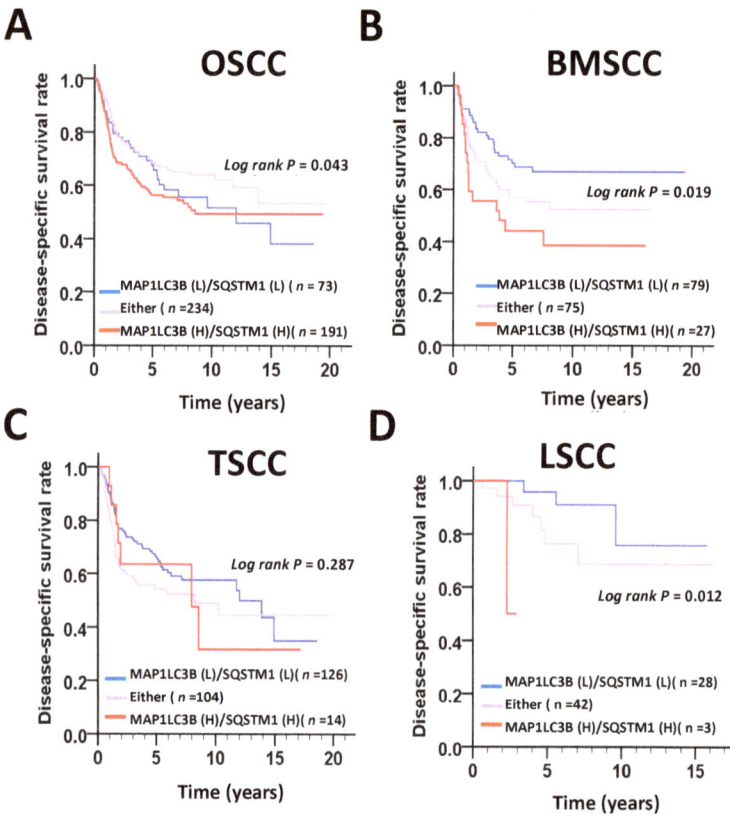

**Figure 3.** DSS survival curves for the coexpression of MAP1LC3B and SQSTM1 in patients with different subsites of OSCC. DSS survival curves for the coexpression of MAP1LC3 and SQSTM1 are shown for OSCC (**A**) and three main subsites, BMSCC (**B**), TSCC (**C**) and LSCC (**D**). The cutoff values for high or low coexpression of MAP1LC3B and SQSTM1 in tumor tissues were based on the receiver operating characteristic (ROC) curve.

**Table 5.** The expression levels of MAP1LC3B and SQSTM1 in disease-specific survival of oral SCC patients.

| Variable (ROC) | | No. (%) | CHR (95% CI) | $p$-value | AHR (95% CI) | $p$-value * |
|---|---|---|---|---|---|---|
| **OSCC** | | | | | | |
| MAP1LC3B expression | Low (0–1) | 116 (23.3) | 1.00 | | 1.00 | |
| | High (2–7) | 382 (76.7) | 0.92 (0.67–1.27) | 0.621 | 0.99 (0.71–1.36) | 0.928 |
| SQSTM1 expression | Low (0–2) | 264 (53.0) | 1.00 | | 1.00 | |
| | High (3–7) | 234 (47.0) | 1.39 (1.05–1.84) | **0.022** | 1.46 (1.10–1.94) | **0.009** |
| MAP1LC3B (L) SQSTM1 (L) | | 73 (14.7) | 1.00 | | 1.00 | |
| either | | 234 (47.0) | 0.71 (0.53–0.94) | **0.017** | 0.78 (0.52–1.18) | 0.235 |
| MAP1LC3B (H) SQSTM1 (H) | | 191 (38.4) | 1.38 (1.04–1.84) | **0.026** | 1.15 (0.76–1.73) | 0.501 |
| **BMSCC** | | | | | | |
| MAP1LC3B expression | Low (0–3) | 101 (55.8) | 1.00 | | 1.00 | |
| | High (4–7) | 80 (44.2) | 1.42 (0.91–2.24) | 0.127 | 1.59 (1.00–2.52) | 0.050 |
| SQSTM1 expression | Low (0–3) | 132 (72.9) | 1.00 | | 1.00 | |
| | High (4–7) | 49 (27.1) | 1.96 (1.22–3.14) | **0.005** | 1.92 (1.19–3.09) | **0.008** |
| MAP1LC3B (L) SQSTM1 (L) | | 79 (43.6) | 1.00 | | 1.00 | |
| either | | 75 (41.4) | 1.23 (0.78–1.94) | 0.367 | 1.59 (0.95–2.67) | 0.077 |
| MAP1LC3B (H) SQSTM1 (H) | | 27 (14.9) | 1.87 (1.07–3.24) | **0.027** | 2.38 (1.27–4.46) | **0.007** |
| **TSCC** | | | | | | |
| MAP1LC3B expression | Low (0–2) | 216 (88.5) | 1.00 | | 1.00 | |
| | High (3–7) | 28 (11.5) | 1.25 (0.71–2.20) | 0.432 | 1.09 (0.62–1.91) | 0.777 |
| SQSTM1 expression | Low (0–2) | 140 (57.4) | 1.00 | | 1.00 | |
| | High (3–7) | 104 (42.6) | 1.27 (0.87–1.85) | 0.223 | 1.36 (0.93–1.98) | 0.117 |
| MAP1LC3B (L) SQSTM1 (L) | | 126 (51.6) | 1.00 | | 1.00 | |
| either | | 104 (42.6) | 1.33 (0.91–1.94) | 0.141 | 1.36 (0.92–2.01) | 0.120 |
| MAP1LC3B (H) SQSTM1 (H) | | 14 (5.7) | 1.11 (0.51–2.38) | 0.795 | 1.27 (0.58–2.80) | 0.553 |
| **LSCC** | | | | | | |
| MAP1LC3B expression | Low (0–5) | 69 (94.5) | 1.00 | | 1.00 | |
| | High (6–7) | 4 (5.5) | 11.40 (1.17–111.09) | **0.036** | 19.93 (1.61–246.87) | **0.020** |
| SQSTM1 expression | Low (0–2) | 29 (39.7) | 1.00 | | 1.00 | |
| | High (3–7) | 44 (60.3) | 2.79 (0.74–10.56) | 0.132 | 2.61 (0.68–10.01) | 0.161 |
| MAP1LC3B (L) SQSTM1 (L) | | 28 (38.4) | 1.00 | | 1.00 | |
| either | | 42 (57.5) | 1.90 (0.55–6.50) | 0.309 | 2.53 (0.65–9.82) | 0.180 |
| MAP1LC3B (H) SQSTM1 (H) | | 3 (4.1) | 11.40 (1.17–111.09) | **0.036** | 20.72 (1.72–250.12) | **0.017** |

Abbreviations: SCC, squamous cell carcinoma; CHR, crude hazard ratio; CI, confidence interval; AHR, adjusted hazard ratio. * $p$-value were adjusted for cell differentiation (moderate + poor vs. well) and AJCC pathological stage (stage III + IV vs. stage I + II) by multiple Cox's regression. Bold values denote statistically significant.

*3.3. Association of the MAP1LC3B and SQSTM1 Expression Levels with Disease-Free Survival (DFS) in OSCC Patients.*

To determine whether MAP1LC3B and SQSTM1 are correlated with relapse in the main subsites of OSCC, we further investigated the relationship of MAP1LC3B and SQSTM1 expression with DFS. The Kaplan–Meier curve showed that a high expression level of MAP1LC3B was notably associated with a poor DFS in BMSCC ($p$ = 0.023, Figure 4) and LSCC ($p$ = 0.009, Figure 4). High expression of SQSTM1 was associated with shorter DFS in only LSCC ($p$ = 0.007) but not at the other two subsites. Likewise, the hazard factor was higher in patients with an elevated expression of MAP1LC3B after adjustment for cell differentiation and AJCC pathological stage following Cox's regression analysis in BMSCC (AHR: 1.90, 95% CI: 0.94–3.85, $p$ = 0.074, Table 6). High SQSTM1 expression had a poor DFS in BMSCC (AHR: 3.77, 95% CI: 1.06–13.38, $p$ = 0.040, Table 6). The combination of high MAP1LC3B and SQSTM1 expression was highly associated with a shorter DFS in patients with BMSCC ($p$ < 0.001, Figure 5) and LSCC ($p$ = 0.003, Figure 5). The adjusted hazard ratios of high coexpression of MAP1LC3B and SQSTM1 in BMSCC and LSCC were also much higher than those with a high single expression of MAP1LC3B or SQSTM1(BMSCC: AHR: 8.19, 95% CI: 2.52–26.64, $p$ < 0.001; LSCC: AHR: 9.49, 95% CI: 2.19–41.08, $p$ = 0.003, Table 6).

**Table 6.** The expression levels of MAP1LC3B and SQSTM1 in disease-free survival of oral SCC patients.

| Variable (ROC) | | No. (%) | CHR (95% CI) | p-value | AHR (95% CI) | p-value * |
|---|---|---|---|---|---|---|
| **OSCC** | | | | | | |
| MAP1LC3B expression | Low (0–1) | 116 (23.3) | 1.00 | | 1.00 | |
| | High (2–7) | 382 (76.7) | 1.01 (0.73–1.40) | 0.960 | 1.09 (0.78–1.52) | 0.620 |
| SQSTM1 expression | Low (0–2) | 264 (53.0) | 1.00 | | 1.00 | |
| | High (3–7) | 234 (47.0) | 1.39 (1.05–1.84) | **0.022** | 1.33 (1.00–1.76) | **0.048** |
| MAP1LC3B (L) SQSTM1 (L) | | 73 (14.7) | 1 | | 1 | |
| either | | 234 (47.0) | 0.77 (0.58–1.03) | 0.075 | 0.93 (0.61–1.43) | 0.737 |
| MAP1LC3B(H) SQSTM1 (H) | | 191 (38.4) | 1.36 (1.03–1.81) | **0.032** | 1.29 (0.84–1.98) | 0.244 |
| **BMSCC** | | | | | | |
| MAP1LC3B expression | Low (0–5) | 168 (92.8) | 1.00 | | 1.00 | |
| | High (6–7) | 13 (7.2) | 2.20 (1.10–4.40) | **0.027** | 1.90 (0.94–3.85) | 0.074 |
| SQSTM1 expression | Low (0–4) | 160 (88.4) | 1.00 | | 1.00 | |
| | High (5–7) | 21 (11.6) | 1.62 (0.88–3.00) | 0.123 | 1.47 (0.79–2.72) | 0.227 |
| MAP1LC3B (L) SQSTM1 (L) | | 150 (82.9) | 1 | | 1 | |
| either | | 28 (15.5) | 1.39 (0.79–2.44) | 0.251 | 1.45 (0.83–2.56) | 0.195 |
| MAP1LC3B(H) SQSTM1 (H) | | 3 (1.7) | 7.66 (2.37–24.75) | **0.001** | 8.19 (2.52–26.64) | **<0.001** |
| **TSCC** | | | | | | |
| MAP1LC3B expression | Low (0–1) | 103 (42.2) | 1.00 | | 1.00 | |
| | High (2–7) | 141 (57.8) | 1.07 (0.71–1.59) | 0.751 | 1.00 (0.67–1.50) | 1.000 |
| SQSTM1 expression | Low (0–2) | 140 (57.4) | 1.00 | | 1.00 | |
| | High (3–7) | 104 (42.6) | 1.38 (0.93–2.06) | 0.109 | 1.35 (0.91–2.01) | 0.137 |
| MAP1LC3B (L) SQSTM1 (L) | | 65 (26.6) | 1 | | 1 | |
| either | | 113 (46.3) | 0.76 (0.51–1.14) | 0.179 | 0.90 (0.55–1.48) | 0.680 |
| MAP1LC3B(H) SQSTM1 (H) | | 66 (27.0) | 1.50 (0.98–2.29) | 0.061 | 1.41 (0.84–2.36) | 0.199 |
| **LSCC** | | | | | | |
| MAP1LC3B expression | Low (0–4) | 60 (82.2) | 1.00 | | 1.00 | |
| | High (5–7) | 13 (17.8) | 3.82 (1.31–11.13) | **0.014** | 2.44 (0.78–7.65) | 0.127 |
| SQSTM1 expression | Low (0–2) | 29 (39.7) | 1.00 | | 1.00 | |
| | High (3–7) | 44 (60.3) | 4.75 (1.37–16.49) | **0.014** | 3.77 (1.06–13.38) | **0.040** |
| MAP1LC3B (L) SQSTM1 (L) | | 28 (38.4) | 1 | | 1 | |
| either | | 33 (45.2) | 1.66 (0.65–4.21) | 0.287 | 3.80 (1.04–13.86) | **0.043** |
| MAP1LC3B(H) SQSTM1 (H) | | 12 (16.4) | 4.01 (1.38–11.66) | **0.011** | 9.49 (2.19–41.08) | **0.003** |

Abbreviations: SCC, squamous cell carcinoma; CHR, crude hazard ratio; CI, confidence interval; AHR, adjusted hazard ratio. * p-value were adjusted for cell differentiation (moderate + poor vs. well) and AJCC pathological stage (stage III + IV vs stage I + II) by multiple Cox's regression. Bold values denote statistically significant.

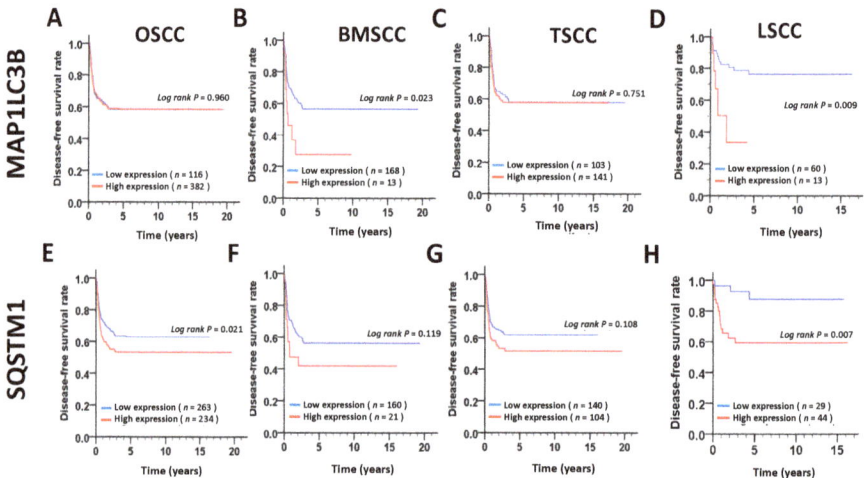

**Figure 4.** DFS survival curves for MAP1LC3B and SQSTM1 expression in patients with different subsites of OSCC. DFS survival curves of MAP1LC3 (**A–D**) and SQSTM1 (**E–H**) are shown for OSCC (**A,E**) and three main subsites, BMSCC (**B,F**), TSCC (**C,G**) and LSCC (**D,H**). The cutoff values for high or low expression of MAP1LC3B and SQSTM1 on tumor tissues were based on the receiver operating characteristic (ROC) curve.

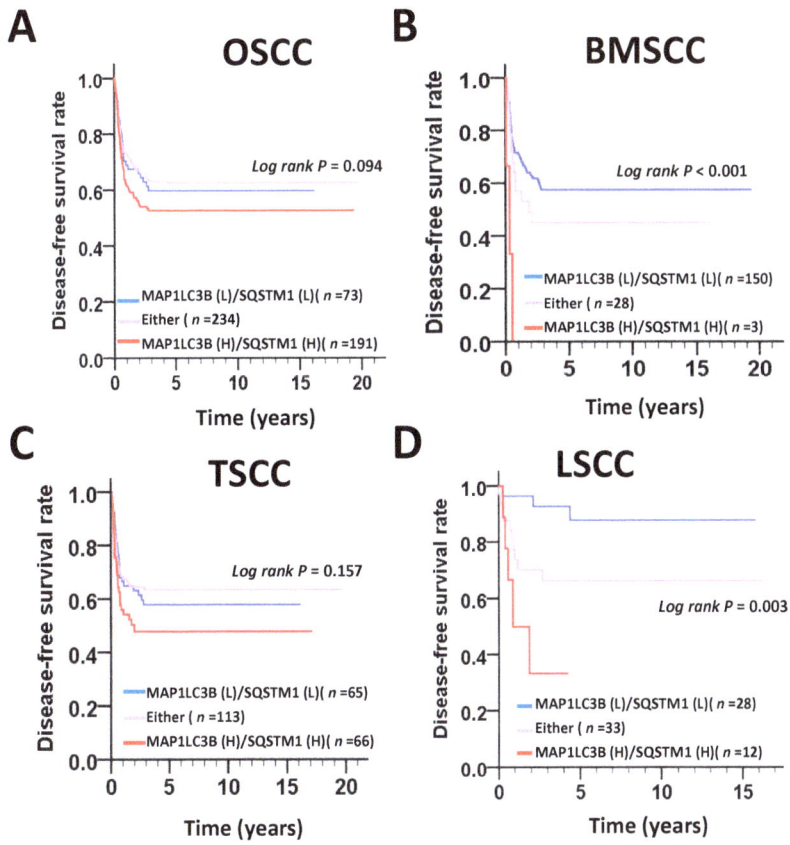

**Figure 5.** DFS survival curves for the coexpression of MAP1LC3B and SQSTM1 in patients with different subsites of OSCC. DFS survival curves for the coexpression of MAP1LC3 and SQSTM1 are shown for OSCC (**A**) and three main subsites, BMSCC (**B**), TSCC (**C**) and LSCC (**D**). The cutoff values for high or low coexpression of MAP1LC3B and SQSTM1 in tumor tissues were based on the receiver operating characteristic (ROC) curve

### 3.4. Involvement of MAP1LC3B and SQSTM1 in the Cell Proliferation and Migration of BMSCC Cells.

According to the clinical results described above, MAP1LC3B and SQSTM1 were more correlated with cancer malignancy in BMSCC and LSCC. Because there was no LSCC cell line available, we further verified the function of MAP1LC3B and SQSTM1 in BMSCC cell lines, including OC3 and TW2.6 (Figure 6A,B). Knockdown of MAP1LC3B resulted in accumulated SQSTM1 in BMSCC cells, while silencing SQSTM1 decreased MAP1LC3B-II flux, implying that deprivation of either MAP1LC3B and SQSTM1 diminished autophagic flux (Figure 6C,D). Similar to treatment with the autophagy inducer ConA, knockdown of MAP1LC3B or SQSTM1 attenuated cell proliferation in both OC3 and TW2.6 cells (Figure 7A). Autophagy is involved in cancer metastasis, and SQSTM1 is associated with lymph node invasion. To determine the effects of MAP1LC3B and SQSTM1 on metastatic characteristics, invasion assays were used. Silencing SQSTM1 inhibited both the invasive ability in highly invasive OC3 cells (OC3-I5, Figure 7B, Wang LH 2017, ROS1). We further mimicked the in vivo status in a tumorsphere culture model for cancer cell stemness (REF) and drug resistance (Figure 7C,D). Interestingly, ablation of MAP1LC3B or SQSTM1 or both decreased tumorsphere formation and enhanced the killing effects of paclitaxel (PTX, Figure 7C,D), implying that MAP1LC3B and SQSTM1 might modulate autophagy for tumor growth and drug resistance in BMSCC cells.

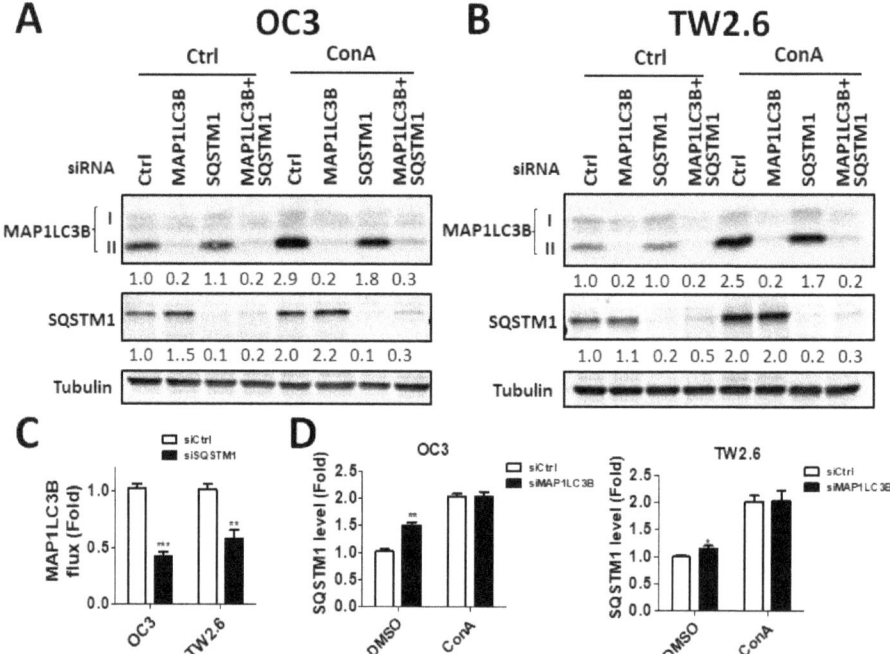

**Figure 6.** Effects of silencing MAP1LC3B and SQSTM1 on autophagy and cell proliferation in BMSCC cells. (**A**) The BMSCC cell lines OC3 and (**B**) TW2.6 were transfected with 5 nM scrambled siRNA or siRNA against MAP1LC3B or SQSTM1 for 48 h and then were treated with ConA for 4 h. The knockdown efficiency was determined by immunoblotting. (**C**) Silencing effects on MAP1LC3B flux and (**D**) SQSTM1 levels were quantified and analyzed.

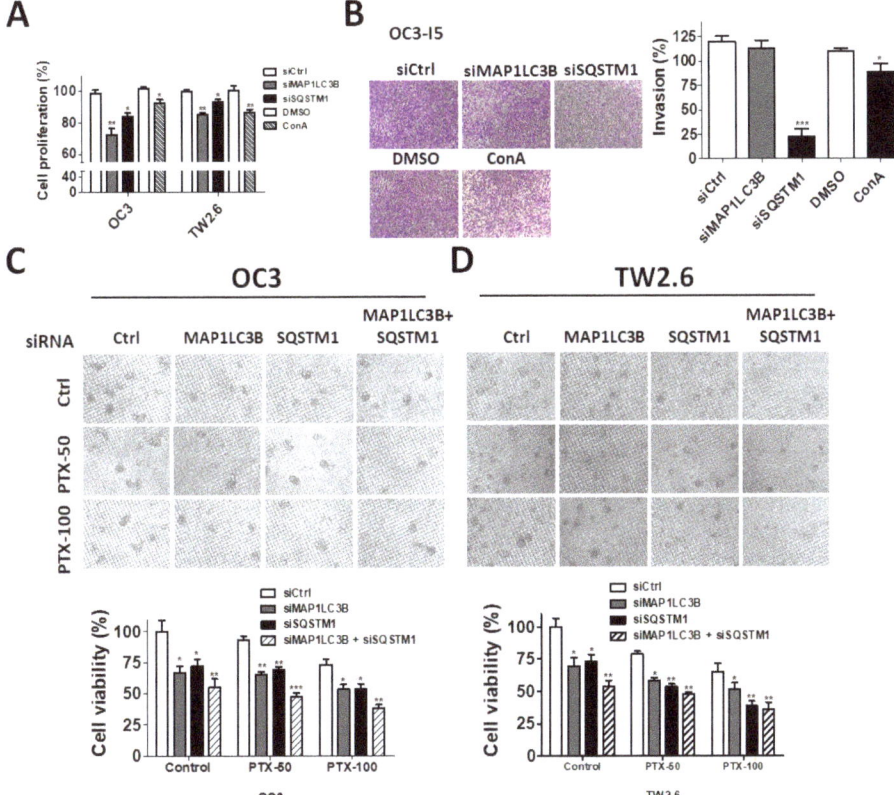

**Figure 7.** Effects of silencing MAP1LC3B and SQSTM1 on metastatic characteristics, tumorsphere formation and paclitaxel sensitivity in BMSCC cells. (**A**) The BMSCC cell lines OC3 and TW2.6 were transfected with 5 nM scrambled siRNA or siRNA against MAP1LC3B or SQSTM1 for 72 h to measure cell proliferation with Cell titer Glo. The cells treated with the autophagy inhibitor ConA for 24 h were used as a control. (**B**) OC3-I5 cells, the highly invasive strain of OC3, were silenced for 48 h and were seeded in Matrigel-coated Transwell filters to assess the cell invasion of BMSCC cells. (**C**) The silenced OC3 and (**D**) TW2.6 cells were cultured in nanoplates to examine tumorsphere formation. The tumorspheres were also treated with or without paclitaxel (PTX, 50 or 100 nM) to determine the effects of genes on drug resistance. The results represented three independent experiments.

## 4. Discussion

MAP1LC3B and SQSTM1 are widely used autophagy markers and adaptors in mammalian cells. Both proteins are essential for the autophagy machinery, and high expression levels of MAP1LC3B and SQSTM1 are significantly associated with an unfavorable clinicopathological outcome in several cancer types, including OSCC. However, the subsite-dependent impact of MAP1LC3B and SQSTM1 on OSCC, such as BMSCC, TSCC and LSCC, is not fully understood. Moreover, the function of MAP1LC3B and SQSTM1 in OSCC remains unclear. In this study, we reported the following findings. First, the expression levels of MAP1LC3B and SQSTM1 were higher in tumor tissues than in adjacent normal tissues at three subsites—BMSCC, TSCC and LSCC. Second, SQSTM1 was correlated with aggressive differentiation in three subsites and was associated with lymph node invasion in BMSCC. Third, SQSTM1 was positively correlated with MAP1LC3B in the tumor tissues of BMSCC, but not in adjacent normal tissues. High coexpression of MAP1LC3B and SQSTM1 was further associated with a poor survival, particularly in BMSCC and LSCC. Fourth, silencing of MAP1LC3B and SQSTM1 diminished autophagy, cell proliferation, and invasion and sensitized BMSCC cells to paclitaxel treatment. Our results suggested that MAP1LC3B and SQSTM1 may modulate autophagy for cancer development, malignancy and relapse in a subsite-dependent manner. To the best of our knowledge, we are the first group to report that the correlation of MAP1LC3B and SQSTM1 with clinicopathological outcomes at certain subsites using the largest cohort, comprising 498 paired tumor and adjacent normal tissues of OSCC.

MAP1LC3B is cleaved and activated by ATG4 to mediate a ubiquitination-like reaction to initiate autophagosome formation [18–20]. MAP1LC3B consists of a soluble form, MAP1LC3B-I, with a molecular weight of 18 KD and a membrane-bound form, MAP1LC3B-II, with a molecular weight of 16 KD. MAP1LC3B-II accumulates on the autophagosome and interacts with SQSTM1 for recruitment to damaged proteins to deliver them to lysosomes [21]. Thus, both MAP1LC3B-II and SQSTM1 can form puncta on autophagosomes during selective autophagy [21]. MAP1LC3B-II and SQSTM1 dot-like staining are shown in tissues and are associated with a poor prognosis in patients with colon cancer [22]. Increased MAP1LC3B puncta is also associated with a poor prognosis in several other cancer types, such as breast cancer and oral cancer [23,24]. However, the puncta of both MAP1LC3B-II and SQSTM1 were very rare in all tissues of our TMA, likely due to the different cancer types or tissues that we used. Moreover, increased MAP1LC3B expression typically shows unfavorable outcomes in lung, melanoma, and pancreatic cancers [25,26], whereas the loss of MAP1LC3B has been reported in several solid tumors, including brain cancer [27], prostate cancer [28], and breast cancer, indicating that MAP1LC3B expression in cancer is still controversial. In our present study, MAP1LC3B expression was higher in tumor tissues than in adjacent normal tissues at three subsites of OSCC. MAP1LC3B was positively correlated with DSS in patients with BMSCC and LSCC, but not in those with TSCC and OSCC. Deprivation of MAP1LC3B with siRNA suppressed cell viability and tumorsphere formation in BMSCC cell lines, implying that MAP1LC3B may contribute to tumorigenesis and malignancy at certain subsites of OSCC, particularly in BMSCC.

Autophagy induction causes SQSTM1 degradation, while defective autophagy leads to SQSTM1 accumulation. Higher SQSTM1 expression is associated with a poor prognosis in gastric cancer [29]. Previous studies have also reported that higher expression of SQSTM1 is correlated with a worse survival in several solid tumors [30,31]. These results suggest that autophagy impairment accumulates SQSTM1, ultimately leading to tumorigenesis by dysregulating the NF-κB signaling transduction pathway and gene expression [14,32]. The interaction of SQSTM1 with tumor necrosis factor receptor-associated factor (TRAF) 6, as well as the degradation of SQSTM1 by autophagy, is important for the role of SQSTM1 in tumorigenesis and cell survival [32]. Nevertheless, the correlation of SQSTM1 with detailed subsites of cancers has never been reported. Our present data show that, at three subsites of OSCC, cytoplasmic SQSTM1 protein expression in TAN tissue was significantly lower than that in tumor tissue. Additionally, SQSTM1 was significantly associated with N classification following Student's t test in BMSCC. Silencing SQSTM1 inhibited cancer cell invasion in BMSCC cells. In the Cox regression method, higher-level expression of cytoplasmic SQSTM1 was associated with a poor prognosis in OSCC, mainly in BMSCC and LSCC, implying that SQSTM1 could be an independent biomarker of the prognosis in BMSCC and LSCC.

The role of autophagy could be switched from a tumor suppressor to an oncogene during tumor progression. Autophagy acts as a tumor suppressor to eliminate abnormal proteins or organelles and reduce the production of reactive oxygen species and DNA damage in the early stage of cancer development [33]. Prodigiosin, a red pigment isolated from gram-negative bacteria, induces autophagic cell death in both lung and oral cancer cells [34,35]. By contrast, autophagy allows cancer cells to survive during metastasis and chemotherapy, which, in turn, results in tumor relapse [36,37]. Autophagic activity is higher in cancer stem cells (CSC) of ovarian cancer than in non-CSC [37]. Pharmacologic inhibition with the autophagy inhibitor chloroquine or genetic ablation with CRISPR/Cas9 knockout for the autophagy essential gene ATG5 significantly reduced the

CSC property and chemoresistance of ovarian cancer cells. Pharmacologic inhibition of the essential autophagy protease ATG4 with clinical drug tioconazole suppresses the tumor size and sensitizes cancer cells to doxorubicin [5]. Moreover, autophagy inhibition decreases metastatic outbreak and increases apoptosis in dormant BC cells [36]. Our study shows that higher cytoplasmic SQSTM1 expression is correlated with lymph node invasion in patients with BMSCC. The silencing of SQSTM1 reduces autophagic flux and invasion in BMSCC cells. SQSTM1 expression was positively correlated with MAP1LC3B expression in tumor tissues of patients with BMSCC. Furthermore, high expression of both MAP1LC3B and SQSTM1 was associated with a shorter DSS and DFS in patients with BMSCC and LSCC, but not in those with TSCC patients. Similar to treatment with autophagy inhibitor, knockdown of these genes repressed autophagy, cell proliferation and chemoresistance in BMSCC cells. Our present results suggested that autophagy may act as a tumor promoter at certain subsites of oral cancer, particularly in BMSCC.

On the other hand, autophagy diminishes the cytotoxic effects of T cells and natural killer (NK) cells against tumor cells [38,39]. PD-L1 inhibits autophagy through activation of MTOR, while the PD-L1 inhibitor attenuates autophagy for cancer cell survival [40]. The anti-malarial drug CQ or HCQ, which blocks autophagosome-lysosome fusion and degradation, has been tested in at least 30 clinical trials for cancer [41]. These results suggest that blocking autophagy might be helpful for cancer therapy of OSCC, which requires further study to evaluate.

**Author Contributions:** Conceptualization, C.W.S.; methodology, P.F.L., H.W.C. and J.S.C.; software, C.H.L.; validation, H.P.L., C.Y.Y., and W.L.T.; formal analysis, J.T.C.; investigation, C.W.S., P.F.L., H.W.C., and L.P.G.; resources, H.W.C.; data curation, Y.J.L.; writing—original draft preparation, P.F.L. and H.W.C.; writing—review and editing, C.W.S.; supervision, C.W.S.; and funding acquisition, C.W.S., P.F.L. and H.W.C.

**Funding:** The work was supported by the Ministry of Science and Technology MOST (106-2311-B-075B-001, 106-2320-B-075B-002, and 107-2311-B-214-003), Kaohsiung Veterans General Hospital (VGHKS106-158) and the Health and Welfare Surcharge of Tobacco Products, the Ministry of Health and Welfare, Taiwan, Republic of China (MOHW107-TDU-B-212-114016).

**Acknowledgments:** We thank Lu-Hai Wang for providing OC3-IV cells and great technical support from Ting-Ying Fu and Chih-Ting Huang.

**Conflicts of Interest:** The authors declare no conflict of interest.

## References

1. Mascolo, M.; Siano, M.; Ilardi, G.; Russo, D.; Merolla, F.; De Rosa, G.; Staibano, S. Epigenetic disregulation in oral cancer. *Int. J. Mol. Sci.* **2012**, *13*, 2331–2353. [CrossRef] [PubMed]
2. Blot, W.J.; McLaughlin, J.K.; Winn, D.M.; Austin, D.F.; Greenberg, R.S.; Preston-Martin, S.; Bernstein, L.; Schoenberg, J.B.; Stemhagen, A.; Fraumeni, J.F., Jr. Smoking and drinking in relation to oral and pharyngeal cancer. *Cancer Res.* **1988**, *48*, 3282–3287. [PubMed]
3. Fu, T.Y.; Wu, C.N.; Sie, H.C.; Cheng, J.T.; Lin, Y.S.; Liou, H.H.; Tseng, Y.K.; Shu, C.W.; Tsai, K.W.; Yen, L.M.; et al. Subsite-specific association of DEAD box RNA helicase DDX60 with the development and prognosis of oral squamous cell carcinoma. *Oncotarget* **2016**, *7*, 85097–85108. [CrossRef] [PubMed]
4. Rivera, C.; Venegas, B. Histological and molecular aspects of oral squamous cell carcinoma (Review). *Oncol. Lett.* **2014**, *8*, 7–11. [CrossRef] [PubMed]
5. Liu, P.F.; Tsai, K.L.; Hsu, C.J.; Tsai, W.L.; Cheng, J.S.; Chang, H.W.; Shiau, C.W.; Goan, Y.G.; Tseng, H.H.; Wu, C.H.; et al. Drug repurposing screening identifies tioconazole as an atg4 inhibitor that suppresses autophagy and sensitizes cancer cells to chemotherapy. *Theranostics* **2018**, *8*, 830–845. [CrossRef] [PubMed]
6. Zhong, Z.; Sanchez-Lopez, E.; Karin, M. Autophagy, inflammation, and immunity: A troika governing cancer and its treatment. *Cell* **2016**, *166*, 288–298. [CrossRef] [PubMed]
7. Monkkonen, T.; Debnath, J. Inflammatory signaling cascades and autophagy in cancer. *Autophagy* **2018**, *14*, 190–198. [CrossRef] [PubMed]
8. Amaravadi, R.; Kimmelman, A.C.; White, E. Recent insights into the function of autophagy in cancer. *Genes Dev.* **2016**, *30*, 1913–1930. [CrossRef] [PubMed]

9. Mizushima, N.; Komatsu, M. Autophagy: Renovation of cells and tissues. *Cell* **2011**, *147*, 728–741. [CrossRef] [PubMed]
10. Guo, J.Y.; Chen, H.Y.; Mathew, R.; Fan, J.; Strohecker, A.M.; Karsli-Uzunbas, G.; Kamphorst, J.J.; Chen, G.; Lemons, J.M.; Karantza, V.; et al. Activated Ras requires autophagy to maintain oxidative metabolism and tumorigenesis. *Genes Dev.* **2011**, *25*, 460–470. [CrossRef] [PubMed]
11. Guo, J.Y.; White, E. Autophagy, metabolism, and cancer. *Cold Spring Harb. Symp. Quant Biol.* **2016**, *81*, 73–78. [CrossRef] [PubMed]
12. Bortnik, S.; Gorski, S.M. Clinical applications of autophagy proteins in cancer: From potential targets to biomarkers. *Int. J. Mol. Sci.* **2017**, *18*, 1496. [CrossRef] [PubMed]
13. Lin, X.; Li, S.; Zhao, Y.; Ma, X.; Zhang, K.; He, X.; Wang, Z. Interaction domains of p62: A bridge between p62 and selective autophagy. *DNA Cell Biol.* **2013**, *32*, 220–227. [CrossRef] [PubMed]
14. Cohen-Kaplan, V.; Livneh, I.; Avni, N.; Fabre, B.; Ziv, T.; Kwon, Y.T.; Ciechanover, A. P62- and ubiquitin-dependent stress-induced autophagy of the mammalian 26S proteasome. *Proc. Natl. Acad. Sci. USA* **2016**, *113*, E7490–E7499. [CrossRef] [PubMed]
15. Rosenfeldt, M.T.; Nixon, C.; Liu, E.; Mah, L.Y.; Ryan, K.M. Analysis of macroautophagy by immunohistochemistry. *Autophagy* **2012**, *8*, 963–969. [CrossRef]
16. Shih, C.H.; Chang, Y.J.; Huang, W.C.; Jang, T.H.; Kung, H.J.; Wang, W.C.; Yang, M.H.; Lin, M.C.; Huang, S.F.; Chou, S.W.; et al. EZH2-mediated upregulation of ROS1 oncogene promotes oral cancer metastasis. *Oncogene* **2017**, *36*, 6542–6554. [CrossRef] [PubMed]
17. Liu, P.F.; Hsu, C.J.; Tsai, W.L.; Cheng, J.S.; Chen, J.J.; Huang, I.F.; Tseng, H.H.; Chang, H.W.; Shu, C.W. Ablation of ATG4B suppressed autophagy and activated AMPK for cell cycle arrest in cancer cells. *Cell Physiol. Biochem.* **2017**, *44*, 728–740. [CrossRef] [PubMed]
18. Tanida, I.; Tanida-Miyake, E.; Ueno, T.; Kominami, E. The human homolog of Saccharomyces cerevisiae Apg7p is a Protein-activating enzyme for multiple substrates including human Apg12p, GATE-16, GABARAP, and MAP-LC3. *J. Biol. Chem.* **2001**, *276*, 1701–1706. [CrossRef] [PubMed]
19. Shu, C.W.; Drag, M.; Bekes, M.; Zhai, D.; Salvesen, G.S.; Reed, J.C. Synthetic substrates for measuring activity of autophagy proteases: Autophagins (Atg4). *Autophagy* **2010**, *6*, 936–947. [CrossRef] [PubMed]
20. Li, M.; Fu, Y.; Yang, Z.; Yin, X.M. Measurement of the activity of the Atg4 cysteine proteases. *Methods Enzymol* **2017**, *587*, 207–225. [PubMed]
21. Yoshii, S.R.; Mizushima, N. Monitoring and measuring autophagy. *Int. J. Mol. Sci.* **2017**, *18*, 1856. [CrossRef] [PubMed]
22. Niklaus, M.; Adams, O.; Berezowska, S.; Zlobec, I.; Graber, F.; Slotta-Huspenina, J.; Nitsche, U.; Rosenberg, R.; Tschan, M.P.; Langer, R. Expression analysis of LC3B and p62 indicates intact activated autophagy is associated with an unfavorable prognosis in colon cancer. *Oncotarget* **2017**, *8*, 54604–54615. [CrossRef] [PubMed]
23. Ladoire, S.; Chaba, K.; Martins, I.; Sukkurwala, A.Q.; Adjemian, S.; Michaud, M.; Poirier-Colame, V.; Andreiuolo, F.; Galluzzi, L.; White, E.; et al. Immunohistochemical detection of cytoplasmic LC3 puncta in human cancer specimens. *Autophagy* **2012**, *8*, 1175–1184. [CrossRef] [PubMed]
24. Liu, J.L.; Chen, F.F.; Lung, J.; Lo, C.H.; Lee, F.H.; Lu, Y.C.; Hung, C.H. Prognostic significance of p62/SQSTM1 subcellular localization and LC3B in oral squamous cell carcinoma. *Br. J. Cancer* **2014**, *111*, 944–954. [CrossRef] [PubMed]
25. Han, C.; Sun, B.; Wang, W.; Cai, W.; Lou, D.; Sun, Y.; Zhao, X. Overexpression of microtubule-associated protein-1 light chain 3 is associated with melanoma metastasis and vasculogenic mimicry. *Tohoku J. Exp. Med.* **2011**, *223*, 243–251. [CrossRef] [PubMed]
26. Karpathiou, G.; Sivridis, E.; Koukourakis, M.I.; Mikroulis, D.; Bouros, D.; Froudarakis, M.E.; Giatromanolaki, A. Light-chain 3A autophagic activity and prognostic significance in non-small cell lung carcinomas. *Chest* **2011**, *140*, 127–134. [CrossRef] [PubMed]
27. Huang, X.; Bai, H.M.; Chen, L.; Li, B.; Lu, Y.C. Reduced expression of LC3B-II and Beclin 1 in glioblastoma multiforme indicates a down-regulated autophagic capacity that relates to the progression of astrocytic tumors. *J. Clin. Neurosci.* **2010**, *17*, 1515–1519. [CrossRef] [PubMed]
28. Giatromanolaki, A.; Sivridis, E.; Mendrinos, S.; Koutsopoulos, A.V.; Koukourakis, M.I. Autophagy proteins in prostate cancer: Relation with anaerobic metabolism and Gleason score. *Urol. Oncol.* **2014**, *32*, 39.e11–39.e18. [CrossRef] [PubMed]

29. Mohamed, A.; Ayman, A.; Deniece, J.; Wang, T.; Kovach, C.; Siddiqui, M.T.; Cohen, C. P62/Ubiquitin IHC expression correlated with clinicopathologic parameters and outcome in gastrointestinal carcinomas. *Front Oncol.* **2015**, *5*, 70. [CrossRef] [PubMed]
30. Ruan, H.; Xu, J.; Wang, L.; Zhao, Z.; Kong, L.; Lan, B.; Li, X. The prognostic value of p62 in solid tumor patients: A meta-analysis. *Oncotarget* **2018**, *9*, 4258–4266. [CrossRef] [PubMed]
31. Iwadate, R.; Inoue, J.; Tsuda, H.; Takano, M.; Furuya, K.; Hirasawa, A.; Aoki, D.; Inazawa, J. High expression of p62 protein is associated with poor prognosis and aggressive phenotypes in endometrial cancer. *Am. J. Pathol.* **2015**, *185*, 2523–2533. [CrossRef] [PubMed]
32. Mathew, R.; Karp, C.M.; Beaudoin, B.; Vuong, N.; Chen, G.; Chen, H.Y.; Bray, K.; Reddy, A.; Bhanot, G.; Gelinas, C.; et al. Autophagy suppresses tumorigenesis through elimination of p62. *Cell* **2009**, *137*, 1062–1075. [CrossRef] [PubMed]
33. Tang, J.Y.; Farooqi, A.A.; Ou-Yang, F.; Hou, M.F.; Huang, H.W.; Wang, H.R.; Li, K.T.; Fayyaz, S.; Shu, C.W.; Chang, H.W. Oxidative stress-modulating drugs have preferential anticancer effects-involving the regulation of apoptosis, DNA damage, endoplasmic reticulum stress, autophagy, metabolism, and migration. *Semin. Cancer Biol.* **2018**. Available online: https://www.sciencedirect.com/science/article/pii/S1044579X18300841 (accessed on 24 August 2018). [CrossRef] [PubMed]
34. Chiu, W.J.; Lin, S.R.; Chen, Y.H.; Tsai, M.J.; Leong, M.K.; Weng, C.F. Prodigiosin-emerged PI3K/Beclin-1-independent pathway elicits autophagic cell death in doxorubicin-sensitive and -resistant lung cancer. *J. Clin. Med.* **2018**, *7*, 321. [CrossRef] [PubMed]
35. Lin, S.R.; Weng, C.F. PG-priming enhances doxorubicin influx to trigger necrotic and autophagic cell death in oral squamous cell carcinoma. *J. Clin. Med.* **2018**, *7*, 375. [CrossRef] [PubMed]
36. Vera-Ramirez, L.; Vodnala, S.K.; Nini, R.; Hunter, K.W.; Green, J.E. Autophagy promotes the survival of dormant breast cancer cells and metastatic tumour recurrence. *Nat. Commun.* **2018**, *9*, 1944. [CrossRef] [PubMed]
37. Pagotto, A.; Pilotto, G.; Mazzoldi, E.L.; Nicoletto, M.O.; Frezzini, S.; Pasto, A.; Amadori, A. Autophagy inhibition reduces chemoresistance and tumorigenic potential of human ovarian cancer stem cells. *Cell Death Dis.* **2017**, *8*, e2943. [CrossRef] [PubMed]
38. Jaboin, J.J.; Hwang, M.; Lu, B. Autophagy in lung cancer. *Method Enzymol.* **2009**, *453*, 287–304.
39. Tittarelli, A.; Janji, B.; Van Moer, K.; Noman, M.Z.; Chouaib, S. The selective degradation of synaptic connexin 43 protein by hypoxia-induced autophagy impairs natural killer cell-mediated tumor cell killing. *J. Biol. Chem.* **2015**, *290*, 23670–23679. [CrossRef] [PubMed]
40. Clark, C.A.; Gupta, H.B.; Curiel, T.J. Tumor cell-intrinsic CD274/PD-L1: A novel metabolic balancing act with clinical potential. *Autophagy* **2017**, *13*, 987–988. [CrossRef] [PubMed]
41. Chude, C.I.; Amaravadi, R.K. targeting autophagy in cancer: Update on clinical trials and novel inhibitors. *Int. J. Mol. Sci.* **2017**, *18*, 1279. [CrossRef] [PubMed]

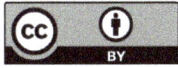

© 2018 by the authors. Licensee MDPI, Basel, Switzerland. This article is an open access article distributed under the terms and conditions of the Creative Commons Attribution (CC BY) license (http://creativecommons.org/licenses/by/4.0/).

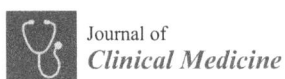 

*Article*

# High Risk of Deep Neck Infection in Patients with Type 1 Diabetes Mellitus: A Nationwide Population-Based Cohort Study

Geng-He Chang [1,2,3,†], Meng-Chang Ding [1,†], Yao-Hsu Yang [2,4,5], Yung-Hsiang Lin [6], Chia-Yen Liu [2], Meng-Hung Lin [2], Ching-Yuan Wu [4,5], Cheng-Ming Hsu [1,5] and Ming-Shao Tsai [1,2,3,*]

1. Department of Otolaryngology, Chiayi Chang Gung Memorial Hospital, Chiayi 613, Taiwan; genghechang@gmail.com (G.-H.C.); tny4646@gmail.com (M.-C.D.); scm00031@gmail.com (C.-M.H.)
2. Health Information and Epidemiology Laboratory, Chiayi Chang Gung Memorial Hospital, Chiayi 613, Taiwan; r95841012@ntu.edu.tw (Y.-H.Y.); qchiayen@gmail.com (C.-Y.L.); mattlin@cgmh.org.tw (M.-H.L.)
3. Graduate Institute of Clinical Medical Sciences, College of Medicine, Chang Gung University, Taoyuan 33302, Taiwan
4. Department of Traditional Chinese Medicine, Chiayi Chang Gung Memorial Hospital, Chiayi 613, Taiwan; smbepigwu77@gmail.com
5. School of Traditional Chinese Medicine, College of Medicine, Chang Gung University, Taoyuan 33302, Taiwan
6. Division of Endocrinology and Metabolism, Chiayi Chang Gung Memorial Hospital, Chiayi 613, Taiwan; bryam1130@gmail.com
* Correspondence: b87401061@cgmh.org.tw; Tel.: +886-975366272; Fax: +886-53623002
† The author contributed equally to this work.

Received: 30 September 2018; Accepted: 23 October 2018; Published: 25 October 2018

**Abstract:** Objective: To investigate the risk of deep neck infection (DNI) in patients with type 1 diabetes mellitus (T1DM). Methods: The database of the Registry for Catastrophic Illness Patients, affiliated to the Taiwan National Health Insurance Research Database, was used to conduct a retrospective cohort study. In total, 5741 patients with T1DM and 22,964 matched patients without diabetes mellitus (DM) were enrolled between 2000 and 2010. The patients were followed up until death or the end of the study period (31 December 2013). The primary outcome was the occurrence of DNI. Results: Patients with T1DM exhibited a significantly higher cumulative incidence of DNI than did those without DM ($p < 0.001$). The Cox proportional hazards model showed that T1DM was significantly associated with a higher incidence of DNI (adjusted hazard ratio, 10.71; 95% confidence interval, 6.02–19.05; $p < 0.001$). The sensitivity test and subgroup analysis revealed a stable effect of T1DM on DNI risk. The therapeutic methods (surgical or nonsurgical) did not differ significantly between the T1DM and non-DM cohorts. Patients with T1DM required significantly longer hospitalization for DNI than did those without DM ($9.0 \pm 6.2$ vs. $4.1 \pm 2.0$ days, $p < 0.001$). Furthermore, the patients with T1DM were predisposed to DNI at a younger age than were those without DM. Conclusions: T1DM is an independent risk factor for DNI and is associated with a 10-fold increase in DNI risk. The patients with T1DM require longer hospitalizations for DNI and are younger than those without DM.

**Keywords:** cervical; cellulitis; abscess; deep neck infection; diabetes mellitus

## 1. Introduction

Deep neck infection (DNI) is a common infectious disease involving the deep neck space; DNI usually requires intensive care and aggressive treatment [1]. The easy availability of antibiotics, improvements in diagnostic technology, and the concept of early surgical debridement have significantly reduced the morbidity and mortality of DNI [2,3]. However, DNI remains a potentially life-threatening disease when lethal complications, such as descending necrotizing mediastinitis, develop [4,5].

A study reported that patients with diabetes mellitus (DM) are at a 1.4-fold higher risk of DNI than those without DM [6]. DNI can cause higher morbidity and mortality among patients with systemic diseases such as DM, end-stage renal disease, liver cirrhosis, and autoimmune diseases [1,4,7–9]. However, the pathogenesis of type 1 DM (T1DM) is different from that of type 2 DM (T2DM). T1DM is characterized by an immune-mediated depletion of beta cells, which causes a lifelong dependence on exogenous insulin [10]. Patients with T1DM, considered to have an immunocompromised status, are expected to be more vulnerable to complicated infection and have a higher infection-related mortality risk than patients with T2DM [11]. Studies investigating the effect of T1DM on DNI are not currently available in the literature. This study investigated the effect of T1DM on DNI occurrence, treatment, and prognosis.

## 2. Methods

### 2.1. Data Source

The government of Taiwan established the National Health Insurance Research Database (NHIRD), which covered 99.6% of Taiwan's population in 2017 [12,13]. The NHIRD provides all medical claims data of all beneficiaries, including disease diagnoses during clinic visits and hospitalization, prescription drugs and doses, examinations, procedures, surgery, payments, resident locations, and income levels, generated during reimbursement for insurance in an electronic format. The diagnostic codes in the NHIRD are based on the International Classification of Diseases, Ninth Revision, Clinical Modification (ICD-9-CM). This study was exempted from obtaining informed consent from the participants because the data were deidentified. All information of the insurants was unidentifiable, and this study did not violate their rights or adversely affect their welfare. The study was approved by the Institutional Review Board of Chang Gung Memorial Hospital (IRB Number: 201601249B1).

### 2.2. Study Cohort

In Taiwan, T1DM is categorized as a "catastrophic illness" in the NHIRD. Patients with T1DM are certified by the government and included in the Registry for Catastrophic Illness Patients (RFCIP). Therefore, they can avail considerable discounts on medical expenses. The certification process requires critical evaluation of medical records, serological, and pathological reports by experts [14]. Therefore, the T1DM diagnosis of the enrolled patients was highly accurate and reliable.

Data regarding patients who received new diagnoses of T1DM between January 2000 and December 2010 in Taiwan were retrieved from the RFCIP (Figure 1). The patients who received T1DM diagnoses in or after 2011 were not included to ensure a follow-up period of at least 3 years. We used the following T1DM-associated ICD-9-CM codes, which were defined for the RFCIP: 250.01, 250.03, 250.11, 250.13, 250.21, 250.23, 250.31, 250.33, 250.41, 250.43, 250.51, 250.53, 250.61, 250.63, 250.71, 250.73, 250.81, 250.83, 250.91, and 250.93 [14]. In addition, patients who received DNI diagnoses before T1DM were excluded. Finally, 6201 patients with T1DM were enrolled in the study cohort.

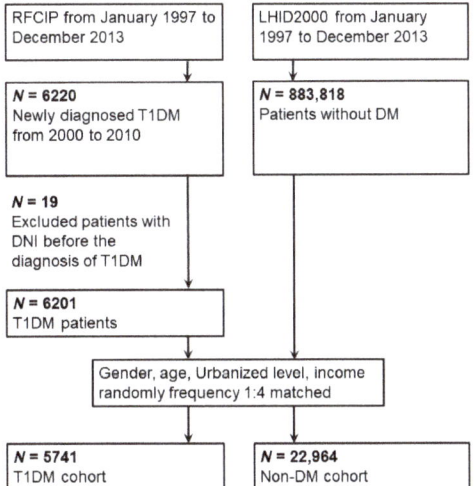

**Figure 1.** Enrollment schema of the study and comparison cohorts. Abbreviations: RFCIP, Registry for Catastrophic Illness Patients; LHID2000, Longitudinal Health Insurance Database 2000; DM, diabetes mellitus; T1DM, type 1 diabetes mellitus; DNI, deep neck infection.

### 2.3. Comparison Cohort

The Longitudinal Health Insurance Database 2000 (LHID2000), a subset database of the NHIRD, consists of 1,000,000 insurants who were randomly statistically selected from all insurants in Taiwan in 2000. Age distribution, sex distribution, or health care costs did not differ significantly between the LHID2000 sample group and all enrollees in the NHIRD, according to a report by the National Health Research Institutes [13]. The LHID2000 has been used in several population-based studies [15,16]. We used the LHID2000 to generate a comparison cohort, which consisted of patients without DM.

### 2.4. Matching Process

For each patient with T1DM, four patients without DM were randomly selected from the LHID2000 database, matched for sex, age, urbanization level, and income level to form a comparison cohort. The index date of the study cohort was the date of registry in the RFCIP for patients with T1DM, and an index date matching that of patients with T1DM was created for the comparison cohort. After the matching process, 5741 T1DM and 22,964 non-DM patients were enrolled in the study.

### 2.5. Main Outcome

The main outcome of this study was the occurrence of DNI, which is defined as hospitalization with the following ICD-9 codes: 528.3 (cellulitis and abscess of oral soft tissues; Ludwig angina), 478.22 (parapharyngeal abscess), 478.24 (retropharyngeal abscess), and 682.1 (cellulitis and abscess of neck) [1,17]. The follow-up period was from the index date to the diagnosis of DNI, death, or the end of 2013.

### 2.6. Comorbidities

Comorbidities were defined using ICD-9-CM codes recorded in the claims data: hypertension (HTN) (ICD-9-CM codes: 401–405), cerebrovascular accident (CVA) (ICD-9-CM codes: 430–438), coronary artery disease (CAD) (ICD-9-CM codes: 410–414), chronic kidney disease (CKD) (ICD-9-CM codes: 403, 404, 585, and 586), systemic autoimmune diseases (SADs) (ICD-9-CM codes: 443.1, 446.0, 446.2, 446.4–446.5, 446.7, 696.0–696.1, 710.0–710.4, and 714.0–714.1), and liver cirrhosis (LC) (ICD-9-CM codes: 571.2, 571.5–571.6) [1,17–19]. Medical comorbidities were included if they appeared at least once in the diagnoses of inpatients or at least thrice in the diagnoses of outpatients.

## 2.7. Treatment Modalities

The treatment methods were divided into two subgroups: "surgical" and "nonsurgical." The patients who received surgical intervention were included in the "surgical" subgroup, whereas those who received antibiotic or abscess aspiration without surgery were included in the "nonsurgical" subgroup [1].

## 2.8. Prognosis Evaluation

For evaluating prognosis, we analyzed the duration of hospitalization, care in intensive care units (ICUs), performance of tracheostomy, and mediastinal complications, which were defined according to the receipt of mediastinal surgery during hospitalization or the diagnostic codes of mediastinitis (ICD-9-CM codes: 510, 513, and 519.2) [1]. Mortality and mediastinitis-related mortality were also investigated in both cohorts. Mortality was defined as death occurring during DNI treatment. Mediastinitis-related mortality was defined as death during DNI treatment accompanied by the diagnosis of mediastinitis [1]. In addition, we analyzed the age distribution of the patients with DNI identified in the T1DM and non-DM cohorts.

## 2.9. Statistical Analysis

The demographic characteristic and comorbidities of the T1DM and non-DM cohorts were compared using the Pearson's chi-square test for categorical variables and the unpaired Student $t$-test for continuous variables. Control variables, such as age, sex, urbanization level, income level, and comorbidities (HTN, CVA, CAD, CKD, SADs, and LC) were included as covariates in the univariate model. Variables in the univariate analysis that showed $p < 0.1$ were included in the multivariate analysis. Kaplan–Meier analysis was used to estimate the cumulative incidence in the two cohorts, and the differences were determined using a two-tailed log-rank test. Multivariable Cox proportional hazard regression models were used to measure the hazard ratio (HR) and 95% confidence interval (CI) of DNI incidence between the T1DM and non-DM cohorts. In addition, the stability of HR was examined using sensitivity testing and subgroup analysis if the interaction effects between the comorbidities and T1DM on DNI were significant. All analyses were performed using SAS software, version 9.4 (SAS Institute, Cary, NC, USA), and the level of statistical significance was set at $p < 0.05$.

## 3. Results

Table 1 illustrates the distribution of sociodemographic characteristics, DNIs, and comorbidities identified in the T1DM and non-DM cohorts. The T1DM cohort exhibited a significantly higher prevalence of DNI, HTN, CVA, CAD, CKD, SADs, and LC. Among the 5741 patients with T1DM, 42 (0.7%) patients with DNI were identified, and the incidence rate was 92.4 per 100,000 person-years in a mean follow-up period of 7.91 ± 2.41 years. By contrast, among the 22,964 controls, 16 (0.1%) patients with DNI were identified in a mean observation period of 8.08 ± 2.29 years, and the incidence rate was 8.6 per 100,000 person-years. The incidence rate ratio was 10.73 with a 95% CI of 6.03–19.08. The incidence of DNI was significantly higher in the T1DM cohort than in the non-DM cohort ($p < 0.001$).

Table 1. Demographic characteristics of the T1DM and non-DM cohorts.

| Characteristic | T1DM N | T1DM % | Non-DM N | Non-DM % | p-Value * |
|---|---|---|---|---|---|
| Total | 5741 | | 22,964 | | |
| Gender | | | | | 1 |
| Male | 2777 | 48.4 | 11,108 | 48.4 | |
| Female | 2964 | 51.6 | 11,856 | 51.6 | |
| Age (years) | | | | | 1 |
| <20 | 2751 | 47.9 | 11,004 | 47.9 | |
| ≥20 | 2990 | 52.1 | 11,960 | 52.1 | |
| Urbanized level | | | | | 1 |
| 1 (City) | 1616 | 28.2 | 6464 | 28.2 | |
| 2 | 2662 | 46.4 | 10,648 | 46.4 | |
| 3 | 867 | 15.1 | 3468 | 15.1 | |
| 4 (Village) | 596 | 10.4 | 2384 | 10.4 | |
| Income (NTD, per month) | | | | | 1 |
| 0 | 4005 | 69.8 | 16,020 | 69.8 | |
| 1–15,840 | 608 | 10.6 | 2432 | 10.6 | |
| 15,841–25,000 | 731 | 12.7 | 2924 | 12.7 | |
| ≥25,001 | 397 | 6.9 | 1588 | 6.9 | |
| Comorbidities | | | | | |
| HTN | 1073 | 18.7 | 1192 | 5.2 | <0.001 |
| CVA | 227 | 4.0 | 350 | 1.5 | <0.001 |
| CAD | 340 | 5.9 | 435 | 1.9 | <0.001 |
| CKD | 332 | 5.8 | 111 | 0.5 | <0.001 |
| SADs | 139 | 2.4 | 388 | 1.7 | <0.001 |
| LC | 118 | 2.1 | 89 | 0.4 | <0.001 |
| DNI | | | | | |
| Total | 42 | 0.7 | 16 | 0.1 | <0.001 |

Abbreviations: T1DM, type 1 diabetes mellitus; NTD, New Taiwan dollar; HTN, hypertension; CVA, cerebrovascular accident; CAD, coronary artery disease; CKD, chronic kidney disease; SADs, systemic autoimmune diseases; LC, liver cirrhosis; DNI, deep neck infection. * Pearson's chi-square test.

Results of the Kaplan–Meier analysis revealed the cumulative incidence of DNI in both the cohorts over a 10-year observation period. The T1DM cohort exhibited a significantly higher incidence of DNI than the non-DM cohort did (log-rank test $p < 0.001$, Figure 2). The Cox proportional hazards model revealed that T1DM was associated with a 10-fold higher risk of DNI (adjusted HR: 10.71, 95% CI: 6.02–19.05, $p < 0.001$, Table 2). In addition, the sensitivity test showed a stable effect of T1DM on DNI risk in the study cohort in the main model with each additional covariate. The results of subgroup analysis showed that T1DM is a risk factor for DNI in all the subgroups.

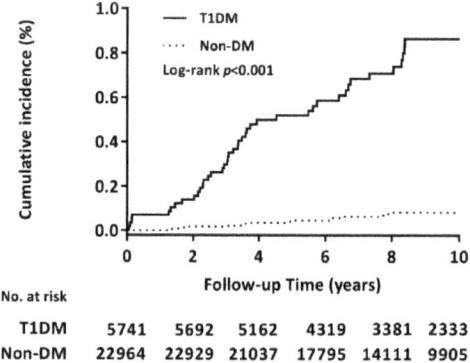

No. at risk

| | | | | | | |
|---|---|---|---|---|---|---|
| T1DM | 5741 | 5692 | 5162 | 4319 | 3381 | 2333 |
| Non-DM | 22964 | 22929 | 21037 | 17795 | 14111 | 9905 |

**Figure 2.** Cumulative incidence of DNI in the T1DM versus non-DM cohorts. Kaplan–Meier analysis demonstrated the cumulative DNI identified in the T1DM and non-DM cohorts during the 10-year follow-up period. The log-rank test revealed a significantly higher cumulative incidence in the T1DM cohort than in the non-DM cohort ($p < 0.001$).

**Table 2.** Multivariable Cox proportional hazards model for associations between DNI and T1DM.

| Variables | HR | 95% CI | p-Value |
|---|---|---|---|
| **Main model \*** | 10.71 | (6.02–19.05) | <0.001 |
| **Additional covariates †** | | | |
| Main model + HTN | 10.20 | (5.66–18.38) | <0.001 |
| Main model + CVA | 10.54 | (5.91–18.77) | <0.001 |
| Main model + CAD | 10.67 | (5.99–19.04) | <0.001 |
| Main model + CKD | 10.36 | (5.79–18.56) | <0.001 |
| Main model + SADs | 10.66 | (5.99–18.97) | <0.001 |
| Main model + LC | 10.27 | (5.75–18.33) | <0.001 |
| **Subgroup effects** | | | |
| **Gender** | | | |
| Male | 4.69 | (2.12–10.38) | <0.001 |
| Female | 24.67 | (8.51–71.52) | <0.001 |
| **Age** | | | |
| <20 | 14.28 | (5.74–35.56) | <0.001 |
| ≥20 | 6.88 | (3.07–15.39) | <0.001 |
| **Without selected comorbidity** | | | |
| HTN | 10.03 | (5.40–18.63) | <0.001 |
| CVA | 9.41 | (5.17–17.14) | <0.001 |
| CAD | 9.34 | (5.13–17.00) | <0.001 |
| CKD | 9.47 | (5.22–17.20) | <0.001 |
| SADs | 9.27 | (5.09–16.88) | <0.001 |
| LC | 9.67 | (5.32–17.56) | <0.001 |

\* Main model was adjusted for sex, age, urbanized level, and income. † The model was adjusted for sex, age, urbanized level, income, and each additional comorbidity. Abbreviations: DNI, deep neck infection; T1DM, type 1 diabetes mellitus; NTD, New Taiwan dollar; HTN, hypertension; CVA, cerebrovascular accident; CAD, coronary artery disease; CKD, chronic kidney disease; SADs, systemic autoimmune diseases; LC, liver cirrhosis.

Table 3 presents the treatment modalities and prognosis of DNI in the patients in both cohorts (Table 3). Although the percentage of patients requiring surgical treatment for DNI was higher in the T1DM cohort than in the non-DM cohort, the difference in the percentages was not significant (T1DM vs. non-DM cohorts = 33.3% vs. 18.8%, $p = 0.276$). DNI in the patients in the T1DM cohort required longer hospitalization durations than did those in the non-DM cohort (T1DM vs. non-DM cohorts: $9.0 \pm 6.2$ vs. $4.1 \pm 2.0$ days, $p < 0.001$). Furthermore, care in ICU and mediastinal complications were only identified in patients with T1DM and DNI (ICU: 6/42, 14.3%; mediastinitis: 1/42, 2.4%). DNI-related mortality was observed in the T1DM cohort (mortality: 2/42, 4.8%) but not in the non-DM cohort.

**Table 3.** Treatment modalities, complications, and prognostic outcomes in patients with DNI.

| Characteristic | T1DM-DNI | | Non-DM-DNI | | p-Value |
|---|---|---|---|---|---|
| | N | % | N | % | |
| Total | 42 | | 16 | | |
| Therapy | | | | | 0.276 [a] |
| Non-surgery | 28 | 66.7 | 13 | 81.3 | |
| Surgery | 14 | 33.3 | 3 | 18.8 | |
| Tracheostomy | 0 | 0.0 | 0 | 0.0 | |
| Hospitalization (day, mean $\pm$ SD) | $9.0 \pm 6.2$ | | $4.1 \pm 2.0$ | | <0.001 [b] |
| ICU care | 6 | 14.3 | 0 | 0.0 | |
| Mediastinitis | 1 | 2.4 | 0 | 0.0 | |
| Mediastinitis-Mortality | 1 | 2.4 | 0 | 0.0 | |
| Mortality * | 2 | 4.8 | 0 | 0.0 | |

* Mortality occurrence after DNI. [a] Pearson's chi-square tests. [b] Student t-tests. Abbreviations: DNI, deep neck infection; SD, standard deviation; ICU, intensive care unit.

Figure 3 presents the age distribution of DNI identified in the T1DM and non-DM cohorts. We divided the age into the following four groups: <10, 10–20, 21–40, and >40 years. Accordingly, the proportions of DNI in the two cohorts (T1DM vs. non-DM) were 2.38% vs. 18.75% (<10 years), 40.47% vs. 18.75% (10–20 years), 42.86% vs. 50% (21–40 years), and 14.28% vs. 12.5% (>40 years). In this study, the peak age of DNI occurrence in the non-DM cohort was 21–40 years, while the T1DM cohort exhibited two peak ages, namely 10–20 and 21–40 years.

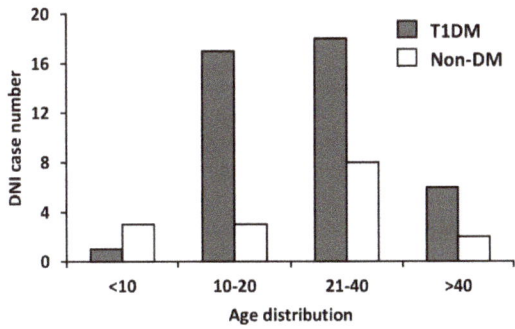

**Figure 3.** Age distribution of DNI in the T1DM and non-DM cohorts. The peak age of DNI occurrence in the non-DM cohort was 21–40 years, while those in the T1DM cohort were 10–20 years and 21–40 years.

## 4. Discussion

Our nationwide study is the first to examine the influence of T1DM on DNI. Our study demonstrated that T1DM is a definite risk factor for DNI. Our results revealed that patients with T1DM are at a 10-fold higher risk of DNI than were those without DM. The higher frequency of infections in patients with T1DM is attributable to hyperglycemia, which results in immune dysfunction, including disrupted neutrophil function, depression of the antioxidant system and humoral immunity, micro- and macroangiopathies, neuropathy, decrease in the antibacterial activity of urine, gastrointestinal and urinary dysmotility, and the need for medical intervention in these patients [20].

Patients with T1DM are more likely to have complicated infections, such as pneumonia, septicemia, and osteomyelitis, than are those without DM [21]. Simonsen et al. reported that the incidence of bacterial infections was significantly higher in patients with T1DM than in those without DM [22]. Muller et al. reported that patients with T1DM and T2DM have an increased risk of infections of the lower respiratory tract, urinary tract, and skin and mucous membranes [23]. In addition, an Australian diabetes register-based study revealed that patients with T1DM exhibited significantly higher infection-related mortality (pneumonia, septicemia, and osteomyelitis) than did those with T2DM [11]. Therefore, T1DM is a risk factor for complicated infections, and it might be associated with higher incidence and severity of infection than T2DM.

Previous studies have reported that surgical treatment was used in 55–80% of patients with DNI [4,9,24–28]. In our study, few patients received surgical treatment in both the cohorts (T1DM: 33.3% and non-DM: 18.7%). This difference in percentage may result from previous studies being conducted in medical centers or tertiary hospitals, which receive and treat patients with severe DNI [4,8,9,24–27]. Hence, patients with severe DNI were more likely accept surgical interventions. However, we enrolled patients from all hospitals in our nationwide study. The distribution of patients with DNI was from primary to tertiary hospitals, and patients with low DNI severity were also included; thus, our study provided a complete spectrum of DNI treatment and prognosis [1]. In general, the use of surgical interventions to treat a DNI indicates that the infection is more severe and life-threatening. In our study, the percentage of surgical treatment for DNI was higher in the T1DM cohort than in the non-DM cohort; however, the difference was not statistically significant.

DNIs in patients with DM have been reported to be associated with long hospitalization durations and numerous complications [4,28–30]. In our study, the duration of hospitalization for DNI was significantly higher in the T1DM than in the non-DM cohort, and this result was consistent with previously reported findings. Patients with T1DM and DNI were reported to exhibit a higher frequency of lethal complications, such as mediastinitis (2.7–10.0%), and higher mortality (1.6–7.5%) than those without DM [4,28,29]. A higher rate of ICU care for DNI was noted in patients with T1DM than with those without DM [1]. In our study, the occurrence of ICU care for DNI, mediastinitis, and DNI-related mortality was higher in the T1DM cohort than in the non-DM cohort, and these results were consistent with those of previous studies.

We analyzed the age distribution of DNI in the T1DM and non-DM cohorts in our study. In the non-DM cohort, the peak age of DNI occurrence was 21–40 years, while in the T1DM cohort, the two peak ages of DNI occurrence were 10–20 years and 21–40 years. In addition, in the T1DM cohort, DNI developed at age 10–20 years. In general, the incidence of DNI was higher at age 20–40 years. Patients with diabetes have been reported to have a late onset of DNI [24,25,28,31]. However, T1DM was characterized by diagnosis at a young age; according to Magliano's report, infection (pneumonia, septicemia, and osteomyelitis) at a young age was more likely to occur in patients with T1DM than in patients with T2DM (T1DM vs. T2DM = 26.9 vs. 60.4 years) [11]. In summary, we believe that patients with T1DM tend to develop DNI at younger age (10–40 years) than do patients without DM (21–40 years) and those with T2DM (>40 years).

Our study has several strengths, including a large number of patients with T1DM representing a nationwide population and a 10-year observation period. In addition, the diagnosis of T1DM was based on data from the RFCIP, a highly accurate and reliable database affiliated to the NHIRD. Nevertheless, the study has some limitations. The diagnoses were based on ICD-9-CM codes and not on original medical records; therefore, it lacked blood sugar level, laboratory data, data from imaging studies, surgical records, and pathologic reports, which are necessary for evaluating disease severity. The bacterial spectrum and drug sensitivity of T1DM-DNI and the difference from non-DM-DNI are important information for clinical management and prescription of antibiotics. However, our database did not contain that information. The effects of the factors omitted in this study on T1DM and DNI should be investigated in future studies. In addition, ICU care, mediastinitis, and mortality were observed only in patients with T1DM; however, the number of patients was insufficient to develop a statistical conclusion. Additional studies including detailed medical records and a large sample size of patients with DNI are needed.

## 5. Conclusions

This nationwide population-based study was the first to investigate the epidemiological data of DNI development and prognosis in patients with T1DM. We concluded that T1DM is a predisposing factor for DNI. The duration of hospitalization for DNI is longer in patients with T1DM than in those without DM. In addition, patients with T1DM are predisposed to developing DNI at a younger age than are those without DM.

**Author Contributions:** Conceptualization, G.-H.C. and M.-S.T.; Methodology, M.-C.D. and Y.-H.Y.; Software, C.-Y.L. and M.-H.L.; Validation, Y.-H.L., C.-Y.W. and C.-M.H.; Formal Analysis, C.-Y.L.; Investigation, G.-H.C. and M.-S.T.; Resources, C.-Y.W. and C.-M.H.; Writing-Original Draft Preparation, G.-H.C. and M.-C.D.; Writing-Review & Editing, M.-S.T.; Supervision, Y.-H.Y. and M.-S.T.

**Funding:** The article did not have any financial support provided by companies toward the completion of the work.

**Acknowledgments:** The authors thank the Health Information and Epidemiology Laboratory (CLRPG6G0041) at the Chiayi Chang Gung Memorial Hospital for the comments and assistance in data analysis. This study was supported by a grant from Chiayi Chang Gung Memorial Hospital (CGRPG6G0011), based on the National Health Insurance Research Database provided by the Central Bureau of National Health Insurance, Department of Health, and managed by the National Health Research Institutes. The interpretation and conclusions contained herein do not represent those of the Bureau of National Health Insurance, Department of Health or National Health Research Institutes. This manuscript was edited by Wallace Academic Editing.

**Data and Material Availability:** The datasets generated and/or analyzed during the current study are available in the Taiwan National Health Insurance Research Database repository [32].

**Conflicts of Interest:** The authors declare that they have no competing interests.

## References

1. Chang, G.H.; Tsai, M.S.; Liu, C.Y.; Lin, M.H.; Tsai, Y.T.; Hsu, C.M.; Yang, Y.H. End-stage renal disease: A risk factor of deep neck infection—A nationwide follow-up study in taiwan. *BMC Infect. Dis.* **2017**, *17*, 424. [CrossRef] [PubMed]
2. Har-El, G.; Aroesty, J.H.; Shaha, A.; Lucente, F.E. Changing trends in deep neck abscess. A Retrospective Study of 110 Patients. *Oral. Surg. Oral. Med. Oral. Pathol.* **1994**, *77*, 446–450. [CrossRef]
3. Sethi, D.S.; Stanley, R.E. Deep neck abscesses—Changing trends. *J. Laryngol. Otol.* **1994**, *108*, 138–143. [CrossRef] [PubMed]
4. Huang, T.T.; Liu, T.C.; Chen, P.R.; Tseng, F.Y.; Yeh, T.H.; Chen, Y.S. Deep Neck Infection: Analysis of 185 Cases. *Head Neck* **2004**, *26*, 854–860. [CrossRef] [PubMed]
5. Sakarya, E.U.; Kulduk, E.; Gundogan, O.; Soy, F.K.; Dundar, R.; Kilavuz, A.E.; Ozbay, C.; Eren, E.; Imre, A. Clinical features of deep neck infection: Analysis of 77 patients. *Kulak Burun Bogaz Ihtis. Derg.* **2015**, *25*, 102–108. [CrossRef] [PubMed]

6. Ko, H.H.; Chien, W.C.; Lin, Y.H.; Chung, C.H.; Cheng, S.J. Examining the correlation between diabetes and odontogenic infection: A nationwide, retrospective, matched-cohort study in Taiwan. *PLoS ONE* **2017**, *12*, e0178941. [CrossRef] [PubMed]
7. Wang, L.F.; Kuo, W.R.; Tsai, S.M.; Huang, K.J. Characterizations of life-threatening deep cervical space infections: A review of one hundred ninety-six cases. *Am. J. Otolaryngol.* **2003**, *24*, 111–117. [CrossRef] [PubMed]
8. Yang, W.; Hu, L.; Wang, Z.; Nie, G.; Li, X.; Lin, D.; Luo, J.; Qin, H.; Wu, J.; Wen, W.; et al. Deep neck infection: A review of 130 cases in southern china. *Medicine* **2015**, *94*, e994. [CrossRef] [PubMed]
9. Bottin, R.; Marioni, G.; Rinaldi, R.; Boninsegna, M.; Salvadori, L.; Staffieri, A. Deep neck infection: A present-day complication. A retrospective review of 83 cases (1998–2001). *Eur. Arch. Otorhinolaryngol.* **2003**, *260*, 576–579. [CrossRef] [PubMed]
10. Chiang, J.L.; Kirkman, M.S.; Laffel, L.M.B.; Peters, A.L. Type 1 diabetes through the life span: A position statement of the american diabetes association. *Diabetes Care* **2014**, *37*, 2034–2054. [CrossRef] [PubMed]
11. Magliano, D.J.; Harding, J.L.; Cohen, K.; Huxley, R.R.; Davis, W.A.; Shaw, J.E. excess risk of dying from infectious causes in those with type 1 and type 2 diabetes. *Diabetes Care* **2015**, *38*, 1274–1280. [CrossRef] [PubMed]
12. Tsai, M.-S.; Lin, M.; Lee, C.; Yang, Y.; Chen, W.; Chang, G.; Tsai, Y.; Chen, P.; Tsai, Y. Chang gung research database: A multi-institutional database consisting of original medical records. *Biomed. J.* **2017**, *40*, 263–269. [CrossRef] [PubMed]
13. Tsai, M.S.; Lee, L.A.; Tsai, Y.T.; Yang, Y.H.; Liu, C.Y.; Lin, M.H.; Hsu, C.M.; Chen, C.K.; Li, H.Y. Sleep apnea and risk of vertigo: A nationwide population-based cohort study. *Laryngoscope* **2018**, *128*, 763–768. [CrossRef] [PubMed]
14. Chou, I.C.; Wang, C.H.; Lin, W.D.; Tsai, F.J.; Lin, C.C.; Kao, C.H. Risk of epilepsy in type 1 diabetes mellitus: A population-based cohort study. *Diabetologia* **2016**, *59*, 1196–1203. [CrossRef] [PubMed]
15. Tsai, M.S.; Yang, Y.H.; Liu, C.Y.; Lin, M.H.; Chang, G.H.; Tsai, Y.T.; Li, H.Y.; Tsai, Y.H.; Hsu, C.M. Unilateral vocal fold paralysis and risk of pneumonia: A nationwide population-based cohort study. *Otolaryngol. Head Neck Surg.* **2018**, *158*, 896–903. [CrossRef] [PubMed]
16. Tsai, Y.T.; Huang, E.I.; Chang, G.H.; Tsai, M.S.; Hsu, C.M.; Yang, Y.H.; Lin, M.H.; Liu, C.Y.; Li, H.Y. Risk of acute epiglottitis in patients with preexisting diabetes mellitus: A population-based case-control study. *PLoS ONE* **2018**, *13*, e0199036. [CrossRef] [PubMed]
17. Liu, C.F.; Weng, S.F.; Lin, Y.S.; Lin, C.S.; Lien, C.F.; Wang, J.J. Increased risk of deep neck infection among hiv-infected patients in the era of highly active antiretroviral therapy—A population-based follow-up study. *BMC Infect. Dis.* **2013**, *13*, 183. [CrossRef] [PubMed]
18. Yen, Y.F.; Chuang, P.H.; Jen, I.A.; Chen, M.; Lan, Y.C.; Liu, Y.L.; Lee, Y.; Chen, Y.H.; Chen, Y.A. Incidence of autoimmune diseases in a nationwide hiv/aids patient cohort in Taiwan, 2000–2012. *Ann. Rheum. Dis.* **2016**, *76*, 661–665. [CrossRef] [PubMed]
19. Shen, T.C.; Lin, C.L.; Chen, C.H.; Tu, C.Y.; Hsia, T.C.; Shih, C.M.; Hsu, W.H.; Chang, Y.J. Increased risk of chronic obstructive pulmonary disease in patients with systemic lupus erythematosus: A population-based cohort study. *PLoS ONE* **2014**, *9*, e91821. [CrossRef] [PubMed]
20. Casqueiro, J.; Casqueiro, J.; Alves, C. Infections in patients with diabetes mellitus: A review of pathogenesis. *Indian J. Endocrinol. Metab.* **2012**, *16*, S27–36. [PubMed]
21. Hidaka, H.; Yamaguchi, T.; Hasegawa, J.; Yano, H.; Kakuta, R.; Ozawa, D.; Nomura, K.; Katori, Y. Clinical and bacteriological influence of diabetes mellitus on deep neck infection: Systematic review and meta-analysis. *Head Neck* **2015**, *37*, 1536–1546. [CrossRef] [PubMed]
22. Simonsen, J.R.; Harjutsalo, V.; Jarvinen, A.; Kirveskari, J.; Forsblom, C.; Groop, P.H.; Lehto, M. FinnDiane Study Group. Bacterial infections in patients with type 1 diabetes: A 14-year follow-up study. *BMJ Open Diabetes Res. Care* **2015**, *3*, e000067. [CrossRef] [PubMed]
23. Muller, L.M.; Gorter, K.J.; Hak, E.; Goudzwaard, W.L.; Schellevis, F.G.; Hoepelman, A.I.; Rutten, G.E. Increased risk of common infections in patients with type 1 and type 2 diabetes mellitus. *Clin. Infect. Dis.* **2005**, *41*, 281–288. [CrossRef] [PubMed]
24. Eftekharian, A.; Roozbahany, N.A.; Vaezeafshar, R.; Narimani, N. Deep neck infections: A retrospective review of 112 cases. *Eur. Arch. Otorhinolaryngol.* **2009**, *266*, 273–277. [CrossRef] [PubMed]

25. Dolezalova, H.; Zemek, J.; Tucek, L. Deep neck infections of odontogenic origin and their clinical significance. A retrospective study from Hradec Kralove, Czech Republic. *Acta Medica* **2015**, *58*, 86–91. [PubMed]
26. Boscolo-Rizzo, P.; Marchiori, C.; Montolli, F.; Vaglia, A.; da Mosto, M.C. Deep neck infections: A constant challenge. *ORL J. Otorhinolaryngol. Relat. Spec.* **2006**, *68*, 259–265. [CrossRef] [PubMed]
27. Bakir, S.; Tanriverdi, M.H.; Gun, R.; Yorgancilar, A.E.; Yildirim, M.; Tekbas, G.; Palanci, Y.; Meric, K.; Topcu, I. Deep neck space infections: A retrospective review of 173 cases. *Am. J. Otolaryngol.* **2012**, *33*, 56–63. [CrossRef] [PubMed]
28. Huang, T.T.; Tseng, F.Y.; Liu, T.C.; Hsu, C.J.; Chen, Y.S. Deep neck infection in diabetic patients: Comparison of clinical picture and outcomes with nondiabetic patients. *Otolaryngol. Head Neck Surg.* **2005**, *132*, 943–947. [CrossRef] [PubMed]
29. Lin, H.T.; Tsai, C.S.; Chen, Y.L.; Liang, J.G. Influence of diabetes mellitus on deep neck infection. *J. Laryngol. Otol.* **2006**, *120*, 650–654. [CrossRef] [PubMed]
30. Lee, J.-K.; Kim, H.; Lim, S. Predisposing factors of complicated deep neck infection: An analysis of 158 cases. *Yonsei Med. J.* **2007**, *48*, 55–62. [CrossRef] [PubMed]
31. Crespo, A.N.; Chone, C.T.; Fonseca, A.S.; Montenegro, M.C.; Pereira, R.; Milani, J.A. Clinical versus computed tomography evaluation in the diagnosis and management of deep neck infection. *Sao Paulo Med. J.* **2004**, *122*, 259–263. [CrossRef] [PubMed]
32. Taiwan National Health Insurance Research Database. Available online: https://nhird.nhri.org.tw/en/How_to_cite_us.html (accessed on 1 September 2018).

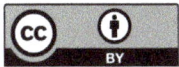

© 2018 by the authors. Licensee MDPI, Basel, Switzerland. This article is an open access article distributed under the terms and conditions of the Creative Commons Attribution (CC BY) license (http://creativecommons.org/licenses/by/4.0/).

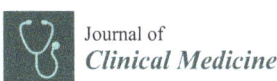 

Article

# PG-Priming Enhances Doxorubicin Influx to Trigger Necrotic and Autophagic Cell Death in Oral Squamous Cell Carcinoma

Shian-Ren Lin and Ching-Feng Weng *

Department of Life Science and Institute of Biotechnology, National Dong Hwa University, Hualien 97401, Taiwan; d9813003@gms.ndhu.edu.tw
* Correspondence: cfweng@gms.ndhu.edu.tw; Tel.: +886-3-8903637

Received: 17 September 2018; Accepted: 18 October 2018; Published: 21 October 2018

**Abstract:** Synergistic effects between natural compounds and chemotherapy drugs are believed to have fewer side effects with equivalent efficacy. However, the synergistic potential of prodigiosin (PG) with doxorubicin (Dox) chemotherapy is still unknown. This study explores the synergistic mechanism of PG and Dox against oral squamous cell carcinoma (OSCC) cells. Three OSCC cell lines were treated with different PG/Dox combinatory schemes for cytotoxicity tests and were further investigated for cell death characteristics by cell cycle flow cytometry and autophagy/apoptosis marker labelling. When OSCC cells were pretreated with PG, the cytotoxicity of the subsequent Dox-treatment was 30% higher than Dox alone. The cytotoxic efficacy of PG-pretreated was found better than those of PG plus Dox co-treatment and Dox-pretreatment. Increase of Sub-G1 phase and caspase-3/LC-3 levels without poly (ADP-ribose) polymeras (PARP) elevation indicated both autophagy and necrosis occurred in OSCC cells. Dox flux after PG-priming was further evaluated by rhodamine-123 accumulation and Dox transporters analysis to elucidate the PG-priming effect. PG-priming autophagy enhanced Dox accumulation according to the increase of rhodamine-123 accumulation without the alterations of Dox transporters. Additionally, the cause of PG-triggered autophagy was determined by co-treatment with endoplasmic reticulum (ER) stress or AMP-activated protein kinase (AMPK) inhibitor. PG-induced autophagy was not related to nutrient deprivation and ER stress was proved by co-treatment with specific inhibitor. Taken together, PG-priming autophagy could sensitize OSCC cells by promoting Dox influx without regulation of Dox transporter. The PG-priming might be a promising adjuvant approach for the chemotherapy of OSCC.

**Keywords:** prodigiosin; doxorubicin; priming; influx; autophagy

## 1. Introduction

Doxorubicin (Adriamycin, Dox), isolated from soil bacteria *Streptomyces peucetius*, is the first member of anthracyclines (including daunorubicin, epirubicin, and idarubicin) [1,2]. The main action of Dox is intercalating within DNA pairs, which leads to the inhibition of topoisomerase IIβ and results in cell cycle blockage [3]. Rendering non-tissue specific characteristics, Dox gets wide indications including leukemia, neuroblastoma, breast carcinoma, ovarian carcinoma, and most recurrent or metastatic cancer [4]. Apart from these, the non-specific characteristics of Dox cause some severe adverse effects in cancer patients including immunosuppression, bone marrow suppression, hepatotoxicity, cardiotoxicity, and mucositis [5,6]. The cause of side effects is from the inhibition of cell division as well as reactive oxygen species (ROS) by-products (doxorubicin-semiquinone, doxorubicinol, dexrazoxane, and 7-deoxy-doxorubicinone) during metabolism of doxorubicin in mitochondria [2,7–9]. As a result, these adverse effects might limit the applicable dosage and cancer treating efficacy of Dox. Accordingly, the alternative approach or new formulation to attenuate Dox side effects and enhance Dox efficacy turns out to be a crucial issue for Dox use in the regimen of chemotherapy. Recently, nanocarriers have exerted a favorable theme and some research has focused on this topic to dissolve these obstacles, such as Dox encapsulated in pH-sensitive, ultrasonic-responsive, or co-capsulated with MDR-1 inhibitor in PEGylated, liposome, or PLGA nano-carrier, which also promote Dox uptake [10–14]. However, cytotoxicity of nanoparticle conjugated Dox was 10 times lower than free-form Dox, which also restricted the use in cancer treatment [15].

A long treatment period with a low dose chemotherapeutic drug might induce chemoresistance within cancer cells and subsequently toxicity could affect its use [16]. Notably, prevailing mechanisms of chemoresistance could be classified into the following seven phases: drug flux, DNA damage repair, cell death inhibition, epithelial-mesenchymal transition (EMT), drug target alteration, drug inactivation, and epigenetics [17]. In Dox resistance, dug efflux would be the most concerning phase [16]. Dox can import into cells through solute carrier family 22 member 16 (SLC22A16, also known organic cation transporter 6, oct-6) and export by ATP-binding cassette transporter family members, in which multidrug-related protein 1 (MDR-1 or p-glycoprotein) and breast cancer resistance protein (BCRP or ABCG2) are involved [3]. These proteins will be regulated (upregulation of exporter and downregulation of importer) during long-term exposure to a non-toxic dose of Dox [18]. Thereby, numerous studies have put more attention to reducing MDR over-expression to reverse multidrug resistance. CRISPER/Cas-9 gene editing, ursodeoxycholic acid, or *Zingiber officinale* Roscoe, have been reported to down-regulate *ABCB1* gene expressions in chemo-resistant cancer cells [19–21].

Prodigiosin (PG, PubChem CID: 5351169) is a red prodiginine pigment isolated from various bacteria including *Serratia marcescens, Pseudoalteromonas rubra, Hahella chejuensis,* and actinomycete bacteria [22–25]. Even though the original biological function in producer bacteria remains unclear, PG has been identified with numerous biological activities including antimicrobial [26–29], antimalarial [26,27,30], and antitumor [26,27,31–34] activities. Moreover, PG showed apoptotic inducing property in many cancer types such as lung cancer [35–37], breast cancer [38,39], colorectal cancer [40–42], leukemia [43,44], and hepatocellular carcinoma [45] without normal cell cytotoxicity [41,46]. Recently, PG has also been identified as an autophagy inducer in OSCC cells [47,48]. However, the application of PG as an adjuvant in chemotherapy is still unknown.

## 2. Experimental Section

### 2.1. Research Aims

This study was conducted to explore the potential of PG combined with doxorubicin in anti-cancer activity by using oral squamous cell carcinoma (OSCC) cells as a test platform. Next, experiments tested the synergistic effects of PG and Dox against OSCC cells to evaluate the adjuvant potential of PG for cancer therapy. Furthermore, the underlying molecular mechanisms of enhanced doxorubicin cytotoxicity under PG-priming were also investigated.

### 2.2. Reagents

Cell-cultured medium and reagents were purchased from Thermo-Fisher (Waltham, MA, USA). Prodigiosin was purified by Dr. Yu-Hsin Chen (Department of Life Science, National Dong-Hwa University, Hualien, Taiwan). Liposome-coated doxorubicin (abbreviated as Dox) was obtained from Dr. Ming-Fang Cheng (Division of Histology and Clinical Pathology, Hualian Army Forces General Hospital, Hualien, Taiwan). Inhibitors used in this study were purchased from Santa Cruz Biotechnology (Dallas, TX, USA). General chemicals were purchased from Sigma Aldrich (Merck KGaA, Darmstadt, Germany). Polyvinylidene difluoride (PVDF) membrane used in Western blotting was obtained from GE Healthcare (Chicago, IL, USA). The antibodies used in this study were obtained from Santa Cruz Biotechnology, as shown in Table 1.

Table 1. Antibodies used in this study.

| Protein | Host | Source | RRID | MW (kDa) | Dilution |
|---|---|---|---|---|---|
| MDR-1 | Human | Mouse | AB_2565004 | 180 | 1:200 |
| PARP1 | Human | Mouse | AB_1127036 | 116 | 1:200 |
| ABCG2 | Human | Mouse | AB_629007 | 80 | 1:200 |
| OCT-6 | Human | Mouse | AB_10989254 | 46 | 1:200 |
| GAPDH | Human | Mouse | AB_1124759 | 37 | 1:1000 |
| Caspase3 | Human | Mouse | AB_1119997 | 32 | 1:200 |
| LC3 I/II | Human | Mouse | AB_2137722 | 15/18 | 1:200 |
| HRP-conjugated 2nd Ab | Mouse | Goat | AB_92635 | | 1:5000 |

MW, molecular weight; RRID, Research Resource Identifiers.

*2.3. Cell Culture*

Cell lines used in this study were obtained from different sources: Human pharynx squamous carcinoma FaDu from Dr. Chun-Shu Lin (Radiation Oncology Department, Tri-Service General Hospital, Taipei, Taiwan), human oral squamous cell carcinoma cell line OECM1 and tongue carcinoma cell line SAS from Professor Ta-Chun Yuan (Department of Life Science, National Dong Hwa University, Hualien, Taiwan), and human bronchus epithelial cell BEAS-2b from American Type Culture Collection (ATCC). OECM1 and SAS were cultured in Roswell Park Memorial Institute medium 1640 (RPMI 1640), FaDu in minimum essential medium (MEM), and BEAS-2b in Dulbecco's Modified Eagle Medium (DMEM) and medium was changed every 2 days. All culture media were mixed with 10% fetal bovine serum (FBS) and 1% antibiotic-antimycotic and cultured within 37 °C, 5% $CO_2$ incubator (Thermo-Fisher). Cells were detached by 0.25% trypsin/ethylenediaminetetraacetic acid (EDTA) for further experiments. All experiments were obtained within 20 passages concerning uniformity and reproducibility.

*2.4. Cytotoxicity Assay*

Cytotoxicity was determined using a colorimetric assay by MTT (3-(4,5-dimethylthiazol-2-yl)-2,5-diphenyltetrazolium bromide) previously described in the literature [48]. The optical density (OD) alteration of mitochondrial enzymatic activity was converted into the cell numbers according to the cell viability or cytotoxicity. Briefly, $1 \times 10^4$ cells per wells were seeded in 96-well plate and incubated in culture conditions overnight. Then, cells were divided into the six following treatment groups: (1) PG-Dox group: treated with PG followed by Dox, (2) Dox-PG group treated with Dox and then PG, and (3) PG + Dox group: treated PG and Dox at the same time, respectively. An additional three groups performed the same treatments with the above-described and replaced Dox with cisplatin. All treatments were carried out in 12 h and 1 mg/mL of MTT solution was added and further incubated for 4 h at 37 °C as treatment finished. Finally, liquid in wells was replaced by dimethyl sulfoxide (DMSO), and the absorbance at 570 nm was measured by Multiskan™ FC microplate photometer (Thermo-Fisher). Cytotoxicity of each treatment was represented by cell viability which calculated from the absorbance ratio at 570 nm between treated and untreated groups.

To understand the cause of PG- and Dox-induced cell death, inhibitor recovering assays were also performed following the above protocol. Autophagy inhibitors (bafilomycin A1 and 3-methyladenine), endoplasmic reticulum (ER) stress inhibitors (tauroursodeoxycholic acid, TUDC), and AMPK inhibitors (dorsomorphin, CC) were cotreated with various concentrations of PG or Dox, respectively.

*2.5. Cell Cycle Analysis*

Cell cycle analysis was carried out by flow cytometry. Firstly, $1 \times 10^6$ cells/well of OSCC were seeded into 6-well plates and incubated in culture condition overnight. To understand drug-pretreated effect, cells were treated with PG for 12 h, Dox for 12 h, or PG for 12 h followed by Dox for additional 12 h, respectively. After treatment, cells including culture medium were collected using trypsin/EDTA and washed by phosphate buffer saline (PBS) twice before being fixed with pre-cooled 70% ethanol/PBS overnight. After fixation, cells were washed twice by PBS and stained with staining buffer (20 µg/mL of propidium iodide, 0.1% Triton X-100, 0.2 mg/mL RNase A) at 37 °C for 1 h. The fluorescent intensity in the cells was measured by a flow cytometer (Cytomics™ FC500, Beckman, Fullerton, CA, USA). Data from $10^4$ cells were collected for each data file. Fluorescent intensities for each cell line were acquiesced and plotted by flow cytometer software. The gating of each phase was based on the acquisition histogram of untreated controls. Phases of each group were collected and the average of each phase was calculated within the groups.

### 2.6. Doxorubicin Flux Analysis

Efflux and influx of Dox was determined by indirect method which used rhodamine 123, a fluorescent Dox transporter substrate, detected as an indicator described previously [49,50]. Briefly, $1 \times 10^4$ cells/well of OSCC were seeded in 96-well plate and incubated in culture condition overnight. After cell confluence, cells were divided into four groups and then treated with various regimens, respectively. For Rhodamine-influx: short-term influx assay: 0.5 µM of PG in full-culture medium was added and incubated for 1 h and replaced culture medium with 2 µM of rhodamine 123 in PBS for additional 1 h; long-term influx assay: the same treatment as short-term influx assay instead the incubation duration of PG from 1 h to 12 h. For Rhodamine-efflux: short-term efflux assay: 2 µM of rhodamine 123 in PBS was firstly incubated for 1 h and followed by 0.5 µM of PG in full-culture medium for additional 1 h; long-term efflux assay: the same as treatment as short-term influx assay instead the incubation duration of PG from 1 h to 12 h. After incubation, cells were trebly washed by PBS and lysed with 0.1% triton X-100 and the fluorescent intensity was determined at 485/538 nm by α-screen multi-plate reader (Perkin Elmer, Waltham, MA, USA). These rhodamine flux studies were used to estimate DOX flux.

### 2.7. Western Blotting

The detail protocol of Western blotting was described in our previous study [51]. In brief, $1 \times 10^6$ cells/well of OSCC cells were seeded into a 6-well plate and treated the same as with cell cycle analysis. Cells were washed by PBS and lysed by radioimmunoprecipitation assay buffer (RIPA). Then, 30 µg of total proteins from cell lysates were electrophoretically separated by sodium dodecyl sulfate polyacrylamide gel electrophoresis (SDS-PAGE) and transferred into polyvinylidene difluoride (PVDF) membrane. Proteins of interest were identified via incubation with appropriate primary followed by horseradish peroxidase (HRP)-conjugated secondary antibodies and exposed to the iBright imaging system (Thermo-Fisher) for monitoring intensity of signals after soaking in enhance chemiluminescent (ECL) reagents. Data acquisition was also performed by the iBright imaging system, and signal intensity was normalized with GAPDH as an internal control.

### 2.8. Statistical Analysis

All quantified results were shown as mean ± standard deviation (SD) of three independent experiments. Significant analysis used a one-way ANOVA, followed by Dunnett's test. A data histogram was built by GraphPad Prism 7.04 (La Jolla, CA, USA).

## 3. Results

### 3.1. Cytotoxicity Change of PG/Dox Treated Strategies

In this study, three combined manners (pretreatment, cotreatment, and posttreatment) of PG/Dox were tested in OSCC. In pretreatment and post-treatment approaches, chemicals were previously treated for 12 h and subsequently washed out, followed by new chemical treatment for additional 12 h. Therefore, the term "PG-pretreatment" would be defined as a "PG-priming" procedure in the subsequent section. The cell viability of all tested OSCC cells were declined in all combined strategies except cotreatment in SAS ($p < 0.05$). In three combined strategies, PG-pretreatment got the highest reducing levels (as compared with Dox alone) than those of the other two strategies, as shown in Figure 1A. This result posed the potential of PG-pretreatment as PG-priming in OSCC. When doubling the concentrations of PG, cell viability was the same as that of single concentration, revealed 0.5 μM of PG, which was the maximum concentration for PG-priming. Also, extending the PG-priming period up to 24 h, the cytotoxicity of Dox failed to exhibit an additive potentiation. These results indicated that 12 h of PG-priming might reach the maximum effect (data not shown). Moreover, with PG-priming in normal cell lines BEAS-2b, the cell viability of Dox treatment did not show the decrease as much as OSCC, even though the concentrations of PG and Dox were twice higher than that of OSCC, as shown in Figure 1B. This result indicated that PG-priming was more effective and less toxic than that of Dox alone. An additional experiment was to investigate whether the PG-priming effect could also be observed in golden chemotherapy drug cisplatin, however, the cytotoxic enhancement in PG/Dox combination could not be found in PG/cisplatin combination, as shown in Figure 1C. Taking all results together, PG-priming could enhance Dox cytotoxicity in OSCC cells through a Dox-related mechanism. In subsequent experiments, the type of cell death triggered by PG-priming and the underlying mechanism were further investigated.

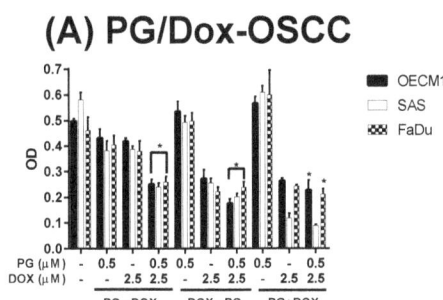
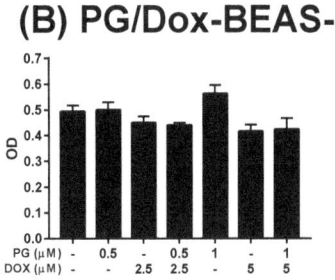
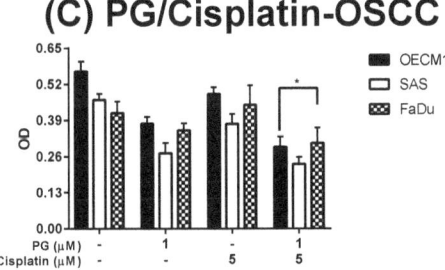

**Figure 1.** Alteration of cytotoxicity in sequential PG (prodigiosin)/Dox (doxorubicin) and PG/cisplatin combination in oral squamous cell carcinoma (OSCC) and BEAS-2b cells. (**A**) OSCC and (**B**) normal bronchus cells-BEAS-2b were treated with various schemes of PG and Dox, and (**C**) Cisplatin substituted Dox for 12 h and analyzed cell viability by 3-(4, 5-dimethylthiazol-2-yl)-2, 5-diphenyltetrazolium bromide (MTT) assay. The results were represented as mean ± SD from three individual experiments. * $p < 0.05$ as compared with Dox alone.

### 3.2. Identification of Cell Death Characteristics

Numerous types of cell death were found in cells, but the most common types were apoptosis and autophagy, respectively. These two cell-death types could be distinguished by analyzing apoptosis and autophagy-related protein and cell markers, and the most obvious marker would be cell cycle analysis.

In cell cycle analysis of SAS, Sub-$G_1$ was significantly increased, but non-cleaved PARP1 and caspase-3 protein levels were not decreased after PG-priming, as shown in Figures 2B and 3B,C. These results revealed that PG-priming prior to Dox treatment would lead to SAS undergoing necrosis. Moreover, while PG combined with autophagic inhibitor (bafilomycin A1 (BA1) and 3-methyladenine (3MA), cell viability of PG-priming could be recovered, as shown in Figure 4. This phenomenon might indicate that both necrosis and autophagy were activated after PG-priming and the autophagy would be a major clue, which was further confirmed by increases in LC3 protein levels, as shown in Figure 3A. In FaDu cells, Sub-$G_1$ phase was not significantly increased after PG/Dox treatment, as shown in Figure 2C. Also, non-cleaved PARP1 and caspase-3 protein levels while PG-priming followed by Dox treatment were decreased when compared with Dox alone, as shown in Figure 3B,C. The results also showed the necrosis activation within FaDu cells similar to SAS cells. Unlike SAS cells, this cell viability could not be recovered by autophagy inhibitor, as shown in Figure 4. In FaDu cells, LC3 protein levels were also significantly increased in the PG/Dox group, as shown in Figure 3A. These results revealed that both necrosis and autophagy were activated in FaDu cells and necrosis would be the main cause of cytotoxicity, whereas OECM1 cells showed different patterns from the above two cells lines. The sub-G1 phase did not significantly increase either in the non-cleaved PARP1 or caspase-3 protein levels, as shown in Figures 2A and 3B,C. Taken together, PG-priming cell death of OECM1 was not related to apoptosis or necrosis. On the other hand, the cell viability of OECM1 after PG-priming could be recovered by autophagy inhibitors, as shown in Figure 4. Also, LC3 protein levels were increased 10-fold, as shown in Figure 3A. These two results gave a clear clue for autophagy in OECM1 by PG-priming. Considering all above results, induced cell death characteristics in three different cell lines by PG-priming illustrated in different configurations. OECM1 showed autophagy, and SAS and FaDu posed both cell death and autophagy. In the subsequent experiments, the potential pathways of PG-enhanced Dox cytotoxicity were under investigation.

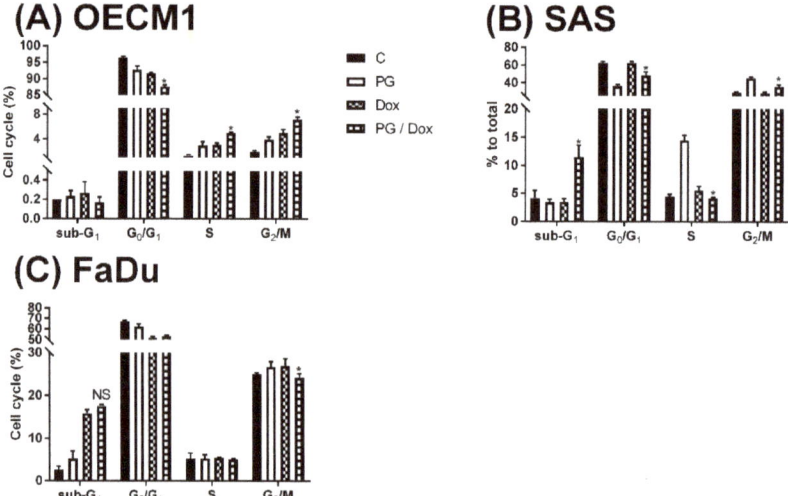

**Figure 2.** Alteration of cell cycle in (**A**) OECM1, (**B**) SAS, and (**C**) FaDu cells. OSCC cells were treated with PG/Dox for 12/12 h prior to staining with propidium iodide (PI) and fluorescent intensity was analyzed by flow cytometry. The results were represented as mean ± SD from three individual experiments. * $p < 0.05$ as compared with DOX alone.

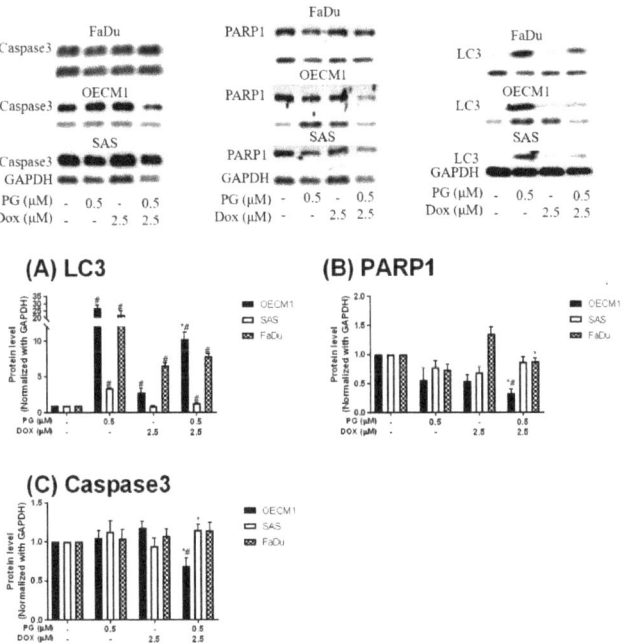

Figure 3. Expression of (A) LC3, (B) PARP1, and (C) Caspase3 in OSCCs after PG-priming. OSCC cells were treated with PG/Dox for 12/12 h and then desired protein levels were analyzed by Western blotting. The results were normalized with GAPDH and represented as mean ± SD from three individual experiments. Molecular weight: PARP1, 116 KDa; GAPDH, 37 KDa; Caspase3, 34 KDa; LC3, 18 KDa. # $p < 0.05$ compared with untreated control; * $p < 0.05$ as compared with Dox alone.

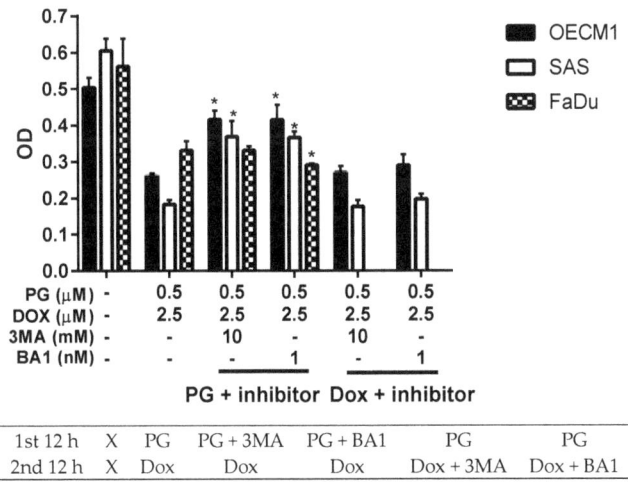

Figure 4. Alteration of cell viability combined with autophagy inhibitor. OSCC cells were treated with PG + inhibitor/DOX or PG/Dox + inhibitor and cell viability was analyzed. Table under figure was the scheme of treatment. "X" meant incubated with complete medium without PG or Dox. The results were represented as mean ± SD from three individual experiments. * $p < 0.05$ as compared with PG/Dox.

## 3.3. Doxorubicin Flux Affected by PG-Induced Autophagy

To measure the possible action of PG-induced autophagy, we examined the Dox flux in PG-priming OSCC cells. This Dox flux was determined by rhodamine-123 (R123) accumulation. R123 is a green fluorescent dye which acts as a Dox-transporter substrate over decades [52]. Accordingly, PG and Dox are all red fluorescence and PG is stronger fluorescence than that of Dox. After PG/Dox combination treatment, PG will interfere with the measurement of Dox fluorescent-intensity. Also, the less cytotoxic nature of R123 could eliminate the interference of cell death caused by Dox. Therefore, R123 was employed as an indicator to indirectly determine the Dox-flux in this study. In short-term priming (1 h), PG-priming did not enhance R123 accumulation, which revealed PG did not allosterically regulate Dox transporter, as shown in Figure 5A. Subsequently, PG-priming showed additional 50–70% of R123 accumulation for long-term priming (12 h). Moreover, the enhancing R123 could be attenuated by autophagy inhibitor, as shown in Figure 5B. This result indicated that PG-priming either enhanced Dox importer expressions or reduced exporter expressions. When checking Dox transporter levels, however, the importer (Oct-6) was not significantly decreased, and exporters (MDR-1 and ABCG2) slightly increased in OECM1 and decreased in SAS and FaDu, as shown in Figure 6. This result was not associated with previous results. It might be postulated as an indication of an unknown but important mechanism of Dox transport.

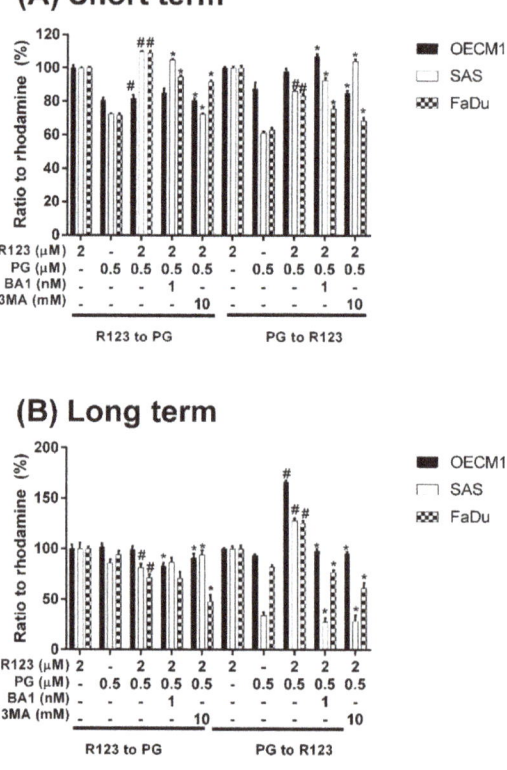

**Figure 5.** Rhodamine 123 accumulation after PG pretreatment. OSCC cells were treated with PG/R123 for (**A**) short term (1/1 h) and (**B**) long term (12/1 h) followed by analyzed fluorescent intensity within cells. The results were represented as mean ± SD from three individual experiments. # $p < 0.05$ as compared with R123 alone; * $p < 0.05$ compared with PG/R123 combination.

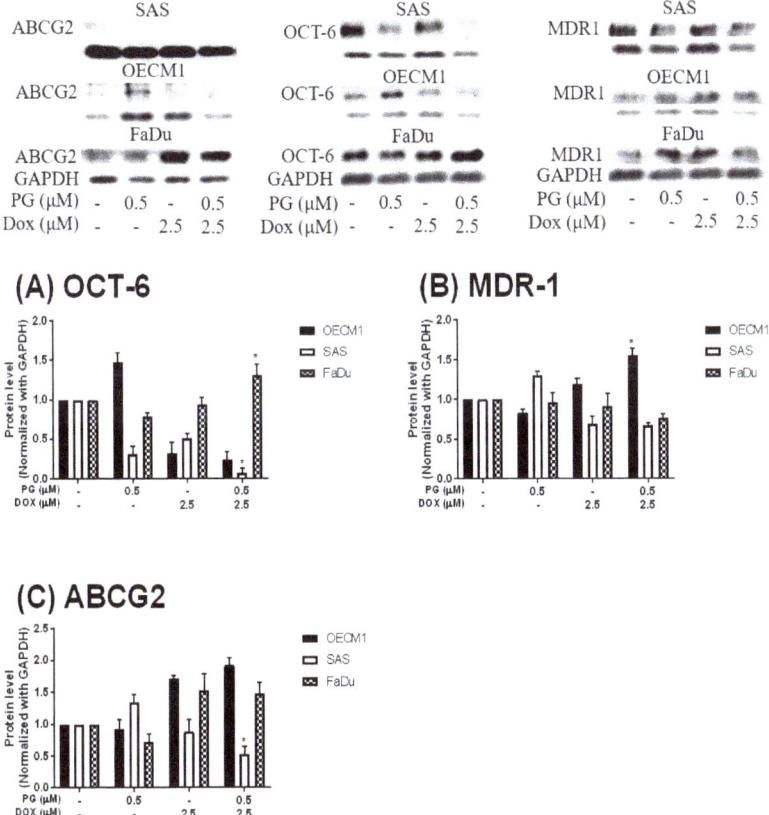

Figure 6. **Protein levels of Doxorubicin-related importer and exporter after PG-priming.** OSCC cells were treated with PG/Dox for 12/12 h and then were analyzed for Importer OCT-6 (**A**) and exporter MDR-1 (**B**) and ABCG2 (**C**) protein levels by Western blotting. The results were normalized with GAPDH and represented as mean ± SD from three individual experiments. Molecular weight: MDR-1, 170 KDa; ABCG2, 72 KDa; OCT-6, 58 KDa; GAPDH, 37 KDa. * $p < 0.05$ compared with Dox alone.

### 3.4. ER Stress and Energy Deprivation Analysis in PG-Priming OSCC Cells

PG could activate autophagy of OSCC cells as proven by the previous section and literature [48]. In this final part, the aim was to find the trigger of PG-induced autophagy in OSCC cells. As we noted, the two known triggers of autophagy are ER stress (unfolded protein response) and energy deprivation, which may be involved in the PG-priming reaction. ER stress was determined by adding ER stress inhibitor TUDC while energy deprivation was blocked by addition of AMPK specific inhibitor CC. When we combined TUDC or CC with PG and Dox treatment, cell viability of three OSCC cells lines were not significantly changed, as shown in Figure 7, (data of FaDu not shown). This result further postulated that PG-induced autophagy and Dox flux increase were not caused by ER stress and energy deprivation.

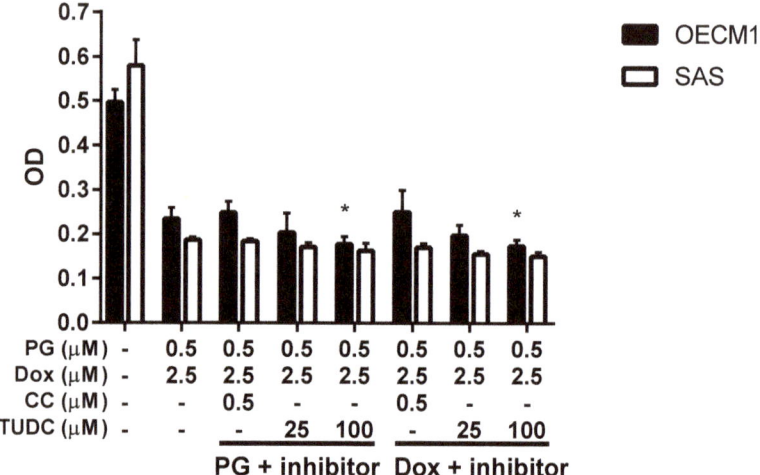

**Figure 7.** Cell viability change when PG/Dox combined with ER stress and energy deprivation inhibitors. OSCC cells were treated with PG + inhibitor/Dox or PG/Dox + inhibitor and were analyzed for cell viability. The inhibitors contained tauroursodeoxycholic acid (TUDC) and dorsomorphin (compound C, CC). The results were represented as mean ± SD from three individual experiments. * $p < 0.05$ compared with PG/Dox.

## 4. Discussion

The present study is the first demonstration of PG-enhanced Dox influx by activating autophagy in OSCC cells. Based on the Dox flux experiments, the enhancing mechanism of Dox influx was neither related to known importers nor exporters. PG could be a potential adjuvant for Dox treatment. Also, this study excluded the characteristics of known autophagy-triggers in PG-induced autophagy, which posed a new site for autophagy triggering mechanisms. In this work, we first report about the autophagy-activating property of Dox, as this activity was known to be inhibited by the intrinsic activation of autophagy.

Due to the non-tissue specific nature and high-cardiotoxicity, several studies have tried to discover natural compounds that could synergistically potentiate the efficacy of Dox without elevating normal cell toxicity. In a previous report, gambogic acid, a xanthonoid from *Garcinia hanburyi*, sensitized ovarian cancer cells toward Dox through accumulation of ROS [53]. Nitidine chloride, an alkaloid, synergized Dox cytotoxicity in breast cancer cell through PI3K/Akt signaling pathway [54]. Gingerol synergized Dox against liver cancer cells, leading to G2/M arrest [55]. Not only pure compounds; phenolic extract of flaxseed oil also promoted Dox efficacy against breast cancer cells [56]. Evodiamine, a major element of *Evodiae fructus*, reversed chemoresistance in multi-drug resistant breast cancer cells through the Ras/MEK/ERK signaling pathway [57]. Additionally, neferine could combat Dox resistance through ROS accumulation and Fas signaling pathway in lung cancer [58]. In gastric cancer, curcumin and formononetin posed different mechanisms to enhance Dox cytotoxicity [59,60]. These natural compounds exhibit potentiation for main applications in cancer treatment, and also play a supporting role in Dox regimen to overcome the limitation of Dox usage [61–66].

The first aim of this study was to explore the synergistic effect within PG/Dox regimen. PG combined with current chemotherapy agents was studied in breast cancer and found that PG could facilitate paclitaxel sensitivity in triple-negative human breast carcinoma cells via down-regulating survivin expression, an anti-apoptotic protein that acts as a caspase inhibitor [67,68]. Our results demonstrated new evidence that PG acts as an adjuvant with conventional chemotherapeutic drugs, such as paclitaxel and Dox as well.

The synergism of natural compounds with Dox could be found in priming fashion, nevertheless the co-treatment is addressed in main efforts [53–60]. While priming with CDK inhibitor in triple-negative breast cancer cell MDA-MB-231, Dox-induced DNA double-strand break would be activated and resulted in cytotoxic enhancement [69]. Cyclophosphamide, a conventional chemotherapeutic drug that acts as an intercalator of DNA, could increase HER2-targeted liposomal Dox accumulation in breast cancer cells [70]. An in vivo study focused on Dox efficacy after mitomycin C and carboplatin (two conventional chemotherapeutic drugs) pretreatment in human metastatic breast cancer-bearing mice. The results showed inhibition growth of xenografted tumors and reducing expressions of p-glycoprotein [71]. In our study, we showed that PG potentiated Dox cytotoxicity only in a pretreatment fashion (as a PG-priming effect), which was the first report of natural compound that primed cancer cells to be sensitized with Dox, and posed the potential of PG as an adjuvant using Dox as a chemotherapeutic agent. The clinical application of PG-priming might provide a great clue for reducing the dosage of Dox and dampening the side effects of Dox.

Due to red fluorescent nature [72], we preliminarily examined PG influx into OSCC cells. The data showed that PG could enter OSCC cells within 1 h and reached saturation after 1.5 h exposure (data not shown). When OSCC cells were primed with PG for 1 h, R123 fluorescent intensity did not significantly accumulate. This gave clear insight into PG action that did not allosterically modulate Dox importer or exporter activity. A previous study has also indicated that PG was not the substrate of multidrug resistance-related protein including MDR-1, BCRP (ABCG2), and MRP2 [73]. Again, our study confirmed that Dox efflux protein was not allosterically activated by PG-priming and further exposed that PG did not allosterically mediate Oct-6 activity.

By R123 accumulation assay, PG did not allosterically control Dox transporter activity but affected transporter expression in long-term priming, as shown in Figure 5. To our best knowledge, the Dox uptake of cells via Oct-6 and excretion of Dox by MDR-1 and ABCG2 have been reported [3,74]. In our study, Dox influx significantly increased in PG-priming for 12 h, which hypothesized that Oct-6 might be up-regulated or MDR-1/ABCG2 down-regulated. However, Oct-6 was down-regulated after PG/Dox treatments in Western blotting. Furthermore, expression levels of MDR-1 and ABCG2 did not show significant reductions. These results proposed a new Dox flux mechanism that needs to be further investigated.

PG was known as apoptotic and autophagic inducer in previous studies [47,75]. According to a recent study, PG induced apoptosis via inhibiting Bcl-2, activating Bak/Bax, intercalating DNA leading to suppress the cell cycle [75]. However, the action of PG-induced autophagy has not been fully explored yet. Remarkably, autophagy was triggered by stresses, such as ER stress (unfolded protein response), nutrient deprivation, and oxidative stress [76–79]. Hence, these cellular stresses would be the trigger clue of PG-induced autophagy. However, our test exposed that using ER stress inhibitor (TUDC) and nutrient deprivation inhibitor (CC) could not restore the cell viability of PG/Dox. Also, our data showed that PG did not elevate ROS level within OSCC cells (data not shown). All-known causes of autophagy, including ER stress, nutrient deprivation, and oxidative stress, were excluded from the trigger clue of PG-induced autophagy in this study, which the new potential mechanism of autophagy activation necessitates to be further elucidated.

During the screening of an autophagic marker, we also found that Dox-induced autophagy in both OECM1 and FaDu cells. It is well known that Dox was an apoptotic inducer via inhibiting cell cycle and producing ROS [80]. The potentiated role of autophagy in Dox treatment is focused on the activation of autophagy to ameliorate cardiotoxicity, and consequently inhibiting autophagy could promote Dox sensitivity in cancer cells [81–84]. The autophagy-activating features of Dox suggested the unclear field of Dox action. In the result of autophagy inhibitor recovery assay, autophagic inhibitors could not recover Dox-induced cell death, which implies that Dox-induced autophagy might not be solely involved in Dox-induced cell death, as shown in Figure 3.

Collectively, a model for the mechanical action of PG-priming autophagy potentiated Dox influx is proposed, as shown in Figure 8. When PG entered OSCC cells, autophagy which was irrelevant to nutrient deprivation, ER stress, and ROS, was activated. Subsequently, PG-induced autophagy could up-regulate Dox importer expression and in terms translocated to cell membrane, and consequently led to the enhancement of Dox influx resulting in cell death.

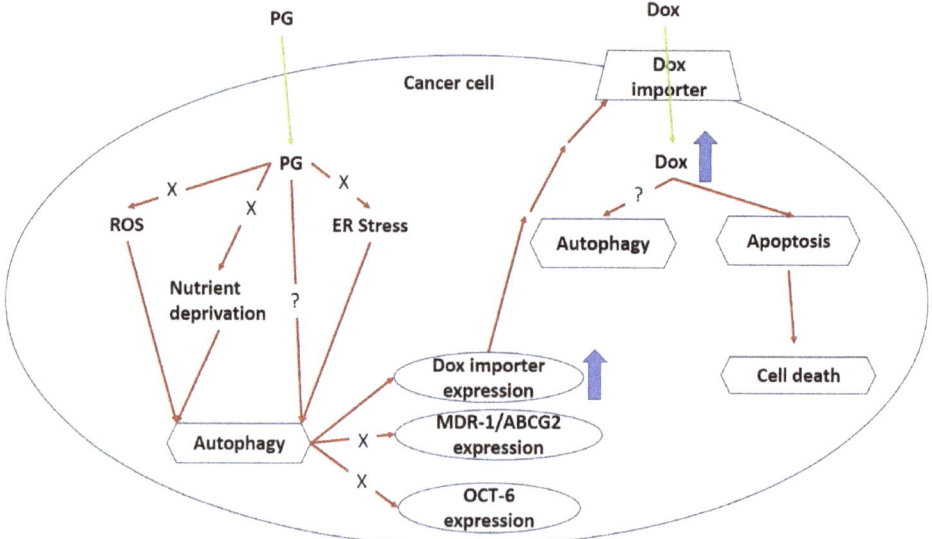

**Figure 8.** Potential mechanism of PG-priming doxorubicin cytotoxicity enhancement. "X" indicates not according to this mechanism. "?" illustrates still unknown. ER, endoplasmic reticulum; ROS, reactive oxygen species.

## 5. Conclusions

The present study firstly demonstrated the potential of PG as an adjuvant for Dox treatment in OSCC cells. PG-induced autophagy was not associated with ER stress, nutrient deprivation, and oxidative stress. Also, the enhancement of Dox influx triggered by PG-primed autophagy did not induce via Dox transporter, such as MDR-1, ABCG2, and OCT-6. The potential mechanism of PG-priming remains unclear and would be a further challenge for PG and Dox investigation.

**Author Contributions:** Conceptualization, S.-R.L. and C.-F.W.; methodology, S.-R.L.; software, C.-F.W.; validation, C.-F.W.; formal analysis, S.-R.L.; investigation, S.-R.L.; writing—original draft preparation, S.-R.L.; writing—review and editing, C.-F.W.; supervision, C.-F.W.; project administration, C.-F.W.; funding acquisition, C.-F.W.

**Funding:** This research was funded by Ministry of Science and Technology, grant number 107-2320-B-259-003 (C.F. Weng).

**Acknowledgments:** We sincerely thank Yu-Tong Chen from Kaoshiung Medical University who gave valuable help in imaging of chemiluminescent Western blotting.

**Conflicts of Interest:** The authors declare no any conflict of interest.

## References

1. McGowan, J.V.; Chung, R.; Maulik, A.; Piotrowska, I.; Walker, J.M.; Yellon, D.M. Anthracycline Chemotherapy and Cardiotoxicity. *Cardiovasc. Drugs Ther.* **2017**, *31*, 63–75. [CrossRef] [PubMed]
2. Damiani, R.M.; Moura, D.J.; Viau, C.M.; Caceres, R.A.; Henriques, J.A.; Saffi, J. Pathways of cardiac toxicity: Comparison between chemotherapeutic drugs doxorubicin and mitoxantrone. *Arch. Toxicol.* **2016**, *90*, 2063–2076. [CrossRef] [PubMed]

3. Thorn, C.F.; Oshiro, C.; Marsh, S.; Hernandez-Boussard, T.; McLeod, H.; Klein, T.E.; Altman, R.B. Doxorubicin pathways: Pharmacodynamics and adverse effects. *Pharmacogenet. Genom.* **2011**, *21*, 440–446. [CrossRef] [PubMed]
4. Johnson-Arbor, K.; Dubey, R. Doxorubicin. In *StatPearls*; StatPearls Publisher: Treasure Island, FL, USA, 2018.
5. Renu, K.; Abilash, V.G.; Pirupathi Pichiah, P.B.; Arunachalam, S. Molecular mechanism of doxorubicin-induced cardiomyopathy—An update. *Eur. J. Pharmacol.* **2018**, *818*, 241–253. [CrossRef] [PubMed]
6. Shafei, A.; El-Bakly, W.; Sobhy, A.; Wagdy, O.; Reda, A.; Aboelenin, O.; Marzouk, A.; El Habak, K.; Mostafa, R.; Ali, M.A.; et al. A review on the efficacy and toxicity of different doxorubicin nanoparticles for targeted therapy in metastatic breast cancer. *Biomed. Pharmacother.* **2017**, *95*, 1209–1218. [CrossRef] [PubMed]
7. Asensio-Lopez, M.C.; Soler, F.; Pascual-Figal, D.; Fernandez-Belda, F.; Lax, A. Doxorubicin-induced oxidative stress: The protective effect of nicorandil on HL-1 cardiomyocytes. *PLoS ONE* **2017**, *12*, e0172803. [CrossRef] [PubMed]
8. Kwatra, M.; Kumar, V.; Jangra, A.; Mishra, M.; Ahmed, S.; Ghosh, P.; Vohora, D.; Khanam, R. Ameliorative effect of naringin against doxorubicin-induced acute cardiac toxicity in rats. *Pharm. Biol.* **2016**, *54*, 637–647. [CrossRef] [PubMed]
9. Meredith, A.M.; Dass, C.R. Increasing role of the cancer chemotherapeutic doxorubicin in cellular metabolism. *J. Pharm. Pharmacol.* **2016**, *68*, 729–741. [CrossRef] [PubMed]
10. Wang, Z.; He, Q.; Zhao, W.; Luo, J.; Gao, W. Tumor-homing, pH- and ultrasound-responsive polypeptide-doxorubicin nanoconjugates overcome doxorubicin resistance in cancer therapy. *J. Control. Release* **2017**, *264*, 66–75. [CrossRef] [PubMed]
11. Tang, J.; Zhang, L.; Gao, H.; Liu, Y.; Zhang, Q.; Ran, R.; Zhang, Z.; He, Q. Co-delivery of doxorubicin and P-gp inhibitor by a reduction-sensitive liposome to overcome multidrug resistance, enhance anti-tumor efficiency and reduce toxicity. *Drug Deliv.* **2016**, *23*, 1130–1143. [CrossRef] [PubMed]
12. Xue, H.; Yu, Z.; Liu, Y.; Yuan, W.; Yang, T.; You, J.; He, X.; Lee, R.J.; Li, L.; Xu, C. Delivery of miR-375 and doxorubicin hydrochloride by lipid-coated hollow mesoporous silica nanoparticles to overcome multiple drug resistance in hepatocellular carcinoma. *Int. J. Nanomed.* **2017**, *12*, 5271–5287. [CrossRef] [PubMed]
13. Gupta, B.; Ramasamy, T.; Poudel, B.K.; Pathak, S.; Regmi, S.; Choi, J.Y.; Son, Y.; Thapa, R.K.; Jeong, J.H.; Kim, J.R.; et al. Development of Bioactive PEGylated Nanostructured Platforms for Sequential Delivery of Doxorubicin and Imatinib to Overcome Drug Resistance in Metastatic Tumors. *ACS Appl. Mater. Interfaces* **2017**, *9*, 9280–9290. [CrossRef] [PubMed]
14. Perillo, E.; Porto, S.; Falanga, A.; Zappavigna, S.; Stiuso, P.; Tirino, V.; Desiderio, V.; Papaccio, G.; Galdiero, M.; Giordano, A.; et al. Liposome armed with herpes virus-derived gH625 peptide to overcome doxorubicin resistance in lung adenocarcinoma cell lines. *Oncotarget* **2016**, *7*, 4077–4092. [CrossRef] [PubMed]
15. Kaminskas, L.M.; McLeod, V.M.; Kelly, B.D.; Sherna, G.; Boyd, B.J.; Williamson, M.; Owen, D.J.; Porter, C.J. A comparison of changes to doxorubicin pharmacokinetics, antitumor activity, and toxicity mediated by PEGylated dendrimer and PEGylated liposome drug delivery systems. *Nanomedicine* **2012**, *8*, 103–111. [CrossRef] [PubMed]
16. Broxterman, H.J.; Gotink, K.J.; Verheul, H.M. Understanding the causes of multidrug resistance in cancer: A comparison of doxorubicin and sunitinib. *Drug Resist. Updat.* **2009**, *12*, 114–126. [CrossRef] [PubMed]
17. Housman, G.; Byler, S.; Heerboth, S.; Lapinska, K.; Longacre, M.; Snyder, N.; Sarkar, S. Drug resistance in cancer: An overview. *Cancers* **2014**, *6*, 1769–1792. [CrossRef] [PubMed]
18. Bradley, G.; Juranka, P.F.; Ling, V. Mechanism of multidrug resistance. *Biochim. Biophys. Acta* **1988**, *948*, 87–128. [CrossRef]
19. Liu, T.; Li, Z.; Zhang, Q.; De Amorim Bernstein, K.; Lozano-Calderon, S.; Choy, E.; Hornicek, F.J.; Duan, Z. Targeting ABCB1 (MDR1) in multi-drug resistant osteosarcoma cells using the CRISPR-Cas9 system to reverse drug resistance. *Oncotarget* **2016**, *7*, 83502–83513. [CrossRef] [PubMed]
20. Komori, Y.; Arisawa, S.; Takai, M.; Yokoyama, K.; Honda, M.; Hayashi, K.; Ishigami, M.; Katano, Y.; Goto, H.; Ueyama, J.; et al. Ursodeoxycholic acid inhibits overexpression of P-glycoprotein induced by doxorubicin in HepG2 cells. *Eur. J. Pharmacol.* **2014**, *724*, 161–167. [CrossRef] [PubMed]
21. Pereira, M.M.; Haniadka, R.; Chacko, P.P.; Palatty, P.L.; Baliga, M.S. Zingiber officinale Roscoe (ginger) as an adjuvant in cancer treatment: A review. *J. BUON* **2011**, *16*, 414–424. [PubMed]

22. Laatsch, H.; Kellner, M.; Weyland, H. Butyl-meta-cycloheptylprodiginine—A revision of the structure of the former ortho-isomer. *J. Antibiot.* **1991**, *44*, 187–191. [CrossRef] [PubMed]
23. Soliev, A.B.; Hosokawa, K.; Enomoto, K. Bioactive pigments from marine bacteria: Applications and physiological roles. *Evid. Based Complement. Alternat. Med.* **2011**, *2011*, 670349. [CrossRef] [PubMed]
24. Chang, C.C.; Chen, W.C.; Ho, T.F.; Wu, H.S.; Wei, Y.H. Development of natural anti-tumor drugs by microorganisms. *J. Biosci. Bioeng.* **2011**, *111*, 501–511. [CrossRef] [PubMed]
25. Marchal, E.; Smithen, D.A.; Uddin, M.I.; Robertson, A.W.; Jakeman, D.L.; Mollard, V.; Goodman, C.D.; MacDougall, K.S.; McFarland, S.A.; McFadden, G.I.; et al. Synthesis and antimalarial activity of prodigiosenes. *Org. Biomol. Chem.* **2014**, *12*, 4132–4142. [CrossRef] [PubMed]
26. Lapenda, J.C.; Silva, P.A.; Vicalvi, M.C.; Sena, K.X.; Nascimento, S.C. Antimicrobial activity of prodigiosin isolated from Serratia marcescens UFPEDA 398. *World J. Microbiol. Biotechnol.* **2015**, *31*, 399–406. [CrossRef] [PubMed]
27. Wang, Y.; Nakajima, A.; Hosokawa, K.; Soliev, A.B.; Osaka, I.; Arakawa, R.; Enomoto, K. Cytotoxic prodigiosin family pigments from *Pseudoalteromonas sp.* 1020R isolated from the Pacific coast of Japan. *Biosci. Biotechnol. Biochem.* **2012**, *76*, 1229–1232. [CrossRef] [PubMed]
28. Kimyon, O.; Das, T.; Ibugo, A.I.; Kutty, S.K.; Ho, K.K.; Tebben, J.; Kumar, N.; Manefield, M. Serratia Secondary Metabolite Prodigiosin Inhibits Pseudomonas aeruginosa Biofilm Development by Producing Reactive Oxygen Species that Damage Biological Molecules. *Front. Microbiol.* **2016**, *7*, 972. [CrossRef] [PubMed]
29. Song, Y.; Liu, G.; Li, J.; Huang, H.; Zhang, X.; Zhang, H.; Ju, J. Cytotoxic and antibacterial angucycline- and prodigiosin-analogues from the deep-sea derived *Streptomyces sp.* SCSIO 11594. *Mar. Drugs* **2015**, *13*, 1304–1316. [CrossRef] [PubMed]
30. Kancharla, P.; Lu, W.; Salem, S.M.; Kelly, J.X.; Reynolds, K.A. Stereospecific synthesis of 23-hydroxyundecylprodiginines and analogues and conversion to antimalarial premarineosins via a Rieske oxygenase catalyzed bicyclization. *J. Org. Chem.* **2014**, *79*, 11674–11689. [CrossRef] [PubMed]
31. Perez-Tomas, R.; Vinas, M. New insights on the antitumoral properties of prodiginines. *Curr. Med. Chem.* **2010**, *17*, 2222–2231. [CrossRef] [PubMed]
32. Sam, S.; Sam, M.R.; Esmaeillou, M.; Safaralizadeh, R. Effective Targeting Survivin, Caspase-3 and MicroRNA-16-1 Expression by Methyl-3-pentyl-6-methoxyprodigiosene Triggers Apoptosis in Colorectal Cancer Stem-Like Cells. *Pathol. Oncol. Res.* **2016**, *22*, 715–723. [CrossRef] [PubMed]
33. Yu, C.J.; Ou, J.H.; Wang, M.L.; Jialielihan, N.; Liu, Y.H. Elevated survivin mediated multidrug resistance and reduced apoptosis in breast cancer stem cells. *J. BUON* **2015**, *20*, 1287–1294. [PubMed]
34. Chiu, W.-J.; Lin, S.-R.; Chen, Y.-H.; Tsai, M.-J.; Leong, M.; Weng, C.-F. Prodigiosin-Emerged PI3K/Beclin-1-Independent Pathway Elicits Autophagic Cell Death in Doxorubicin-Sensitive and -Resistant Lung Cancer. *J. Clin. Med.* **2018**, *7*, 321. [CrossRef] [PubMed]
35. Llagostera, E.; Soto-Cerrato, V.; Montaner, B.; Perez-Tomas, R. Prodigiosin induces apoptosis by acting on mitochondria in human lung cancer cells. *Ann. N.Y. Acad. Sci.* **2003**, *1010*, 178–181. [CrossRef] [PubMed]
36. Llagostera, E.; Soto-Cerrato, V.; Joshi, R.; Montaner, B.; Gimenez-Bonafe, P.; Perez-Tomas, R. High cytotoxic sensitivity of the human small cell lung doxorubicin-resistant carcinoma (GLC4/ADR) cell line to prodigiosin through apoptosis activation. *Anticancer Drugs* **2005**, *16*, 393–399. [CrossRef] [PubMed]
37. Zhou, W.; Jin, Z.X.; Wan, Y.J. Apoptosis of human lung adenocarcinoma A549 cells induced by prodigiosin analogue obtained from an entomopathogenic bacterium Serratia marcescens. *Appl. Microbiol. Biotechnol.* **2010**, *88*, 1269–1275. [CrossRef] [PubMed]
38. Soto-Cerrato, V.; Llagostera, E.; Montaner, B.; Scheffer, G.L.; Perez-Tomas, R. Mitochondria-mediated apoptosis operating irrespective of multidrug resistance in breast cancer cells by the anticancer agent prodigiosin. *Biochem. Pharmacol.* **2004**, *68*, 1345–1352. [CrossRef] [PubMed]
39. Monge, M.; Vilaseca, M.; Soto-Cerrato, V.; Montaner, B.; Giralt, E.; Perez-Tomas, R. Proteomic analysis of prodigiosin-induced apoptosis in a breast cancer mitoxantrone-resistant (MCF-7 MR) cell line. *Investig. New Drugs* **2007**, *25*, 21–29. [CrossRef] [PubMed]
40. Montaner, B.; Perez-Tomas, R. Prodigiosin-induced apoptosis in human colon cancer cells. *Life Sci.* **2001**, *68*, 2025–2036. [CrossRef]

41. Dalili, D.; Fouladdel, S.; Rastkari, N.; Samadi, N.; Ahmadkhaniha, R.; Ardavan, A.; Azizi, E. Prodigiosin, the red pigment of Serratia marcescens, shows cytotoxic effects and apoptosis induction in HT-29 and T47D cancer cell lines. *Nat. Prod. Res.* **2012**, *26*, 2078–2083. [PubMed]
42. Hassankhani, R.; Sam, M.R.; Esmaeilou, M.; Ahangar, P. Prodigiosin isolated from cell wall of *Serratia marcescens* alters expression of apoptosis-related genes and increases apoptosis in colorectal cancer cells. *Med. Oncol.* **2015**, *32*, 366. [CrossRef] [PubMed]
43. Sam, M.R.; Pourpak, R.S. Regulation of p53 and survivin by prodigiosin compound derived from Serratia marcescens contribute to caspase-3-dependent apoptosis in acute lymphoblastic leukemia cells. *Hum. Exp. Toxicol.* **2018**, *37*, 608–617. [CrossRef] [PubMed]
44. Campas, C.; Dalmau, M.; Montaner, B.; Barragan, M.; Bellosillo, B.; Colomer, D.; Pons, G.; Perez-Tomas, R.; Gil, J. Prodigiosin induces apoptosis of B and T cells from B-cell chronic lymphocytic leukemia. *Leukemia* **2003**, *17*, 746–750. [CrossRef] [PubMed]
45. Yenkejeh, R.A.; Sam, M.R.; Esmaeillou, M. Targeting survivin with prodigiosin isolated from cell wall of Serratia marcescens induces apoptosis in hepatocellular carcinoma cells. *Hum. Exp. Toxicol.* **2017**, *36*, 402–411. [CrossRef] [PubMed]
46. Chang, C.C.; Wang, Y.H.; Chern, C.M.; Liou, K.T.; Hou, Y.C.; Peng, Y.T.; Shen, Y.C. Prodigiosin inhibits gp91(phox) and iNOS expression to protect mice against the oxidative/nitrosative brain injury induced by hypoxia-ischemia. *Toxicol. Appl. Pharmacol.* **2011**, *257*, 137–147. [CrossRef] [PubMed]
47. Lin, S.R.; Fu, Y.S.; Tsai, M.J.; Cheng, H.; Weng, C.F. Natural Compounds from Herbs that can Potentially Execute as Autophagy Inducers for Cancer Therapy. *Int. J. Mol. Sci.* **2017**, *18*, e1412. [CrossRef] [PubMed]
48. Cheng, M.F.; Lin, C.S.; Chen, Y.H.; Sung, P.J.; Lin, S.R.; Tong, Y.W.; Weng, C.F. Inhibitory Growth of Oral Squamous Cell Carcinoma Cancer via Bacterial Prodigiosin. *Mar. Drugs* **2017**, *15*, e224. [CrossRef] [PubMed]
49. McGrail, D.J.; Khambhati, N.N.; Qi, M.X.; Patel, K.S.; Ravikumar, N.; Brandenburg, C.P.; Dawson, M.R. Alterations in ovarian cancer cell adhesion drive taxol resistance by increasing microtubule dynamics in a FAK-dependent manner. *Sci. Rep.* **2015**, *5*, 9529. [CrossRef] [PubMed]
50. Nabekura, T.; Hiroi, T.; Kawasaki, T.; Uwai, Y. Effects of natural nuclear factor-kappa B inhibitors on anticancer drug efflux transporter human P-glycoprotein. *Biomed. Pharmacother.* **2015**, *70*, 140–145. [CrossRef] [PubMed]
51. Thiyagarajan, V.; Lin, S.X.; Lee, C.H.; Weng, C.F. A focal adhesion kinase inhibitor 16-hydroxy-cleroda-3,13-dien-16,15-olide incorporated into enteric-coated nanoparticles for controlled anti-glioma drug delivery. *Colloids Surf. B Biointerfaces* **2016**, *141*, 120–131. [CrossRef] [PubMed]
52. Kessel, D. Exploring multidrug resistance using rhodamine 123. *Cancer Commun.* **1989**, *1*, 145–149. [PubMed]
53. Wang, J.; Yuan, Z. Gambogic acid sensitizes ovarian cancer cells to doxorubicin through ROS-mediated apoptosis. *Cell Biochem. Biophys.* **2013**, *67*, 199–206. [CrossRef] [PubMed]
54. Sun, M.; Zhang, N.; Wang, X.; Cai, C.; Cun, J.; Li, Y.; Lv, S.; Yang, Q. Nitidine chloride induces apoptosis, cell cycle arrest, and synergistic cytotoxicity with doxorubicin in breast cancer cells. *Tumour Biol.* **2014**, *35*, 10201–10212. [CrossRef] [PubMed]
55. Al-Abbasi, F.A.; Alghamdi, E.A.; Baghdadi, M.A.; Alamoudi, A.J.; El-Halawany, A.M.; El-Bassossy, H.M.; Aseeri, A.H.; Al-Abd, A.M. Gingerol Synergizes the Cytotoxic Effects of Doxorubicin against Liver Cancer Cells and Protects from Its Vascular Toxicity. *Molecules* **2016**, *21*, 886. [CrossRef] [PubMed]
56. Guerriero, E.; Sorice, A.; Capone, F.; Storti, G.; Colonna, G.; Ciliberto, G.; Costantini, S. Combining doxorubicin with a phenolic extract from flaxseed oil: Evaluation of the effect on two breast cancer cell lines. *Int. J. Oncol.* **2017**, *50*, 468–476. [CrossRef] [PubMed]
57. Wang, S.; Wang, L.; Shi, Z.; Zhong, Z.; Chen, M.; Wang, Y. Evodiamine synergizes with doxorubicin in the treatment of chemoresistant human breast cancer without inhibiting P-glycoprotein. *PLoS ONE* **2014**, *9*, e97512. [CrossRef] [PubMed]
58. Poornima, P.; Kumar, V.B.; Weng, C.F.; Padma, V.V. Doxorubicin induced apoptosis was potentiated by neferine in human lung adenocarcima, A549 cells. *Food Chem. Toxicol.* **2014**, *68*, 87–98. [CrossRef] [PubMed]
59. Liu, Q.; Sun, Y.; Zheng, J.M.; Yan, X.L.; Chen, H.M.; Chen, J.K.; Huang, H.Q. Formononetin sensitizes glioma cells to doxorubicin through preventing EMT via inhibition of histone deacetylase 5. *Int. J. Clin. Exp. Pathol.* **2015**, *8*, 6434–6441. [PubMed]
60. Yu, L.L.; Wu, J.G.; Dai, N.; Yu, H.G.; Si, J.M. Curcumin reverses chemoresistance of human gastric cancer cells by downregulating the NF-kappaB transcription factor. *Oncol. Rep.* **2011**, *26*, 1197–1203. [PubMed]

61. Mansingh, D.P.; O, J.S.; Sali, V.K.; Vasanthi, H.R. [6]-Gingerol-induced cell cycle arrest, reactive oxygen species generation, and disruption of mitochondrial membrane potential are associated with apoptosis in human gastric cancer (AGS) cells. *J. Biochem. Mol. Toxicol.* **2018**, *10*, e22206. [CrossRef] [PubMed]
62. Chen, S.; Yang, L.; Feng, J. Nitidine chloride inhibits proliferation and induces apoptosis in ovarian cancer cells by activating the Fas signalling pathway. *J. Pharm. Pharmacol.* **2018**, *70*, 778–786. [CrossRef] [PubMed]
63. Zhu, M.; Wang, M.; Jiang, Y.; Wu, H.; Lu, G.; Shi, W.; Cong, D.; Song, S.; Liu, K.; Wang, H. Gambogic Acid Induces Apoptosis of Non-Small Cell Lung Cancer (NSCLC) Cells by Suppressing Notch Signaling. *Med. Sci. Monit.* **2018**, *24*, 7146–7151. [CrossRef] [PubMed]
64. Wang, R.; Deng, D.; Shao, N.; Xu, Y.; Xue, L.; Peng, Y.; Liu, Y.; Zhi, F. Evodiamine activates cellular apoptosis through suppressing PI3K/AKT and activating MAPK in glioma. *Onco Targets Ther.* **2018**, *11*, 1183–1192. [CrossRef] [PubMed]
65. Park, S.; Bazer, F.W.; Lim, W.; Song, G. The O-methylated isoflavone, formononetin, inhibits human ovarian cancer cell proliferation by sub G0/G1 cell phase arrest through PI3K/AKT and ERK1/2 inactivation. *J. Cell. Biochem.* **2018**, *119*, 7377–7387. [CrossRef] [PubMed]
66. Luo, Z.; Li, D.; Luo, X.; Li, L.; Gu, S.; Yu, L.; Ma, Y. Curcumin may serve an anticancer role in human osteosarcoma cell line U-2 OS by targeting ITPR1. *Oncol. Lett.* **2018**, *15*, 5593–5601. [CrossRef] [PubMed]
67. Ho, T.F.; Peng, Y.T.; Chuang, S.M.; Lin, S.C.; Feng, B.L.; Lu, C.H.; Yu, W.J.; Chang, J.S.; Chang, C.C. Prodigiosin down-regulates survivin to facilitate paclitaxel sensitization in human breast carcinoma cell lines. *Toxicol. Appl. Pharmacol.* **2009**, *235*, 253–260. [CrossRef] [PubMed]
68. Sah, N.K.; Khan, Z.; Khan, G.J.; Bisen, P.S. Structural, functional and therapeutic biology of survivin. *Cancer Lett.* **2006**, *244*, 164–171. [CrossRef] [PubMed]
69. Jabbour-Leung, N.A.; Chen, X.; Bui, T.; Jiang, Y.; Yang, D.; Vijayaraghavan, S.; McArthur, M.J.; Hunt, K.K.; Keyomarsi, K. Sequential Combination Therapy of CDK Inhibition and Doxorubicin Is Synthetically Lethal in p53-Mutant Triple-Negative Breast Cancer. *Mol. Cancer Ther.* **2016**, *15*, 593–607. [CrossRef] [PubMed]
70. Geretti, E.; Leonard, S.C.; Dumont, N.; Lee, H.; Zheng, J.; De Souza, R.; Gaddy, D.F.; Espelin, C.W.; Jaffray, D.A.; Moyo, V.; et al. Cyclophosphamide-Mediated Tumor Priming for Enhanced Delivery and Antitumor Activity of HER2-Targeted Liposomal Doxorubicin (MM-302). *Mol. Cancer Ther.* **2015**, *14*, 2060–2071. [CrossRef] [PubMed]
71. Ihnat, M.A.; Nervi, A.M.; Anthony, S.P.; Kaltreider, R.C.; Warren, A.J.; Pesce, C.A.; Davis, S.A.; Lariviere, J.P.; Hamilton, J.W. Effects of mitomycin C and carboplatin pretreatment on multidrug resistance-associated P-glycoprotein expression and on subsequent suppression of tumor growth by doxorubicin and paclitaxel in human metastatic breast cancer xenografted nude mice. *Oncol. Res.* **1999**, *11*, 303–310. [PubMed]
72. Tenconi, E.; Guichard, P.; Motte, P.; Matagne, A.; Rigali, S. Use of red autofluorescence for monitoring prodiginine biosynthesis. *J. Microbiol. Methods* **2013**, *93*, 138–143. [CrossRef] [PubMed]
73. Elahian, F.; Moghimi, B.; Dinmohammadi, F.; Ghamghami, M.; Hamidi, M.; Mirzaei, S.A. The Anticancer Agent Prodigiosin Is Not a Multidrug Resistance Protein Substrate. *DNA Cell Biol.* **2013**, *32*, 90–97. [CrossRef] [PubMed]
74. Okabe, M.; Unno, M.; Harigae, H.; Kaku, M.; Okitsu, Y.; Sasaki, T.; Mizoi, T.; Shiiba, K.; Takanaga, H.; Terasaki, T.; et al. Characterization of the organic cation transporter SLC22A16: A doxorubicin importer. *Biochem. Biophys. Res. Commun.* **2005**, *333*, 754–762. [CrossRef] [PubMed]
75. Darshan, N.; Manonmani, H.K. Prodigiosin and its potential applications. *J. Food Sci. Technol.* **2015**, *52*, 5393–5407. [CrossRef] [PubMed]
76. Anding, A.L.; Baehrecke, E.H. Autophagy in Cell Life and Cell Death. *Apoptosis Dev.* **2015**, *114*, 67–91. [CrossRef]
77. Parzych, K.R.; Klionsky, D.J. An overview of autophagy: Morphology, mechanism, and regulation. *Antioxid. Redox Signal.* **2014**, *20*, 460–473. [CrossRef] [PubMed]
78. Lee, W.S.; Yoo, W.H.; Chae, H.J. ER Stress and Autophagy. *Curr. Mol. Med.* **2015**, *15*, 735–745. [CrossRef] [PubMed]
79. Filomeni, G.; De Zio, D.; Cecconi, F. Oxidative stress and autophagy: The clash between damage and metabolic needs. *Cell Death Differ.* **2015**, *22*, 377–388. [CrossRef] [PubMed]
80. Tacar, O.; Sriamornsak, P.; Dass, C.R. Doxorubicin: An update on anticancer molecular action, toxicity and novel drug delivery systems. *J. Pharm. Pharmacol.* **2013**, *65*, 157–170. [CrossRef] [PubMed]

81. Dirks-Naylor, A.J. The role of autophagy in doxorubicin-induced cardiotoxicity. *Life Sci.* **2013**, *93*, 913–916. [CrossRef] [PubMed]
82. Zhao, D.; Yuan, H.; Yi, F.; Meng, C.; Zhu, Q. Autophagy prevents doxorubicininduced apoptosis in osteosarcoma. *Mol. Med. Rep.* **2014**, *9*, 1975–1981. [CrossRef] [PubMed]
83. Gomes, L.R.; Vessoni, A.T.; Menck, C.F. Three-dimensional microenvironment confers enhanced sensitivity to doxorubicin by reducing p53-dependent induction of autophagy. *Oncogene* **2015**, *34*, 5329–5340. [CrossRef] [PubMed]
84. Zilinyi, R.; Czompa, A.; Czegledi, A.; Gajtko, A.; Pituk, D.; Lekli, I.; Tosaki, A. The Cardioprotective Effect of Metformin in Doxorubicin-Induced Cardiotoxicity: The Role of Autophagy. *Molecules* **2018**, *23*, E1184. [CrossRef] [PubMed]

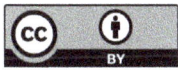

© 2018 by the authors. Licensee MDPI, Basel, Switzerland. This article is an open access article distributed under the terms and conditions of the Creative Commons Attribution (CC BY) license (http://creativecommons.org/licenses/by/4.0/).

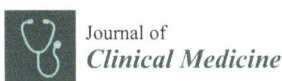 

Article

# Predictive Value of the Pretreatment Neutrophil-to-Lymphocyte Ratio in Head and Neck Squamous Cell Carcinoma

Miao-Fen Chen [1,2,*,†], Ming-Shao Tsai [2,3,†], Wen-Cheng Chen [1,2] and Ping-Tsung Chen [2,4]

1. Department of Radiation Oncology, Chang Gung Memorial Hospital, Chiayi 61363, Taiwan; rto_chen@yahoo.com.tw
2. Chang Gung University College of Medicine, Taoyuan 33302, Taiwan; b87401061@cgmh.org.tw (M.-S.T.); chencgmh@gmail.com (P.-T.C.)
3. Department of Otolaryngology & Head and Neck Surgery, Chang Gung Memorial Hospital, Chiayi 61363, Taiwan
4. Department of Hematology and Oncology, Chang Gung Memorial Hospital, Chiayi 61363, Taiwan
* Correspondence: miaofen@adm.cgmh.org.tw
† These two authors contributed equally to this work.

Received: 21 August 2018; Accepted: 18 September 2018; Published: 20 September 2018

**Abstract:** This study assessed the significance of the neutrophil-to-lymphocyte ratio (NLR) in head and neck squamous cell carcinoma (HNSCC), and the relationships of the NLR with the aldehyde dehydrogenase 1 (ALDH1) level in tumors and the proportion of myeloid-derived suppressor cells (MDSCs) in the peripheral circulation. In total, 227 HNSCC patients who had received curative treatment at our hospital were enrolled into the present study. The NLR of each HNSCC patient before treatment was calculated. The associations of NLR with various clinicopathological parameters and prognoses were then examined. In addition, correlations between the proportion of MDSCs and level of ALDH1 with the NLR were assessed. Our data revealed that an elevated NLR was significantly correlated with the risk of developing locoregional recurrence and with a reduced overall survival in HNSCC patients. Multivariate analyses revealed that the NLR pretreatment and surgical resection were significantly correlated with the rate of treatment failure and the overall survival rate in HNSCC patients. Furthermore, the levels of ALDH1 in tumors and MDSCs in the peripheral circulation were significantly correlated with the prognosis of HNSCC, and the NLR was positively correlated with MDSC levels in the circulation and ALDH1 staining intensity in tumor specimens. In conclusion, the NLR has power in predicting the expression of ALDH1 in tumors, the circulating level of MDSCs, and the prognosis in HNSCC. We suggest that the NLR is an important biomarker that can assist the clinician and patient in making informed decisions regarding treatment options for HNSCC patients.

**Keywords:** head and neck squamous cell carcinoma (HNSCC); neutrophil-to-lymphocyte ratio (NLR); myeloid-derived suppressor cells (MDSC); aldehyde dehydrogenase 1 (ALDH1); prognosis

## 1. Introduction

Head and neck squamous cell carcinoma (HNSCC) is a heterogeneous disease occurring in various sites, including the oral cavity, oropharynx, and hypopharynx [1]. Treatment failure and locoregional recurrence are common and account for the majority of deaths [2]. Identification of potential molecular markers predicting aggressive tumor growth and treatment response is important for the effective management and prognosis of HNSCC.

Abundant epidemiological data have revealed a strong correlation between inflammation and cancer incidence. Systemic inflammation is a recognized characteristic of malignancy, and numerous inflammatory markers have been investigated as prognostic indicators for cancer patients [3,4]. Host inflammatory responses were reported to play an important role in tumor development and progression [5]. The neutrophil-to-lymphocyte ratio (NLR) is an inflammatory- and immunologically-based index [6,7]. The NLR may reflect host inflammatory responses and changes in the tumor microenvironment [8]. An elevated NLR in many solid tumors, including HNSCC, has been associated with reduced survival [8–10]. However, the predictive value of the NLR in the immune and treatment responses of HNSCC is still unclear. Myeloid-derived suppressor cells (MDSCs) have been reported to attenuate immune surveillance and induce an immunosuppressive tumor microenvironment to promote cancer metastasis [11,12]. We previously reported that the recruitment of MDSCs is significantly associated with a poor prognosis in patients with HNSCC [13]. Furthermore, one of the main causes of treatment failure is the emergence of resistant cancer cells after therapy, which can be partly explained by cancer stem cells (CSCs) [14,15]. CSCs produce immunosuppressive molecules that attenuate the immune system and recruit or activate cells that suppress the immune system, such as MDSCs [16–18]. Aldehyde dehydrogenase 1 (ALDH1), a novel CSC-like cell marker, was reported to play important roles in the treatment response and tumor-promoting microenvironment in squamous cell carcinomas (SCCs) of the aerodigestive tract [19–21]. Accordingly, in the present study, we examined the predictive role of an elevated NLR in the prognosis and relationships of the NLR with the ALDH1 level in tumors, and the proportion of MDSCs in the peripheral circulation of patients with HNSCC.

## 2. Materials and Methods

### 2.1. Study Population and Study Design

The study protocol was approved by the institutional review board of Chang Gung Memorial hospital (No. 1035434B). Written informed consent was obtained from all patients. A total of 227 patients with a histologically confirmed diagnosis of HNSCC who received curative treatment were enrolled in our study. The planned treatments included definitive radiotherapy and chemotherapy (CCRT) or surgery +/− adjuvant treatment for patients with HNSCC, according to the guidelines proposed by the oncology team at our hospital. We included patient demographics (age and sex), diagnosis, clinical stage, and treatment characteristics (Table 1). In addition, the patients enrolled in the study had available data regarding ALDH1 levels in tumor specimens and/or the percentage of MDSCs in the peripheral circulation. The NLR was calculated by dividing the absolute neutrophil count by the absolute lymphocyte count. The mean absolute neutrophil count was $5.77 \pm 3.29 \times 10^3/\mu L$, and the mean absolute lymphocyte count was $1.55 \pm 0.85 \times 10^3/\mu L$. To assess the predictive value of the NLR, NLR was redefined as a binary variable by finding the value from a receiver operating characteristic (ROC) curve that maximized the percentage correctly classified for predicting tumor recurrence after treatment. The optimal cut-offs for NLR was 3. Accordingly, all HNSCC patients were divided into two groups according to the pretreatment NLR: high (NLR $\geq$ 3) and low (NLR < 3) groups.

Table 1. Characteristics of head and neck squamous cell carcinoma (HNSCC) patients with curative-intent treatment.

|  | Number of Patients | | p-Value |
| --- | --- | --- | --- |
|  | NLR < 3 | NLR $\geq$ 3 |  |
| Patient | 108 | 119 |  |
| Age |  |  |  |
| <55 (median) | 52 | 53 | 0.58 |
| $\geq$55 | 56 | 66 |  |
| Differentiation |  |  | 0.38 |
| Well differentiated | 39 | 39 |  |

Table 1. Cont.

|  | Number of Patients | | p-Value |
|---|---|---|---|
|  | NLR < 3 | NLR ≥ 3 |  |
| Moderately differentiated | 38 | 41 |  |
| Poorly differentiated | 23 | 32 |  |
| Unknown | 8 | 7 |  |
| Tumor stage |  |  | 0.073 |
| ≤T2 | 61 | 53 |  |
| T3–T4 | 47 | 66 |  |
| Clinical LN involvement |  |  | 0.87 |
| Negative | 42 | 45 |  |
| Positive | 66 | 74 |  |
| Tx policy |  |  | 0.98 |
| Definite CCRT | 31 | 34 |  |
| Surgery +/− neoadjuvant/adjuvant Tx | 77 | 85 |  |
| Location |  |  | 0.23 |
| Oral cavity | 72 | 88 |  |
| Pharynx (Oro-Hypo) | 36 | 31 |  |
| Loco-regional recurrence |  |  | <0.001 * |
| Control | 88 | 65 |  |
| Failure | 20 | 54 |  |
| Distant metastasis |  |  | 0.146 |
| Negative | 102 | 108 |  |
| Positive | 6 | 13 |  |
| Status |  |  | <0.001 * |
| Alive | 86 | 66 |  |
| Dead | 22 | 53 |  |

NLR: neutrophil-to-lymphocyte ratio; CCRT: radiotherapy and chemotherapy; LN: lymph node; Tx: treatment; *: Statistically significant covariate; T: tumor.

### 2.2. Immunohistochemical (IHC) Staining

Formalin-fixed and paraffin-embedded tissues, collected at diagnosis from 227 patients with HNSCC who had completed curative treatment, were subjected to IHC analysis (Table 2). The IHC data were assessed using the semiquantitative immunoreactive score, and positive staining was defined as an immunoreactive score ≥ 2 [21]. The clinical end points were overall survival (OS), disease-free survival, and failure pattern. Disease failure was defined as documented locoregional recurrence and/or distant metastases.

Table 2. Characteristics of head and neck squamous cell carcinoma (HNSCC) patients with curative-intent treatment.

|  | Number of Patients | | p-Value |
|---|---|---|---|
|  | ALDH1 (−) | ALDH1 (+) |  |
| Patients | 118 | 109 |  |
| Age |  |  |  |
| <55 (median) | 56 | 49 | 0.71 |
| ≥55 | 62 | 60 |  |
| Differentiation |  |  | 0.38 |
| Well differentiated | 44 | 34 |  |
| Moderately differentiated | 39 | 40 |  |
| Poorly differentiated | 27 | 28 |  |
| Unknown | 8 | 7 |  |

Table 2. Cont.

|  | Number of Patients | | p-Value |
| --- | --- | --- | --- |
|  | ALDH1 (−) | ALDH1 (+) |  |
| Tumor stage |  |  | 0.13 |
| ≤T2 | 65 | 49 |  |
| T3–T4 | 53 | 60 |  |
| Clinical LN involvement |  |  | 0.016 * |
| Negative | 54 | 33 |  |
| Positive | 64 | 76 |  |
| Tx policy |  |  | 0.42 |
| Definite CCRT | 35 | 34 |  |
| Surgery +/− neoadjuvant/adjuvant Tx | 83 | 75 |  |
| Location |  |  | 0.96 |
| Oral cavity | 72 | 77 |  |
| Pharynx (Oro-Hypo) | 36 | 32 |  |
| NLR |  |  | <0.001 * |
| <3 | 89 | 19 |  |
| ≥3 | 29 | 90 |  |
| Loco-regional recurrence |  |  | <0.001 * |
| Control | 104 | 49 |  |
| Failure | 14 | 60 |  |
| Distant metastasis |  |  | 0.019 * |
| Negative | 113 | 95 |  |
| Positive | 5 | 14 |  |
| Status |  |  | <0.001 * |
| Alive | 96 | 56 |  |
| Dead | 22 | 53 |  |

ALDH1. aldehyde dehydrogenase 1; *: Statistically significant covariate.

### 2.3. MDSC Isolation and Flow Cytometry Analysis

Peripheral blood samples were obtained from 118 patients with pathologically and clinically confirmed HNSCC (Table 3). To assess the proportion of MDSCs among peripheral blood mononuclear cells (PBMCs), multicolor fluorescence-activated cell sorting (FACS) was performed using the FACS Caliber flow cytometer (BD Biosciences, San Jose, CA, USA). Human low-density neutrophils and granulocytic MDSCs are closely related, and presently there is no generally accepted consensus on mutually exclusive definitions for these cell types [22]. In the majority of oncological studies, human granulocytic MDSCs are characterized as CD14$^-$CD15$^+$CD11b$^+$HLA-DR$^-$ cells [7]. Accordingly, the human MDSC subset characterized as CD11b$^+$CD14$^-$HLA-DR$^-$ cells was sorted from the peripheral blood. The leukocytes were separated from the peripheral blood using a Ficoll gradient before analysis or sorting. Multicolor cell analysis was performed using the following antibodies: PerCP-Cy5.5-conjugated CD14, polyethylene (PE)-conjugated CD11b, and fluorescein isothiocyanate-conjugated HLA-DR. The percentage of MDSCs was measured using multicolor flow cytometry, and isotype-specific antibodies were used as negative controls.

**Table 3.** Characteristics of head and neck squamous cell carcinoma (HNSCC) patients with curative-intent treatment.

|  | Number of Patients | | p-Value |
|---|---|---|---|
|  | MDSC (Low) | MDSC (High) |  |
| Patients | 59 | 59 |  |
| Age |  |  |  |
| <55 (median) | 28 | 26 | 0.72 |
| ≥55 | 31 | 33 |  |
| Differentiation |  |  | 0.15 |
| Well differentiated | 12 | 9 |  |
| Moderately differentiated | 24 | 18 |  |
| Poorly differentiated | 17 | 23 |  |
| Unknown | 6 | 9 |  |
| Tumor stage |  |  | 0.005 * |
| ≤T2 | 35 | 20 |  |
| T3–T4 | 24 | 39 |  |
| Clinical LN involvement |  |  | 0.018 * |
| Negative | 25 | 13 |  |
| Positive | 34 | 46 |  |
| Tx policy |  |  | 0.016 * |
| Definite CCRT | 26 | 39 |  |
| Surgery +/− neoadjuvant/adjuvant Tx | 33 | 20 |  |
| Location |  |  | 0.19 |
| Oral cavity | 29 | 22 |  |
| Pharynx (Oro-Hypo) | 30 | 37 |  |
| NLR |  |  | <0.001 * |
| <3 | 51 | 13 |  |
| ≥3 | 8 | 46 |  |
| ALDH1 staining |  |  | <0.001 * |
| Negative | 55 | 9 |  |
| Positive | 4 | 50 |  |
| Disease failure |  |  | <0.001 * |
| Negative | 52 | 26 |  |
| Positive | 7 | 33 |  |
| Status |  |  | <0.001 * |
| Alive | 54 | 34 |  |
| Dead | 5 | 25 |  |

MDSC: myeloid-derived suppressor cell; *: Statistically significant covariate.

*2.4. Statistical Analysis*

The Kaplan–Meier method was used to plot survival curves, and the log-rank test was used to determine differences in the survival curves between the two groups. The Cox proportional hazard model was used to compute hazard ratios with 95% confidence intervals (CI) after adjustment for esophageal cancer treatment and clinical characteristics. All analyses were conducted using SAS statistical software, version 9.2 (SAS Institute, Cary, NC, USA).

## 3. Results

*3.1. Correlations Between the Pretreatment NLR and Clinicopathological Characteristics of HNSCC Patients*

A total of 227 patients with HNSCC were enrolled in this study (Table 1). The median follow-up time was 25.6 months (range 1.37–148 months). There were 114 (50%) patients with clinical tumor stage T1/T2 disease and 140 (62%) with clinical lymph node involvement. Of these patients, 162 (71%)

received surgery with or without adjuvant treatment, and the others received definitive RT and chemotherapy. The pretreatment NLR was calculated as the ratio of the absolute neutrophil count to the lymphocyte count. The median pretreatment NLR of the overall cohort was 3.12 (range 0.5 to 31.8). At baseline, 119 (52%) patients had a high NLR of three or higher and 108 (48%) a low NLR less than three. The relationships between the clinicopathological variables and the pretreatment NLR values are shown in Table 1 and Figure 1a. A high NLR at baseline was significantly associated with locoregional recurrence ($p < 0.001$) and a higher risk of death during follow-up ($p < 0.001$). To further examine whether the pretreatment NLR was associated with the outcomes of HNSCC patients after curative treatment, Kaplan–Meier survival analysis was used to compare the low and high NLR subgroups. Patients with a high pretreatment NLR had a shorter overall survival (OS) time ($p < 0.001$; Figure 1b). As shown in Figure 1c,d, a high NLR was significantly associated with a reduced OS rate in both oro/hypopharyngeal cancer ($p < 0.001$) and oral cancer patients ($p = 0.047$). The results of multivariate analyses (Tables 4 and 5) revealed that the pretreatment NLR and surgical resection were significantly correlated with the risk of developing disease failure after treatment and with the OS rate. We further analyzed the predictive value of the NLR according to treatment modality. The data revealed that high NLR was associated with shorter disease-specific survival (DSS) time in patients treated with CCRT and those treated with surgery (Figure 1e,f). Moreover, in the subgroup of surgery, a high NLR was the significant predictor independent of clinical T-stage. In the subgroup of CCRT, a high NLR was associated with shorter disease-specific survival time in patients with advanced tumor stage ($p = 0.021$), but not in those with early tumor stage ($p = 0.053$).

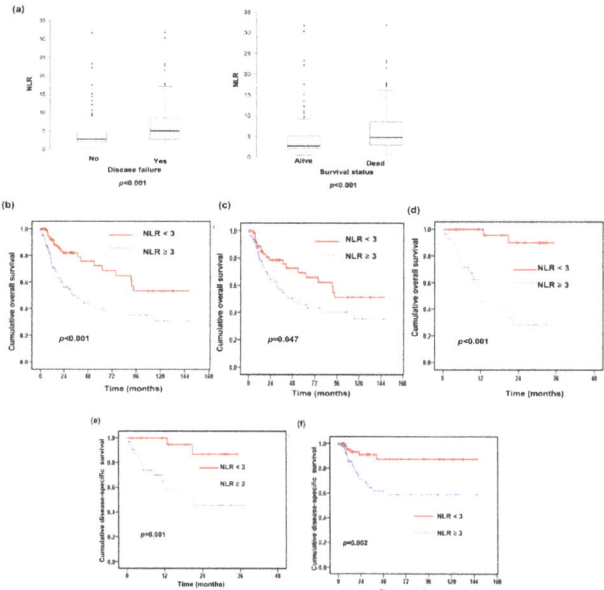

**Figure 1.** Correlations between the baseline neutrophil-to-lymphocyte ratio (NLR) and the prognosis for patients with head and neck squamous cell carcinoma (HNSCC). (**a**) The pretreatment NLR in HNSCC patients. Box-plot showing NLR at baseline was elevated in patients with locoregional recurrence and having higher risk of death during follow-up. The data showed the third quartile (Q3) and first quartile (Q1) range of the data and data outliers. Lines indicate the median values. The survival differences are according to the pre-treatment NLR (NLR $\geq$ 3 vs. NLR < 3) in (**b**) all, (**c**) subgroup of oral cancer patients, and (**d**) the subgroup of patients with oro-hypopharyngeal cancer. In addition, the differences of disease-specific survival (DSS) are according to the pre-treatment NLR in (**e**) the subgroup of definite CCRT, and (**f**) the subgroup of surgery.

**Table 4.** Adjusted hazard ratio (HR) of determining factors associated with overall survival (OS) of patients with head and neck squamous cell carcinoma (HNSCC).

| Variable | HR | 95% CI | p-Value |
|---|---|---|---|
| Age | | | |
| <50 | Ref | | |
| ≥50 | 1.51 | 0.92–2.47 | 0.1 |
| Differentiation | | | |
| Well–Moderately differentiated | Ref | | |
| Poorly differentiated. | 0.77 | 0.43–1.36 | 0.36 |
| Clinical T stage | | | |
| ≥T2 | Ref | | |
| T3–T4 | 0.85 | 0.54–1.36 | 0.5 |
| Clinical N stage | | | |
| N 0 | Ref | | |
| N (+) | 1.49 | 0.9–2.47 | 0.12 |
| NLR | | | |
| <3 | Ref | | |
| ≥3 | 2.69 | 1.62–4.46 | <0.001 * |
| Treatment | | | |
| Definite CCRT | Ref | | |
| Surgery +/− neoadjuvant/adjuvant Tx | 0.44 | 0.24–0.79 | 0.006 * |

CI: Confidence Interval; Ref: Reference Group; N: Lymph node staging; *: Statistically significant covariate.

**Table 5.** Adjusted hazard ratio (HR) of determining factors associated with disease failure of patients with head and neck squamous cell carcinoma (HNSCC).

| Variable | HR | 95% CI | p-Value |
|---|---|---|---|
| Age | | | |
| <50 | Ref | | |
| ≥50 | 1.26 | 0.8–1.99 | 0.314 |
| Differentiation | | | |
| Well–Moderately differentiated | Ref | | |
| Poorly differentiated | 0.87 | 0.52–0.47 | 0.61 |
| Clinical T stage | | | |
| ≤T2 | Ref | | |
| T3–T4 | 0.94 | 0.61–1.45 | 0.77 |
| Clinical N stage | | | |
| N 0 | Ref | | |
| N (+) | 1.6 | 0.99–2.58 | 0.057 |
| NLR | | | |
| < 3 | Ref | | |
| ≥ 3 | 2.71 | 1.69–4.38 | <0.001 * |
| Treatment | | | |
| Definite CCRT | Ref | | |
| Surgery +/− neoadjuvant/adjuvant Tx | 0.37 | 0.22–0.63 | <0.001 * |

*: Statistically significant covariate.

*3.2. Relationships of ALDH1 Expression with the Pretreatment NLR and Clinical Outcome*

We previously reported that positive ALDH1 staining was significantly related to a poor treatment response and higher disease failure rate in oral squamous cell carcinoma (SCC) [21]. Accordingly, we analyzed the predictive role of ALDH1 levels in the clinical outcome and its correlation with the pretreatment NLR in the 227 HNSCC patients. Figure 2a shows representative slides of positive and negative ALDH1 staining in HNSCC specimens at diagnosis. IHC revealed ALDH1 overexpression in 109 (48%) in these patients. As shown in Table 2, positive ALDH1 staining was significantly associated with the risk of lymph node involvement ($p = 0.016$), a higher rate of locoregional failure ($p < 0.001$), and distant metastasis ($p = 0.019$). As shown in Figure 2b,c, positive staining of ALDH1 was significantly associated with a higher locoregional failure rate and lower OS rate. In the multivariate analysis, positive staining of ALDH1 was significantly associated with a higher risk of developing disease failure and a shorter OS time in HNSCC (Tables 6 and 7). Furthermore, the distribution of the pretreatment NLR was significantly associated with ALDH1 staining in tumor specimens (Table 2 and Figure 2d). Based on the results, we suggest that positive staining of ALDH1 is an independent predictor of shorter survival and a higher rate of disease failure, and a high pretreatment NLR plays a role in predicting ALDH1 expression levels and subsequently a poor prognosis in HNSCC.

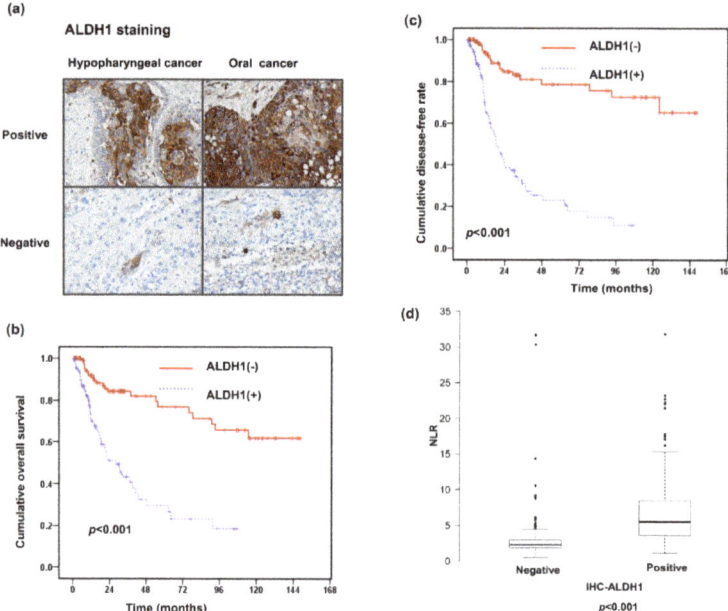

**Figure 2.** Relationships between NLR, aldehyde dehydrogenase 1 (ALDH1) expression level, and clinical outcome. (**a**) Representative images of immunohistochemical (IHC) staining with anti-ALDH1 antibodies of oral cancer and hypopharyngeal cancer specimens. Survival differences demonstrated according to the staining of ALDH1 in (**b**) overall survival rate and (**c**) disease failure-free rate. (**d**) NLR levels in the groups of HNSCC patients with and without ALDH1 positive staining in tumor specimens. The data show the third quartile (Q3) and first quartile (Q1) range of the data and data outlier. Lines indicate the median values.

**Table 6.** Adjusted hazard ratio (HR) of determining factors associated with overall survival (OS) of patients with head and neck squamous cell carcinoma (HNSCC).

| Variable | HR | 95% CI | $p$-Value |
|---|---|---|---|
| Age | | | |
| <50 | Ref | | |
| ≥50 | 1.36 | 0.84–2.12 | 0.21 |
| Differentiation | | | |
| Well–Moderately differentiated | Ref | | |
| Poorly differentiated | 0.79 | 0.45–1.39 | 0.42 |
| Clinical T stage | | | |
| ≤T2 | Ref | | |
| T3–T4 | 1.01 | 0.62–1.60 | 0.98 |
| Clinical N stage | | | |
| N 0 | Ref | | |
| N (+) | 1.17 | 0.71–1.93 | 0.53 |
| ALDH1 | | | |
| Negative | Ref | | |
| Positive | 4.1 | 2.43–6.92 | <0.001 * |
| Treatment | | | |
| Definite CCRT | Ref | | |
| Surgery +/− neoadjuvant/adjuvant Tx | 0.48 | 0.27–0.87 | 0.015 * |

*: Statistically significant covariate.

**Table 7.** Adjusted hazard ratio (HR) of determining factors associated with disease failure of patients with head and neck squamous cell carcinoma (HNSCC).

| Variable | HR | 95% CI | $p$-Value |
|---|---|---|---|
| Age | | | |
| <50 | Ref | | |
| ≥50 | 1.12 | 0.71–1.77 | 0.62 |
| Differentiation | | | |
| Well–Moderately differentiated | Ref | | |
| Poorly differentiated | 0.88 | 0.53–1.47 | 0.63 |
| Clinical T stage | | | |
| ≤T2 | Ref | | |
| T3–T4 | 1.1 | 0.70–1.71 | 0.68 |
| Clinical N stage | | | |
| N 0 | Ref | | |
| N (+) | 1.26 | 0.78–2.03 | 0.35 |
| ALDH1 | | | |
| Negative | Ref | | |
| Positive | 5.92 | 3.46–10.11 | <0.001 * |
| Treatment | | | |
| Definite CCRT | Ref | | |
| Surgery +/− neoadjuvant/adjuvant Tx | 0.42 | 0.25–0.71 | 0.001 * |

*: Statistically significant covariate.

*3.3. Predictive Role of Pretreatment NLR on Levels of $CD11b^+CD14^-HLA-DR^-$ Cells in Peripheral Circulation*

Accumulating evidence indicates that MDSCs, a population of cells with suppressive activity, contribute to the negative regulation of immune responses and subsequently to tumor promotion [11]. We previously reported that circulating MDSC levels were significantly increased in patients with HNSCC, and this was associated with the clinical tumor burden [13]. In the present study, the percentage of CD11b⁺CD14⁻HLA-DR⁻ cells, a subset of MDSCs, in the peripheral circulation of 118 patients with HNSCC was evaluated by flow cytometry. Representative flow cytometry data from two HNSCC patients are shown in Figure 3a. The mean percentage of CD11b⁺CD14⁻HLA-DR⁻ cells in the peripheral blood mononuclear cells of the 118 HSCC patients was 11.6 ± 7.4%. As shown Figure 3b,c, the percentage of CD11b⁺CD14⁻HLA-DR⁻ cells was significantly correlated with the risk of developing disease failure and death after treatment ($p < 0.001$). An increased MDSC level was reported to be associated with attenuating immune surveillance noted in CSC tumors [16,17,21]. Figure 3d shows that the level of MDSCs was significantly higher in the ALDH1-positive group than in the ALDH1-negative group ($p < 0.001$). The 118 patients were further divided into two groups according to the mean CD11b⁺CD14⁻HLA-DR⁻ cell percentage at diagnosis (11.6%): high (≥11.6%) and low (<11.6%) groups. As shown in Table 3, a high percentage of CD11b⁺CD14⁻HLA-DR⁻ cells was associated with a more advanced clinical tumor stage (T3/T4, $p = 0.005$), lymph node involvement ($p = 0.018$), a higher pretreatment NLR, and shorter survival compared with a low CD11b⁺CD14⁻HLA-DR⁻ cell percentage. In the multivariate analysis, a higher percentage of circulating MDSCs was significantly associated with a higher risk of developing disease failure and a shorter survival in patients with HNSCC (Tables 8 and 9). We further assessed the usefulness of the NLR in predicting the CD11b⁺CD14⁻HLA-DR⁻ cell percentage. A strong correlation was found between the pretreatment NLR and the percentage of CD11b⁺CD14⁻HLA-DR⁻ cells in peripheral circulation of HNSCC patients (Figure 3e).

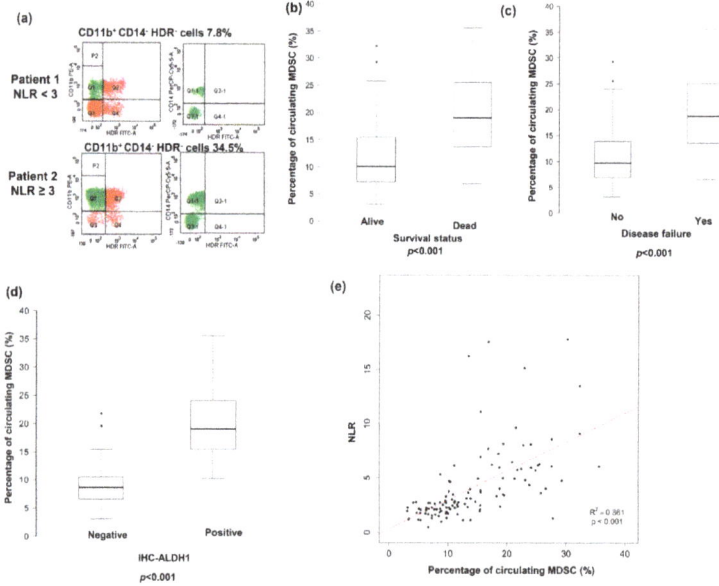

**Figure 3.** Correlation between pre-treatment NLR in the levels of circulating CD11b⁺CD14⁻HLA-DR⁻ cells and ALDH1. (**a**) Flow cytometric analysis of circulating CD11b⁺CD14⁻HLA-DR⁻ cells in isolated peripheral blood mononuclear cells (PBMCs). HLA-DR−CD11b+ cells were gated, and the CD14 negative population was then selected. Representative data from two cancer patients are shown (upper row, the patient with pretreatment NLR < 3; lower row, the patient with pretreatment NLR ≥ 3). Elevated circulating levels of CD11b⁺CD14⁻HLA-DR⁻ cells associated with the higher risk of death (**b**), disease recurrence after treatment (**c**), and ALDH1 positive staining (**d**). (**e**) Positive correlation between the levels of CD11b⁺CD14⁻HLA-DR⁻ cells and pre-treatment NLR in the peripheral circulation.

**Table 8.** Adjusted hazard ratio (HR) of determining factors associated with overall survival (OS) of patients with neck squamous cell carcinoma (HNSCC).

| Variable | HR | 95% CI | p-Value |
|---|---|---|---|
| Age | | | |
| <50 | Ref | | |
| ≥50 | 0.71 | 0.32–1.55 | 0.39 |
| Differentiation | | | |
| Well–Moderately differentiated | Ref | | |
| Poorly differentiated | 0.44 | 0.18–1.06 | 0.07 |
| Clinical T stage | | | |
| ≤T2 | Ref | | |
| T3–T4 | 1.04 | 0.44–2.48 | 0.93 |
| Clinical N stage | | | |
| N 0 | Ref | | |
| N (+) | 1.19 | 0.49–2.90 | 0.70 |
| MDSC | | | |
| Low | Ref | | |
| High | 6.19 | 2.34–18.0 | <0.001 * |
| Treatment | | | |
| Definite CCRT | Ref | | |
| Surgery +/− neoadjuvant/adjuvant Tx | 0.43 | 0.19–0.98 | 0.044 * |

*: Statistically significant covariate.

**Table 9.** Adjusted hazard ratio (HR) of determining factors associated with disease failure of patients with neck squamous cell carcinoma (HNSCC).

| Variable | HR | 95% CI | p-Value |
|---|---|---|---|
| Age | | | |
| <50 | Ref | | |
| ≥50 | 0.70 | 0.34–1.40 | 0.31 |
| Differentiation | | | |
| Well–Moderately differentiated | Ref | | |
| Poorly differentiated | 0.61 | 0.29–1.25 | 0.18 |
| Clinical T stage | | | |
| ≤T2 | Ref | | |
| T3–T4 | 1.28 | 0.60–2.76 | 0.52 |
| Clinical N stage | | | |
| N 0 | Ref | | |
| N (+) | 1.59 | 0.68–3.75 | 0.29 |
| ALDH1 | | | |
| Negative | Ref | | |
| Positive | 5.31 | 2.23–12.62 | <0.001 * |
| Treatment | | | |
| Definite CCRT | Ref | | |
| Surgery +/− neoadjuvant/adjuvant Tx | 0.39 | 0.19–0.82 | 0.012 * |

*: Statistically significant covariate.

## 4. Discussion

The tumor microenvironment plays an important role in cancer development and progression and may be associated with systemic inflammation [23]. Neutrophils form the first line of host immune defense against bacterial and fungal infections [24]. Compared with their role in host defenses, which is relatively well established, we are just beginning to learn about the precise role of neutrophils in cancer [25,26]. Many recent studies suggested that an elevated NLR is associated with poor survival of subjects with cancer [8,27], including head and neck cancer [10,28]. In the present study, an advantage of our analyses was that the results were based on a relatively large population of HNSCC patients from a single institute, with available information regarding staging and primary treatment details. Based on the analyses of 227 HNSCC patients who received curative treatment, an elevated pretreatment NLR was significantly associated with higher loco-regional recurrence rate and reduced OS rate. According to univariate and multivariate analyses, a pretreatment NLR of three or higher was associated with a shorter OS compared with a NLR below three. Treatment policy included surgery with or without adjuvant treatment for oral cancers and definitive radiation and chemotherapy for oropharyngeal and hypopharyngeal cancers. We further analyzed the predictive value of the NLR according to treatment modality. The data revealed that an increased NLR was a significant predictor for poor prognosis in patients treated with CCRT and those treated with surgery. Based on these results, the NLR is a useful baseline variable for assessing prognosis in HNSCC patients considered for curative treatment.

Circulating blood contains several types of immune cells that participate in the immune response. The interactions among the various populations of immune cells have been recognized as critical in forming the immune microenvironment, which provides the milieu for the anti-cancer immune response to occur [29–32]. MDSCs constitute an immature population of myeloid cells thought to be an important subset of cells that contribute to an immunosuppressive tumor microenvironment, and MDSC numbers are significantly increased in cancer patients [33,34]. Increasing evidence has demonstrated an association between suppressive neutrophils and granulocytic MDSCs related to immune suppression and their relevance to disease [35]. Many of the pro-tumor features of suppressive neutrophils are shared with granulocytic MDSCs, and the distinction between these two cell populations is a matter of intensive debate. We previously found that MDSC recruitment provided a microenvironment conducive to tumor growth and the development of treatment resistance in HNSCC [13]. To date, granulocytic MDSCs have been defined mainly as $CD11b^+CD14^-HLA-DR^-$ cell lineages in human cancers [7,22,35]. Accordingly, we characterized the proportions of $CD11b^+CD14^-HLA-DR^-$ myeloid cells in a cohort of HNSCC patients. FACS analyses revealed that the percentage of these MDSCs was correlated with the clinical tumor burden, disease status, and survival. We further demonstrated a positive correlation between the NLR and circulating $CD11b^+CD14^-HLA-DR^-$ cell level in HNSCC patients. In the present study, we showed that the pretreatment NLR was related to the circulating $CD11b^+CD14^-HLA-DR^-$ cell level and disease progression.

Much of the relationship between immune cells, either circulating or within tumors, and disease outcome in cancer can probably be explained by the inflammatory response that is secondary to the cancer. CSCs are becoming recognized as being responsible for metastasis and treatment resistance [36,37]. ALDH1, a detoxifying enzyme, has been identified as a novel CSC-like cell marker and is relevant to the prognosis of cancers [19,20,38,39]. Immune evasion was reported to play a role in the contribution of CSCs in tumor promotion [16,40]. CSCs can recruit cells that suppress the immune system, such as the activation of myeloid-derived suppressor cells (MDSCs), to attenuate immune surveillance [16–18,41–43]. Our previous data revealed correlations between ALDH1 expression levels and treatment resistance, CSC-like properties, higher circulating MDSC levels, and poor prognosis in oral SCC. Accordingly, we further examined the predictive value of ALDH1 for HNSCC prognosis and the correlations of the ALDH1 level with the MDSC level and NLR. By analyzing the clinical outcomes of 227 patients with HNSCC, the elevated expression of ALDH1 was correlated with a higher incidence of lymph node involvement, higher disease failure rate, and lower survival rate. Moreover, there were significant correlations among ALDH1 IHC staining, the levels of circulating MDSCs, and NLR. Patients with a higher NLR had a higher ALDH1 level in their tumors and more MDSCs in the peripheral circulation, which are associated with poor prognosis of HNSCC. The current study is limited by the inherent nature of investigating a hospital-based registry and the nonrandomized approach to treatment selection. Furthermore, we could not account for potential unmeasured selection biases regarding performance status, comorbidity, access to health care, or other patient-related factors.

## 5. Conclusions

With the increasing use of personalized therapy, patient selection has become an important issue in assessing efficacy. The targeted therapy of CSCs may enhance the treatment response, thereby resulting in improved clinical outcomes in patients with HNSCC. In addition, MDSCs have been suggested to be a novel target for multiple cancers, and numerous clinically available agents have been developed [34]. Thus, it is imperative to identify clinically feasible parameters highly relevant to the characteristics of CSC and the level of MDSCs. The NLR is a cheaper and faster laboratory measure compared with other biomarkers, and it does not involve any additional cost. In the present study, we showed that the NLR was relevant to ALDH1 and MDSC levels and a strong prognostic indicator for HNSCC patients. Discussions based on pretreatment NLR results may help the patient decide whether the side effects of curative treatments are worth the risk. We suggest the NLR to be an important biomarker for patients that can assist the clinician and patient to make informed decisions regarding treatment options.

**Author Contributions:** Conceptualization, M.-F.C., M.-S.T. and W.-C.C.; Data curation, M.-S.T.; Formal analysis, P.-T.C.; Funding acquisition, M.-F.C.; Investigation, M.-F.C.; Methodology, W.-C.C.; Writing—original draft, M.-S.T.; Writing—review & editing, M.-F.C.

**Funding:** The grant was support by Chang Gung Memorial Hospital, Taiwan, grant CMRPG6E0372-3.

**Acknowledgments:** The authors would like to thank the Health Information and Epidemiology Laboratory (CLRPG6G0041) for their comments and assistance in data analysis.

**Conflicts of Interest:** The authors declare that they have no competing interests. All authors read and approved the final manuscript.

## References

1. Gillison, M.L.; D'Souza, G.; Westra, W.; Sugar, E.; Xiao, W.; Begum, S.; Viscidi, R. Distinct risk factor profiles for human papillomavirus type 16-positive and human papillomavirus type 16-negative head and neck cancers. *J. Natl. Cancer Inst.* **2008**, *100*, 407–420. [CrossRef] [PubMed]
2. Leemans, C.R.; Tiwari, R.; Nauta, J.J.; van der Waal, I.; Snow, G.B. Recurrence at the primary site in head and neck cancer and the significance of neck lymph node metastases as a prognostic factor. *Cancer* **1994**, *73*, 187–190. [CrossRef]
3. Hanahan, D.; Weinberg, R.A. Hallmarks of cancer: The next generation. *Cell* **2011**, *144*, 646–674. [CrossRef] [PubMed]
4. McMillan, D.C. The systemic inflammation-based Glasgow Prognostic Score: A decade of experience in patients with cancer. *Cancer Treat. Rev.* **2013**, *39*, 534–540. [CrossRef] [PubMed]
5. Grivennikov, S.I.; Greten, F.R.; Karin, M. Immunity, inflammation, and cancer. *Cell* **2010**, *140*, 883–899. [CrossRef] [PubMed]
6. Houghton, A.M. The paradox of tumor-associated neutrophils: Fueling tumor growth with cytotoxic substances. *Cell Cycle* **2010**, *9*, 1732–1737. [CrossRef] [PubMed]
7. Dumitru, C.A.; Moses, K.; Trellakis, S.; Lang, S.; Brandau, S. Neutrophils and granulocytic myeloid-derived suppressor cells: Immunophenotyping, cell biology and clinical relevance in human oncology. *Cancer Immunol. Immunother.* **2012**, *61*, 1155–1167. [CrossRef] [PubMed]
8. Guthrie, G.J.; Charles, K.A.; Roxburgh, C.S.; Horgan, P.G.; McMillan, D.C.; Clarke, S.J. The systemic inflammation-based neutrophil-lymphocyte ratio: Experience in patients with cancer. *Crit. Rev. Oncol. Hematol.* **2013**, *88*, 218–230. [CrossRef] [PubMed]
9. Yodying, H.; Matsuda, A.; Miyashita, M.; Matsumoto, S.; Sakurazawa, N.; Yamada, M.; Uchida, E. Prognostic significance of neutrophil-to-lymphocyte ratio and platelet-to-lymphocyte ratio in oncologic outcomes of esophageal cancer: A systematic review and meta-analysis. *Ann. Surg. Oncol.* **2016**, *23*, 646–654. [CrossRef] [PubMed]
10. Takenaka, Y.; Oya, R.; Kitamiura, T.; Ashida, N.; Shimizu, K.; Takemura, K.; Yamamoto, Y.; Uno, A. Prognostic role of neutrophil-to-lymphocyte ratio in head and neck cancer: A meta-analysis. *Head Neck* **2018**, *40*, 647–655. [CrossRef] [PubMed]

11. Bunt, S.K.; Sinha, P.; Clements, V.K.; Leips, J.; Ostrand-Rosenberg, S. Inflammation induces myeloid-derived suppressor cells that facilitate tumor progression. *J. Immunol.* **2006**, *176*, 284–290. [CrossRef] [PubMed]
12. Smyth, M.J.; Cretney, E.; Kershaw, M.H.; Hayakawa, Y. Cytokines in cancer immunity and immunotherapy. *Immunol. Rev.* **2004**, *202*, 275–293. [CrossRef] [PubMed]
13. Chen, W.C.; Lai, C.H.; Chuang, H.C.; Lin, P.Y.; Chen, M.F. Inflammation-induced myeloid-derived suppressor cells associated with squamous cell carcinoma of the head and neck. *Head Neck* **2017**, *39*, 347–355. [CrossRef] [PubMed]
14. Krause, M.; Dubrovska, A.; Linge, A.; Baumann, M. Cancer stem cells: Radioresistance, prediction of radiotherapy outcome and specific targets for combined treatments. *Adv. Drug Deliv. Rev.* **2017**, *109*, 63–73. [CrossRef] [PubMed]
15. Frank, N.Y.; Schatton, T.; Frank, M.H. The therapeutic promise of the cancer stem cell concept. *J. Clin. Investig.* **2010**, *120*, 41–50. [CrossRef] [PubMed]
16. Silver, D.J.; Sinyuk, M.; Vogelbaum, M.A.; Ahluwalia, M.S.; Lathia, J.D. The intersection of cancer, cancer stem cells, and the immune system: Therapeutic opportunities. *Neuro. Oncol.* **2016**, *18*, 153–159. [CrossRef] [PubMed]
17. Qi, Y.; Li, R.M.; Kong, F.M.; Li, H.; Yu, J.P.; Ren, X.B. How do tumor stem cells actively escape from host immunosurveillance? *Biochem. Biophys. Res. Commun.* **2012**, *420*, 699–703. [CrossRef] [PubMed]
18. Parsa, A.T.; Waldron, J.S.; Panner, A.; Crane, C.A.; Parney, I.F.; Barry, J.J.; Cachola, K.E.; Murray, J.C.; Tihan, T.; Jensen, M.C.; et al. Loss of tumor suppressor PTEN function increases B7-H1 expression and immunoresistance in glioma. *Nat. Med.* **2007**, *13*, 84–88. [CrossRef] [PubMed]
19. Qian, X.; Wagner, S.; Ma, C.; Coordes, A.; Gekeler, J.; Klussmann, J.P.; Hummel, M.; Kaufmann, A.M.; Albers, A.E. Prognostic significance of ALDH1A1-positive cancer stem cells in patients with locally advanced, metastasized head and neck squamous cell carcinoma. *J. Cancer Res. Clin. Oncol.* **2014**, *140*, 1151–1158. [CrossRef] [PubMed]
20. Xu, J.; Muller, S.; Nannapaneni, S.; Pan, L.; Wang, Y.; Peng, X.; Wang, D.; Tighiouart, M.; Chen, Z.; Saba, N.F.; et al. Comparison of quantum dot technology with conventional immunohistochemistry in examining aldehyde dehydrogenase 1A1 as a potential biomarker for lymph node metastasis of head and neck cancer. *Eur. J. Cancer* **2012**, *48*, 1682–1691. [CrossRef] [PubMed]
21. Tsai, M.S.; Chen, W.C.; Lai, C.H.; Chen, Y.Y.; Chen, M.F. Epigenetic therapy regulates the expression of ALDH1 and immunologic response: Relevance to the prognosis of oral cancer. *Oral Oncol.* **2017**, *73*, 88–96. [CrossRef] [PubMed]
22. Brandau, S.; Moses, K.; Lang, S. The kinship of neutrophils and granulocytic myeloid-derived suppressor cells in cancer: Cousins, siblings or twins? *Semin. Cancer Biol.* **2013**, *23*, 171–182. [CrossRef] [PubMed]
23. De Vlaeminck, Y.; Gonzalez-Rascon, A.; Goyvaerts, C.; Breckpot, K. Cancer-Associated Myeloid Regulatory Cells. *Front. Immunol.* **2016**, *7*, 113. [CrossRef] [PubMed]
24. Borregaard, N. Neutrophils, from marrow to microbes. *Immunity* **2010**, *33*, 657–670. [CrossRef] [PubMed]
25. Uribe-Querol, E.; Rosales, C. Neutrophils in cancer: Two sides of the same coin. *J. Immunol. Res.* **2015**, *2015*. [CrossRef] [PubMed]
26. Swierczak, A.; Mouchemore, K.A.; Hamilton, J.A.; Anderson, R.L. Neutrophils: Important contributors to tumor progression and metastasis. *Cancer Metastasis Rev.* **2015**, *34*, 735–751. [CrossRef] [PubMed]
27. Templeton, A.J.; McNamara, M.G.; Seruga, B.; Vera-Badillo, F.E.; Aneja, P.; Ocana, A.; Leibowitz-Amit, R.; Sonpavde, G.; Knox, J.J.; Tran, B.; et al. Prognostic role of neutrophil-to-lymphocyte ratio in solid tumors: A systematic review and meta-analysis. *J. Natl. Cancer Inst.* **2014**, *106*. [CrossRef] [PubMed]
28. Yu, Y.; Wang, H.; Yan, A.; Wang, H.; Li, X.; Liu, J.; Li, W. Pretreatment neutrophil to lymphocyte ratio in determining the prognosis of head and neck cancer: A meta-analysis. *BMC Cancer* **2018**, *18*, 383–392. [CrossRef] [PubMed]
29. Zamarron, B.F.; Chen, W. Dual roles of immune cells and their factors in cancer development and progression. *Int. J. Biol. Sci.* **2011**, *7*, 651–658. [CrossRef] [PubMed]
30. Tanaka, A.; Sakaguchi, S. Regulatory T cells in cancer immunotherapy. *Cell Res.* **2017**, *27*, 109–118. [CrossRef] [PubMed]
31. Treffers, L.W.; Hiemstra, I.H.; Kuijpers, T.W.; van den Berg, T.K.; Matlung, H.L. Neutrophils in cancer. *Immunol. Rev.* **2016**, *273*, 312–328. [CrossRef] [PubMed]

32. Schupp, J.; Krebs, F.K.; Zimmer, N.; Trzeciak, E.; Schuppan, D.; Tuettenberg, A. Targeting myeloid cells in the tumor sustaining microenvironment. *Cell Immunol.* **2017**. [CrossRef] [PubMed]
33. Moses, K.; Brandau, S. Human neutrophils: Their role in cancer and relation to myeloid-derived suppressor cells. *Semin. Immunol.* **2016**, *28*, 187–196. [CrossRef] [PubMed]
34. Najjar, Y.G.; Finke, J.H. Clinical perspectives on targeting of myeloid derived suppressor cells in the treatment of cancer. *Front. Oncol.* **2013**, *3*, 49–58. [CrossRef] [PubMed]
35. Pillay, J.; Tak, T.; Kamp, V.M.; Koenderman, L. Immune suppression by neutrophils and granulocytic myeloid-derived suppressor cells: Similarities and differences. *Cell. Mol. Life Sci.* **2013**, *70*, 3813–3827. [CrossRef] [PubMed]
36. Koch, U.; Krause, M.; Baumann, M. Cancer stem cells at the crossroads of current cancer therapy failures—radiation oncology perspective. *Semin. Cancer Biol.* **2010**, *20*, 116–124. [CrossRef] [PubMed]
37. Gerweck, L.E.; Wakimoto, H. At the crossroads of cancer stem cells; radiation biology; and radiation oncology. *Cancer Res.* **2016**, *76*, 994–998. [CrossRef] [PubMed]
38. Clay, M.R.; Tabor, M.; Owen, J.H.; Carey, T.E.; Bradford, C.R.; Wolf, G.T.; Wicha, M.S.; Prince, M.E. Single-marker identification of head and neck squamous cell carcinoma cancer stem cells with aldehyde dehydrogenase. *Head Neck* **2010**, *32*, 1195–1201. [CrossRef] [PubMed]
39. Ginestier, C.; Hur, M.H.; Charafe-Jauffret, E.; Monville, F.; Dutcher, J.; Brown, M.; Jacquemier, J.; Viens, P.; Kleer, C.G.; Liu, S.; et al. ALDH1 is a marker of normal and malignant human mammary stem cells and a predictor of poor clinical outcome. *Cancer Res.* **2007**, *1*, 555–567. [CrossRef] [PubMed]
40. Cho, R.W.; Clarke, M.F. Recent advances in cancer stem cells. *Curr. Opin. Genet. Dev.* **2008**, *18*, 48–53. [CrossRef] [PubMed]
41. Aguirre-Ghiso, J.A. Models, mechanisms and clinical evidence for cancer dormancy. *Nat. Rev. Cancer* **2007**, *7*, 834–846. [CrossRef] [PubMed]
42. Codony-Servat, J.; Rosell, R. Cancer stem cells and immunoresistance: Clinical implications and solutions. *Transl. Lung Cancer Res.* **2015**, *4*, 689–703. [PubMed]
43. Sica, A.; Porta, C.; Amadori, A.; Pasto, A. Tumor-associated myeloid cells as guiding forces of cancer cell stemness. *Cancer Immunol. Immunother.* **2017**, *66*, 1025–1036. [CrossRef] [PubMed]

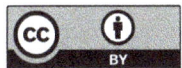

© 2018 by the authors. Licensee MDPI, Basel, Switzerland. This article is an open access article distributed under the terms and conditions of the Creative Commons Attribution (CC BY) license (http://creativecommons.org/licenses/by/4.0/).

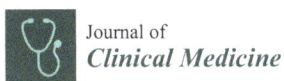 

Article

# The Role of Diffusion-Weighted Magnetic Resonance Imaging in the Differentiation of Head and Neck Masses

Lutfi Kanmaz [1] and Erdal Karavas [2,*]

[1] Department of Otorhinolaryngology—Head and Neck Surgery, Pazarcık State Hospital, Kahramanmaraş 46700, Turkey; lutfikanmaz@gmail.com
[2] Department of Radiology, Faculty of Medicine, Erzincan University, Erzincan 24100, Turkey
* Correspondence: erdalkaravas@hotmail.com; Tel.: +90-446-212-2222

Received: 22 April 2018; Accepted: 21 May 2018; Published: 29 May 2018

**Abstract:** The purpose of this study was to evaluate the value of diffusion-weighted MRI (DW-MRI) in differentiating benign and malignant head and neck masses by comparing their apparent diffusion coefficient (ADC) values. The study included 32 patients with a neck mass >1 cm in diameter who were examined with echo planar DW-MRI. Two different diffusion gradients (b values of b = 0 and b = 1000 s/mm$^2$) were applied. DWI and ADC maps of 32 neck masses in 32 patients were obtained. Mean ADC values of benign and malignant neck lesions were measured and compared statistically. A total of 15 (46.9%) malignant masses and 17 (53.1%) benign masses were determined. Of all the neck masses, the ADC value of cystic masses was the highest and that of lymphomas was the lowest. The mean ADC values of benign and malignant neck masses were $1.57 \times 10^{-3}$ mm$^2$/s and $0.90 \times 10^{-3}$ mm$^2$/s, respectively. The difference between mean ADC values of benign and malignant neck masses was significant ($p < 0.01$). Diffusion-weighted MRI with ADC measurements can be useful in the differential diagnosis of neck masses.

**Keywords:** neck mass; diffusion-weighted MRI; apparent diffusion coefficient

## 1. Introduction

Quick and accurate diagnosis directly affects treatment success for patients with a neck mass, which is a common finding in ENT clinics. Inadequate or late diagnosis of a malignant mass increases the morbidity and mortality of a disease.

The rapid development of diagnostic imaging technology has provided clinical practice with new facilities for the evaluation of neck masses. These new methods are gaining importance with the advantageous factors of cost and ease of use. At present, ultrasonography (USG) and/or computed tomography (CT) are used as conventional methods for the evaluation of neck lesions.

If necessary, magnetic resonance imaging (MRI) is used for the characterization of neck masses. MRI evaluates the morphology, signal intensity and enhancement pattern of lesions. However, none of these methods can accurately differentiate benign from malignant lesions. This has led to the necessity of researching new diagnostic methods. Diffusion-weighted magnetic resonance imaging (DW-MRI) is a non-contrast enhanced technique that can be obtained during a single breath-hold. In the literature, DW-MRI was first used in the early diagnosis of stroke in neuroradiology [1,2]. In the early period, the use of this technique was limited in the central nervous system due to its sensitivity to cardiac, respiratory, and peristaltic movements. However, following improvements in the echo planar imaging technique as a fast MRI sequence, it became possible to successfully apply diffusion-weighted echo planar MRI even in other areas with high-susceptibility artifacts. DW-MRI was first applied to head and neck lesions in 2001 and promising results have been achieved [3]. Subsequent studies showed that

DW-MRI appeared to be helpful in differentiating epidermoid carcinoma and malignant lymphoma, staging neck nodal disease, and distinguishing radiotherapy-induced tissue changes from persistent or recurrent cancer. In these studies, apparent diffusion coefficient (ADC) values of tissues and lesions are calculated using diffusion-weighted images and different values in the differential diagnosis. Moreover, with the use of this imaging technique, the creation of an ADC map is an excellent method for differentiation between the viable and necrotic parts of head and neck tumors. Thus, the ADC map can be used to select the best biopsy site and to detect tumor viability in the post-treatment follow-up of patients after radiation therapy. The technique may also be useful in characterizing thyroid nodules and salivary gland neoplasms.

The purpose of this study was to evaluate the value of DW-MRI in differentiating benign and malignant head and neck masses by comparing their ADC values.

## 2. Materials and Methods

This prospective study was performed on 43 consecutive patients who underwent MRI for a diagnosis of head and neck lesions in our center. All patients were examined with contrast-enhanced MRI and DW-MRI. The study was conducted in the Department of Otorhinolaryngology, Bakırköy Dr. Sadi Konuk Training and Research Hospital, in the period of June 2009 to June 2010.

Institutional Ethics Committee approval was obtained for the study.

*2.1. Subjects*

A total of 11 patients were excluded from the study; four patients with neck masses <1 cm in the greatest minimal transverse diameter, two who had undergone biopsy, three due to distortion artifacts, and two with a final diagnosis of neck metastasis of a thyroid carcinoma.

Thus the final study population of 32 consecutive patients with neck masses >1 cm in diameter consisted of 12 females (37.5%) and 20 males (62.5%) with a mean age of $45.13 \pm 17.08$ years (range, 9–78 years). All patients were questioned in detail about age, location, and duration of the mass, associated symptoms, and then routine blood tests such as serological tests were applied. Within the head and neck examination, diagnostic pan-endoscopy of the nasal cavity, nasopharynx, oropharynx, hypopharynx, and larynx was also performed. All clinical evaluations were documented.

When patients had multiple neck masses with the same histological diagnosis, only the largest one was used for calculation of ADC values. Thus, the diffusion-weighted images and ADC maps of 32 neck masses in 32 patients were studied.

Localization of the lesions was classified according to the lymph node regions and neck facial spaces. The final diagnosis of the patients was made by histopathological examination of surgical specimens. A diagnosis of tuberculosis lymphadenitis was made by histology and culture, two undifferentiated nasopharyngeal carcinoma metastases by primary tumor biopsy and FNAB, neck metastasis in five patients with NHL diagnosed by excisional lymph node biopsy, and one adenocarcinoma metastasis by FNAB. A diagnosis of SCC metastasis was confirmed with neck dissection. Diagnosis of carotid body paraganglioma in one patient was established with MR angiography and DSA (digital subtraction angiography) before excision.

*2.2. MR Imaging Techniques*

All the MR examinations were performed with a 1.5 Tesla MR unit (Siemens Avanto, Erlangen, Germany). Routine examination consisted of T2-weighted fast spin-echo images (with a section thickness of 4 mm, an interslice gap of 1–2 mm, a field of view (FOV) of 25–30 cm and an acquisition matrix of $256 \times 224$) and DW-MRIs. Before DW-MRI, T2-weighted images were obtained in the axial plane. A total of 14 transverse images covering the lesions were obtained. DW-MRIs were obtained at the section level where the largest transverse section of the lesion was detected on the MRIs which were obtained before administration of contrast material. DW-MRI was obtained using multi-slice spin-echo single-shot echo planar imaging in the axial plane. For each patient, diffusion-weighted images and ADC maps were obtained by applying diffusion-sensitive gradients in three orthogonal directions (x, y, and z) and two different b-values (0 and 1000 s/mm$^2$). ADC maps of the images were automatically reconstructed on the main console. Then, the region of interest (ROI) was defined by a radiologist measuring the signal intensity of the lesion. ROIs were determined on the solid appearing parts for the solid masses and on the cystic areas for the cystic lesions. The ADC values of the lesions were calculated with an ROI >1 cm$^2$.

*2.3. Statistical Analysis*

Statistical analyses of the study data were performed using NCSS (Number Cruncher Statistical System) 2007 and PASS (Power Analysis and Sample Size) 2008 Statistical Software (HyLown Consulting LLC., Atlanta, GA, USA). The Student's *t*-test was used to compare data between two groups. Results were stated as the mean and standard deviation. Qualitative data were compared using the chi-square test. The receiver operating characteristic (ROC) curve was applied to determine the cut-off point with the highest accuracy and sensitivity. The value of $p < 0.05$ was considered statistically significant at a 95% confidence level.

## 3. Results

This study was performed on 32 consecutive patients with head and neck masses who underwent echo planar DW-MRI from June 2009 to June 2010. The patients consisted of 12 females (37.5%) and 20 males (62.5%) with a mean age of 45.13 ± 17.08 years (range, 9–78 years).

Malignant masses were determined in 15 (46.9%) cases and benign masses in 17 (53.1%). The benign masses consisted of five pleomorphic adenoma originating from major salivary glands, three reactive lymphadenopathies, two branchial cleft cysts, two cervical sympathetic chain schwannomas, two Whartin's tumors, one glomus tumor, one tbc lymphadenitis, and one thyroglossal duct cyst. The malignant masses were five Non-Hodgkin's lymphoma, three larynx SCC met., two undifferentiated carcinoma met., two oropharynx SCC met., one GIS adeno ca met., one primary unknown carcinoma met., and one tonsil SCC met. The diagnoses of the patients are listed in Table 1.

Of the total neck masses, the ADC value of cystic masses was the highest ($1.98 \times 10^{-3}$ mm$^2$/s) and that of lymphomas ($0.80 \times 10^{-3}$ mm$^2$/s) was the lowest. The mean ADC values of benign and malignant neck masses were $1.57 \times 10^{-3}$ mm$^2$/s and $0.90 \times 10^{-3}$ mm$^2$/s, respectively. The difference between the mean ADC value of benign and malignant neck masses was statistically significant ($p < 0.01$). The localizations of the masses are listed in Table 1. The numbers of malignant and benign masses were 15 (46.9%) and 17 (53.1%), respectively. The mean ADC value of benign masses with high signal intensity was statistically significantly higher than that of malignant masses with low signal intensity ($p < 0.01$) (Table 2). Malignant masses were classified in two categories as malignant lymphomas (33.3%) and carcinomas (66.7%, squamous cell carcinoma or adenocarcinoma). There was no statistically significant difference between the two categories in the malignant group ($p > 0.05$) (Table 2). When an ADC value of $1.13 \times 10^{-3}$ mm$^2$/s or less was used to predict malignancy, the best results were achieved with high accuracy, with sensitivity of 93.33%, specificity of 82.35%, positive predictive value of 82.35%, and a negative predictive value of 93.33% (Table 3).

The ROC curve was used to evaluate the diagnostic capability of the ADC value to differentiate benign from malignant masses. When $1.13 \times 10^{-3}$ mm$^2$/s was used as a threshold value in differentiating benign from malignant masses, the area under the curve was 0.918 (Table 4, Figure 1).

**Table 1.** Diagnosis and localization of 32 head and neck masses.

| Diagnosis | n | % |
|---|---|---|
| Pleomorphic adenoma | 5 | 15.6 |
| Reactive lymphadenitis | 3 | 9.4 |
| Branchial cleft cyst | 2 | 6.3 |
| Schwannoma | 2 | 6.3 |
| Whartin tumor | 2 | 6.3 |
| Glomus tumor | 1 | 3.1 |
| Tbc lymphadenitis | 1 | 3.1 |
| Thyroglossal duct cyst | 1 | 3.1 |
| Non-hodgkin's lymphoma | 5 | 15.6 |
| Larynx SCC metastasis | 3 | 9.4 |
| Undifferentiated carcinoma metastasis | 2 | 6.3 |
| Oropharynx SCC metastasis | 2 | 6.3 |
| GIS adenocarcinoma metastasis | 1 | 3.1 |
| Primary unknown carcinoma met. | 1 | 3.1 |
| Tonsil SCC metastasis | 1 | 3.1 |
| **Localizations** | **n** | **%** |
| Anterior cervical | 1 | 3.1 |
| Superior lateral cervical | 9 | 28.1 |
| Middle lateral cervical | 3 | 9.4 |
| Posterior cervical | 1 | 3.1 |
| Sup-mid lateral cervical | 2 | 6.3 |
| Parapharyngeal area | 3 | 9.4 |
| Parotid area | 7 | 21.9 |
| Submandibular area | 5 | 15.6 |
| Supraclavicular area | 1 | 3.1 |

**Table 2.** Pathological diagnosis and distribution of mean ADC values in the examined groups.

| Pathology | n | % | ADC ($\times 10^{-3}$ mm$^2$/s) Ave. $\pm$ SD. | +p |
|---|---|---|---|---|
| Malignant | 15 | 46.9 | 0.90 $\pm$ 0.17 | 0.001 ** |
| Benign | 17 | 53.1 | 1.57 $\pm$ 0.42 | |
| Lymphoma | 5 | 33.3 | 0.80 $\pm$ 0.14 | 0.100 |
| Carcinoma | 10 | 66.7 | 0.96 $\pm$ 0.17 | |

+ Student $t$ test; ** $p \leq 0.001$.

**Table 3.** Calculating the threshold value.

| Value | Sensitivity | Specificity | Positive Predictive Value | Negative Predictive Value | Accuracy | Relative Risk |
|---|---|---|---|---|---|---|
| 0.95 | 66.67 | 88.24 | 83.33 | 75.00 | 78.13 | 3.33 |
| 0.98 | 66.67 | 82.35 | 76.92 | 73.68 | 75.00 | 2.92 |
| 1.05 | 80.00 | 82.35 | 80.00 | 82.35 | 81.25 | 4.53 |
| 1.12 | 86.67 | 82.35 | 81.25 | 87.50 | 84.38 | 6.50 |
| 1.13 | 93.33 | 82.35 | 82.35 | 93.33 | 87.50 | 12.35 |
| 1.20 | 100.00 | 82.35 | 83.33 | 100.00 | 90.63 | - |
| 1.21 | 100.00 | 76.47 | 78.95 | 100.00 | 87.50 | - |
| 1.34 | 100.00 | 70.59 | 75.00 | 100.00 | 84.38 | - |

**Table 4.** Area under the curve (AUC).

| Area under the Curve | | | | | |
|---|---|---|---|---|---|
| Area | Std. Error (a) | p | 95% Confidence Interval | |
| | | | Upper | Lower |
| 0.918 | 0.05 | 0.001 | 0.819 | 1.016 |

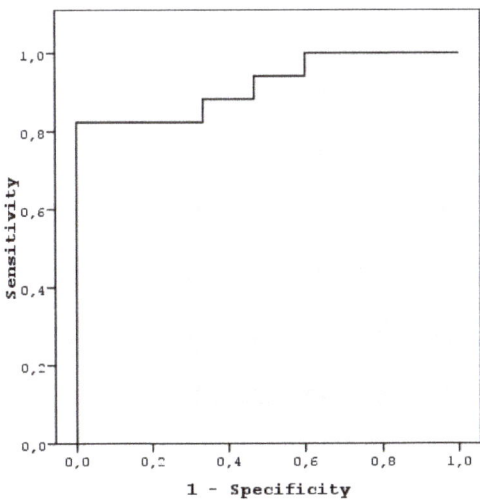

**Figure 1.** Receiver operating characteristic (ROC) curve of the ADC value.

## 4. Discussion

Diffusion is defined as the randomized microscopic movement of water molecules and is used as a sensitive parameter for the characterization of tissue at a microscopic level. Today, in vivo measurement of diffusion is possible with DW-MRI and ADC measurements. As a result of new technological developments, MRI has become sensitive to the diffusion of water protons in biological tissues and diffusion-weighted imaging can be obtained. Intracellular and extracellular water balance is also shown in a way that is important for diagnosis and follow-up of stroke. Initially, the use of this technique was limited to brain studies because of technical problems regarding motion artifact due to cardiac, respiratory, and peristaltic movements. However, following improvements in echo planar imaging techniques, an echo planar DW-MRI can now be successfully performed even in areas with high susceptibility artifacts [4]. This technique was first used in neuroradiological imaging for diagnosis of early cerebral ischemia and has become a diagnostic tool in this area [1,5].

In 1994, Muller et al. measured the ADC of water in liver, spleen, kidney, and muscle and showed that in vivo diffusion measurements of abdominal organs obtained with MRI could prove helpful in the identification and classification of abdominal disease [6]. Subsequently, in several studies, DW-MRI has been shown to be able to be used in the differential diagnosis of lesions in the liver, kidney, and other abdominal organs with the measurement of ADCs [7,8].

In the literature, DW-MRI has also been seen to have an application area in the different regions of the head and neck. The characterization of head and neck lesions with echo planar DW-MRI by Wang et al. [3] was the first study in this area. They found that the mean ADC value of the benign lesions was statistically significantly different than that of malignant lesions. In 2003, Sumi et al. [9] studied the differential diagnosis of metastatic lymph nodes with diffusion-weighted MR imaging. Over several years, further studies have been made in this area. In another study on neck lymph nodes, ADC maps, as a new technique, have been used to determine the necrotic and non-necrotic solid areas of malignant lesions [10]. Eida et al. [11] reported that preoperative tissue characterization of salivary gland tumors could be made with ADC map construction. In another study, Abdel Razek et al. reported that the mean ADC value of malignant thyroid nodules was statistically significantly lower than that of benign ones [12]. The diffusion technique involves the diffusion motion of water protons in the tissues. According to the diffusion of tissue, the diffusion of water molecules varies in the different regions of tissue. Therefore, the diffusion coefficient of the tissue varies depending on any change in the proportion of extracellular to intracellular water molecules. Thus, diffusion-weighted MR imaging produces different contrast and ADC values according to the microstructure of the tissues [3].

In the current study, the mean ADC value of benign masses with high signal intensity was significantly (Figure 2) higher than that of malignant (Figure 3) masses with low signal intensity. These differences in ADC values may be explained by the differences in the histopathological characteristics of benign and malignant tumors. Generally, malignant tumors show hypercellularity and have enlarged nuclei, and hyperchromatism. These histopathological characteristics reduce the diffusion space of water protons in the extracellular and intracellular regions [13,14].

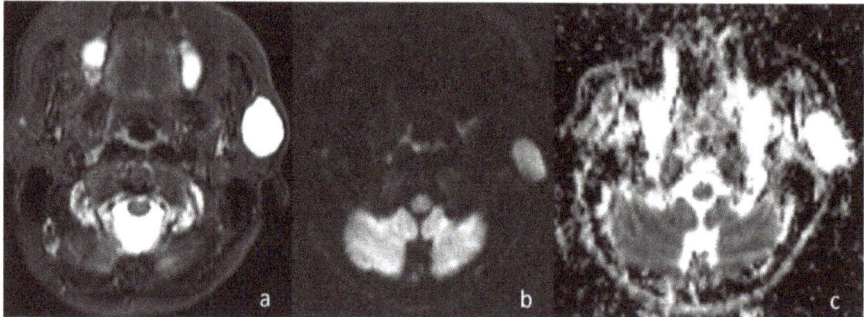

**Figure 2.** Pleomorphic adenoma of the parotid gland. (**a**) Axial T2-weighted image (T2WI) shows a mass in the left parotid gland; (**b**) the lesion shows low signal intensity on DWI; and (**c**) the mass is hyperintense on the ADC map (ADC value of $1.55 \times 10^{-3}$ mm$^2$/s).

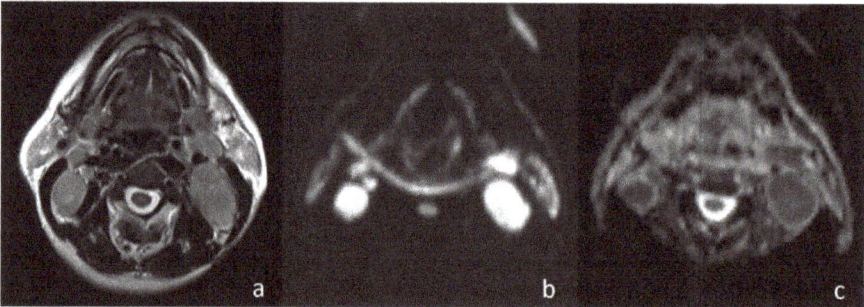

**Figure 3.** Undifferentiated nasopharyngeal carcinoma. (**a**) Axial T2WI shows bilateral metastatic cervical lymph nodes; (**b**) lymph node, on the left side of the neck, shows high signal intensity on DWI; and (**c**) the mass is hypointense on the ADC map (ADC value of $0.91 \times 10^{-3}$ mm$^2$/s).

Apparently higher ADC values for benign cystic masses may be expected because of the relatively freer mobility of water protons in the fluid. In the current study, cystic masses were not grouped separately due to low numbers. However, consistent with previous studies, the mean ADC value of three cystic masses (Figure 4) ($1.98 \times 10^{-3}$ mm$^2$/s) was higher than that of other benign solid masses (ADC = $1.48 \times 10^{-3}$ mm$^2$/s). In addition, the differences in ADC values among cystic masses could be explained by the different protein concentrations. A high protein level restricts the movement of water molecules by increasing the viscosity [15].

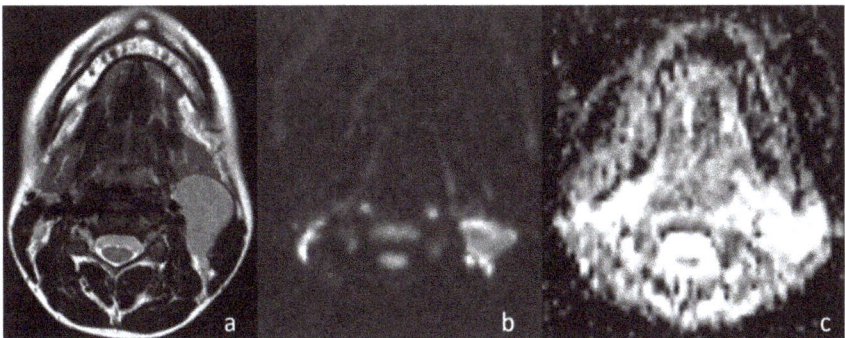

**Figure 4.** Second branchial cleft cyst. (**a**) Axial T2WI shows a unilocular cystic mass in the left carotid space; (**b**) the lesion shows low signal intensity on DWI; and (**c**) the lesion is hyperintense on the ADC map (ADC value of $2.02 \times 10^{-3}$ mm$^2$/s).

Sumi et al. [16] reported that the mean ADC value of lymphomas is lower than that of metastatic lymph nodes of carcinomas due to the difference in cellular density. Maeda et al. [17] also reported that carcinomas could contain small foci of necrosis on histopathological examination that was not identifiable on conventional MRI. This investigation has also been used to explain the higher ADC values of SCCs than those of lymphomas. In the current study, although there was no statistically significant difference, the mean ADC value of lymphomas (Figure 5) ($0.80 \times 10^{-3}$ mm$^2$/s) was lower than that of the other malignant tumors ($0.96 \times 10^{-3}$ mm$^2$/s). In the malignant group, larynx SCC metastasis with the value of $1.15 \times 10^{-3}$ mm$^2$/s showed the highest values.

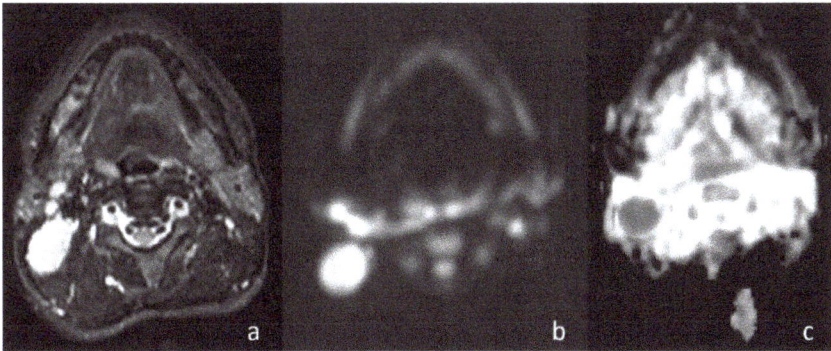

**Figure 5.** Non-Hodgkin lymphoma. (**a**) Axial T2WI shows metastatic cervical lymph node nearby SCM; (**b**) the lymph node, on the right side of the neck at level of lateral cervical region, shows high signal intensity on DWI; and (**c**) the mass is hypointense on the ADC map (ADC value of $0.62 \times 10^{-3}$ mm$^2$/s).

One of the considerations that must be taken into account when using diffusion-weighted MRI for the differential diagnosis of masses is the recognition of the fact that some malignant masses behave like a benign tumor independently of the 'cut-off' ADC value obtained at the end of the study. These masses are some primary or metastatic SCC and thyroid carcinoma metastases [3]. In the current study, a case with diagnosis of larynx SCC metastasis in the ADC value of $1.20 \times 10^{-3}$ mm$^2$/s showed the feature of a benign tumor. The reason that the high ADC values are non-standardized might be the presence of small foci of micronecrosis and the hypervascular tumor portions that escalate the perfusion effect in some malignant tumors and of dense extracellular fluid in follicular components in thyroid carcinomas [3]. Considering this situation, the macroscopic solid portions were determined using MRI observations and the ADC measurements were made, and the cases with neck masses of thyroid origin were excluded from the study. Although DW-MRI is more reliable than that of other MR imaging techniques to identify micronecrosis of primary or metastatic tumors, [18–20] the differentiation between the viable and necrotic parts of head and neck tumors with DW-MRI by reconstructing ADC maps is possible for accurate biopsy results [21]. In addition, DW-MRI with ADC measurement may be used for differentiating residual or recurrent head and neck tumors from postoperative or postradiation changes [22].

With concern for inaccurate ADC measurements in small lesions according to the susceptibility artifacts and image distortions as a limitation of this imaging technique, neck masses <1 cm in the greatest minimal transverse diameter on MRI were excluded from the study. In a study by Chen et al., performed to compare periodically rotated overlapping parallel lines with enhanced reconstruction (PROPELLER) DW-MRI and echo planar DW-MRI techniques, it was suggested that it was possible to reduce the distortion of head and neck masses through PROPELLER diffusion-weighted MRI to a large extent [23].

One of the limitations of the current study was the area of necrosis that showed falsely higher ADC values, especially in the center of metastatic neck masses [10]. Therefore, ADC values were measured by selecting the solid portions of tumors.

In the study, three masses in the benign group indicated lower ADC values than the cut-off value in accordance with the malignant mass. In one of these masses, which was tuberculous lymphadenopathy (ADC = $0.92 \times 10^{-3}$ mm$^2$/s); restriction of diffusion could be explained by the presence of inflammatory cells in the pus that reduced the diffusion space of water protons [24]. In another study, this situation was explained by the thickness of the caseous material of granulomatous lesions [25]. Whartin tumor (ADC = $0.88 \times 10^{-3}$ mm$^2$/s) was the other case that was falsely diagnosed as a malignant tumor (Figure 6). Intense lymphoid accumulation in the stroma and proliferation of the epithelial component could be the reason for the limited motion of the water protons in the extracellular space [3]. Reactive lymphadenitis was the third case. A varying amount of fibrosis in the stroma of inflammatory cells could have resulted in the low ADC value by restriction of the diffusion of water molecules [3].

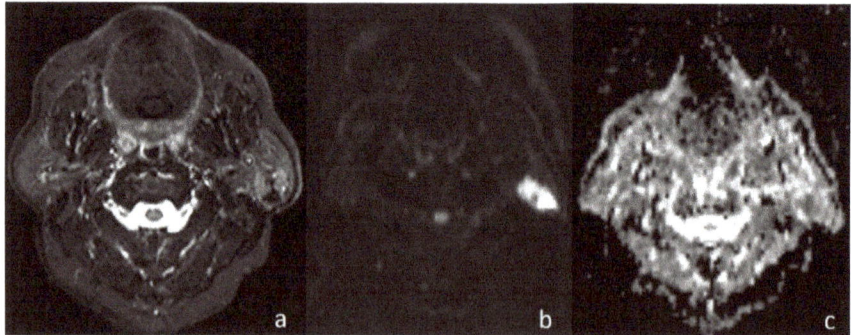

**Figure 6.** Warthin tumor. (**a**) Axial T2WI showing the mass localised in the superficial lobe and spreading into the deep lobe of the left parotid gland; (**b**) the lesion shows high signal intensity on DWI; and (**c**) the lesion is hypointense on the ADC map (ADC value of $0.88 \times 10^{-3}$ mm$^2$/s) and the tumor was falsely diagnosed as a malignant lesion.

In the current study, in cases with malignant diseases, the mass appeared hyperintense on diffusion images (obtained at b = 1000 s/mm$^2$) and with low signal intensity on ADC maps and, conversely, benign masses appeared hypointense and hyperintense, respectively. There was a statistically significant difference in ADC values between the malignant masses and benign lesions ($p < 0.01$). When an ADC value of $1.13 \times 10^{-3}$ mm$^2$/s or less was used to predict malignancy, the best results were achieved with high accuracy, with 93.33% sensitivity, 82.35% specificity, 82.35% positive predictive value, and 93.33% negative predictive value.

In this study, the patient groups were heterogeneous with different histopathological entities and there was a limited number of cases in each benign or malignant group. Further investigations of a larger series with a specific group of the same pathological diagnosis are necessary.

## 5. Conclusions

In summary, DW-MRI seems to be a promising non-invasive imaging technique for characterization of head and neck masses or for any other subjects as discussed above. It can be concluded that further studies on larger series and advances of diffusion MR techniques to improve the image quality would help DW-MRI to become a routine imaging technique.

**Author Contributions:** L.K. conceived and designed the experiments; L.K. and E.K. performed the experiments; L.K. analyzed the data; L.K. and E.K. contributed reagents/materials/analysis tools; and L.K. wrote the paper.

**Acknowledgments:** The authors would like to thank Filiz Saçan for help and technical support. The authors declare that this study has not received any financial support.

**Conflicts of Interest:** The authors declare no conflict of interest.

## References

1. Warach, S.; Chien, D.; Li, W.; Ronthal, M.; Edelman, R.R. Fast magnetic resonance diffusion-weighted imaging of acute human stroke. *Neurology* **1992**, *9*, 1717–1723. [CrossRef]
2. Lutsep, H.L.; Albers, G.W.; DeCrespigny, A.; Kamat, G.N.; Marks, M.P.; Moseley, M.E. Clinical utility of diffusion-weighted magnetic resonance imaging in the assessment of ischemic stroke. *Ann. Neurol.* **1997**, *5*, 574–580. [CrossRef] [PubMed]
3. Wang, J.; Takashima, S.; Takayama, F.; Kawakami, S.; Saito, A.; Matsushita, T.; Momose, M.; Ishiyama, T. Head and neck lesions: Characterization with diffusion-weighted echo planar MR imaging. *Radiology* **2001**, *3*, 621–630. [CrossRef] [PubMed]
4. Reimer, P.; Saini, S.; Hahn, P.F.; Brady, T.J.; Cohen, M.S. Clinical application of abdominal echo planar imaging (EPI): Optimization using a retrofitted EPI system. *J. Comput. Assist. Tomogr.* **1994**, *5*, 673–679. [CrossRef]
5. Yoo, A.J.; Barak, E.R.; Copen, W.A.; Kamalian, S.; Gharai, L.R.; Pervez, M.A.; Schwamm, L.H.; González, R.G.; Schaefer, P.W. Combining acute diffusion-weighted imaging and mean transmit time lesion volumes with National Institutes of Health Stroke Scale Score improves the prediction of acute stroke outcome. *Stroke* **2010**, *8*, 1728–1735. [CrossRef] [PubMed]
6. Müller, M.F.; Prasad, P.; Siewert, B.; Nissenbaum, M.A.; Raptopoulos, V.; Edelman, R.R. Abdominal diffusion mapping with use of a whole-body echo planar system. *Radiology* **1994**, *2*, 475–483.
7. Kim, T.; Murakami, T.; Takahashi, S.; Hori, M.; Tsuda, K.; Nakamura, H. Diffusion-weighted single-shot echo planar MR imaging for liver disease. *AJR Am. J. Roentgenol.* **1999**, *2*, 393–398. [CrossRef] [PubMed]
8. Namimoto, T.; Yamashita, Y.; Mitsuzaki, K.; Nakayama, Y.; Tang, Y.; Takahashi, M. Measurement of the apparent diffusion coefficient in diffuse renal disease by diffusion weighted echo planar MR imaging. *J. Magn. Reson. Imaging* **1999**, *6*, 832–837. [CrossRef]
9. Sumi, M.; Sakihama, N.; Sumi, T.; Morikawa, M.; Uetani, M.; Kabasawa, H.; Shigeno, K.; Hayashi, K.; Takahashi, H.; Nakamura, T. Discrimination of metastatic cervical lymph nodes with diffusion-weighted MR imaging in patients with head and neck cancer. *AJNR Am. J. Neuroradiol.* **2003**, *8*, 1627–1634.
10. Abdel Razek, A.A.; Soliman, N.Y.; Elkhamary, S.; Alsharaway, M.K.; Tawfik, A. Role of diffusion-weighted MR imaging in cervical lymphadenopathy. *Eur. Radiol.* **2006**, *7*, 1468–1477. [CrossRef] [PubMed]
11. Eida, S.; Sumi, M.; Sakihama, N.; Takahashi, H.; Nakamura, T. Apparent diffusion coefficient mapping of salivary gland tumors: Prediction of the benignancy and malignancy. *AJNR Am. J. Neuroradiol.* **2007**, *1*, 116–121.

12. Razek, A.A.; Sadek, A.G.; Kombar, O.R.; Elmahdy, T.E.; Nada, N. Role of apparent diffusion coefficient values in differentiation between malignant and benign solitary thyroid nodules. *AJNR Am. J. Neuroradiol.* **2008**, *3*, 563–568. [CrossRef] [PubMed]
13. Thoeny, H.C.; De Keyzer, F. Extracranial applications of diffusion-weighted magnetic resonance imaging. *Eur. Radiol.* **2007**, *6*, 1385–1393. [CrossRef] [PubMed]
14. Herrington, C.S. Tumours: Cancer and Benign Tumours. In *Muir's Textbook of Pathology*, 15th ed.; Herrington, C.S., Ed.; CRC Press: Boca Raton, FL, USA, 2014; pp. 77–101.
15. Kim, Y.J.; Chang, K.H.; Song, I.C.; Kim, H.D.; Seong, S.O.; Kim, Y.H.; Han, M.H. Brain abscess and necrotic or cystic brain tumor: Discrimination with signal intensity on diffusion weighted MR imaging. *AJR Am. J. Roentgenol.* **1998**, *6*, 1487–1490. [CrossRef] [PubMed]
16. Sumi, M.; Van Cauteren, M.; Nakamura, T. MR microimaging of benign and malignant nodes in the neck. *AJR Am. J. Roentgenol.* **2006**, *3*, 749–757. [CrossRef] [PubMed]
17. Maeda, M.; Kato, H.; Sakuma, H.; Maier, S.E.; Takeda, K. Usefulness of the apparent diffusion coefficient in line scan diffusion-weighted imaging for distinguishing between squamous cell carcinomas and malignant lymphomas of the head and neck. *AJNR Am. J. Neuroradiol.* **2005**, *5*, 1186–1192.
18. Yousem, D.M.; Montone, K.T. Head and neck lesions: Radiologic-pathologic correlations. *Radiol. Clin. N. Am.* **1998**, *5*, 983–1014. [CrossRef]
19. Van den Brekel, M.W.; Stel, H.V.; Castelijns, J.A.; Nauta, J.J.; van der Waal, I.; Valk, J.; Meyer, C.J.; Snow, G.B. Cervical lymph node metastasis: Assessment of radiologic criteria. *Radiology* **1990**, *2*, 379–384. [CrossRef] [PubMed]
20. Lang, P.; Wendland, M.F.; Saeed, M.; Gindele, A.; Rosenau, W.; Mathur, A.; Gooding, C.A.; Genant, H.K. Osteogenic sarcoma: Noninvasive in vivo assessment of tumor necrosis with diffusion-weighted MR imaging. *Radiology* **1998**, *1*, 227–235. [CrossRef] [PubMed]
21. Razek, A.A.; Megahed, A.S.; Denewer, A.; Motamed, A.; Tawfik, A.; Nada, N. Role of diffusion-weighted magnetic resonance imaging in differentiation between the viable and necrotic parts of head and neck tumors. *Acta Radiol.* **2008**, *3*, 364–370. [CrossRef] [PubMed]
22. Hermans, R. Diffusion-weighted MRI in head and neck cancer. *Curr. Opin. Otolaryngol. Head Neck Surg.* **2010**, *2*, 72–78. [CrossRef] [PubMed]
23. Chen, X.; Xian, J.; Wang, X.; Wang, Y.; Zhang, Z.; Guo, J.; Li, J. Role of periodically rotated overlapping parallel lines with enhanced reconstruction diffusion-weighted imaging in correcting distortion and evaluating head and neck masses using 3 T MRI. *Clin. Radiol.* **2014**, *4*, 403–409. [CrossRef] [PubMed]
24. Perrone, A.; Guerrisi, P.; Izzo, L.; D'Angeli, I.; Sassi, S.; Mele, L.L.; Marini, M.; Mazza, D.; Marini, M. Diffusion-weighted MRI in cervical lymph nodes: Differentiation between benign and malignant lesions. *Eur. J. Radiol.* **2011**, *2*, 281–286. [CrossRef] [PubMed]
25. Abdel Razek, A.A.; Gaballa, G.; Elhawarey, G. Characterization of pediatric head and neck masses with diffusion-weighted MR imaging. *Eur. Radiol.* **2008**, *1*, 201–208. [CrossRef] [PubMed]

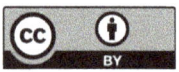

© 2018 by the authors. Licensee MDPI, Basel, Switzerland. This article is an open access article distributed under the terms and conditions of the Creative Commons Attribution (CC BY) license (http://creativecommons.org/licenses/by/4.0/).

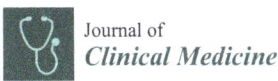 

Article

# Canaloplasty in Corticosteroid-Induced Glaucoma. Preliminary Results

Paolo Brusini [1,*], Claudia Tosoni [1] and Marco Zeppieri [2]

1 Department of Ophthalmology, "Città di Udine" Health Center, Viale Venezia, 410, 33100 Udine, Italy; c.tosoni@libero.it
2 Department of Ophthalmology, "Azienda Ospedaliero-Universitaria" "Santa Maria della Misericordia" Hospital of Udine, P.le S. Maria della Misericordia, 15, 33100 Udine, Italy; markzeppieri@hotmail.com
* Correspondence: brusini@libero.it; Tel.: +3-943-223-9371; Fax: +3-943-254-5400

Received: 11 December 2017; Accepted: 7 February 2018; Published: 11 February 2018

**Abstract:** Purpose: to present the mid-term results of canaloplasty in a small cohort of corticosteroid glaucoma patients. Material and Methods: Nine eyes from seven patients with various types of corticosteroid glaucoma in maximum medical therapy underwent canaloplasty. Patients underwent complete ophthalmic examination every six months. Success was defined as: post-operative intraocular pressure (IOP) $\leq$ 21 mmHg and $\leq$ 16 mmHg without ("complete success"), and with/without medical treatment ("qualified success"). The IOP reduction had to be $\geq$ 20. The number of medications before and after surgery was considered. The follow-up mean period was 32.7 $\pm$ 20.8 months (range 14–72 months). Results: The pre-operative mean IOP was 30.7 $\pm$ 7.2 mmHg (range: 24–45). The mean IOP at 6 and 12-month follow-up was 13.1 $\pm$ 2.6 mmHg, and 13.7 $\pm$ 1.9 mmHg, respectively. Qualified and complete success at 6 and 12 months was 100% for both of the two definitions. The number of medications used preoperatively and at the 12-month follow-up was 4.3 $\pm$ 0.7, and 0.2 $\pm$ 1.0, respectively. No serious complication was observed. Conclusions: The mid-term results of canaloplasty in patients with corticosteroid-induced glaucoma appear to be very promising. Canaloplasty should be considered as a possible alternative to filtering surgery in this form of glaucoma, when medical therapy is not sufficient to maintain the IOP within reasonable limits.

**Keywords:** canaloplasty; non-perforating surgical procedures; corticosteroid-induced glaucoma; Schlemm's canal

## 1. Introduction

Corticosteroid-induced glaucoma is a quite common form of secondary glaucoma due to either systemic or, more frequently, topical, peri- or intraocular administration of glucocorticoids in predisposed subjects [1–5]. It is known that corticosteroids raise intraocular pressure (IOP) by lowering the facility of aqueous outflow. Quite a high percentage of normal subjects (ranging from 5% to over 40% depending on the definition of corticosteroid-responders [6,7] may undergo a significant increase of IOP after using topical corticosteroids for several days. The increasing use of intravitreal injections of triamcinolone acetonide and intravitreal implants of dexamethasone for exudative maculopathies will probably exacerbate this problem. A secondary glaucoma can develop in some cases, even though for most patients the IOP returns to baseline after ceasing steroid use. If traditional medical therapy is not able to lower IOP within the safe range, structural and functional damage can quickly develop. In these cases, a laser trabeculoplasty can be attended [8–10], but more often a surgical treatment must be performed before serious visual impairment occurs. Trabeculectomy with intra-operative antimetabolites is still considered to be the gold standard surgical procedure for different types of glaucoma, including corticosteroid-induced glaucoma [11,12]. This technique is simple to perform and effective, however, several early and late potentially serious complications can occur. In particular, problems related to the subconjunctival bleb, and the frequent development of a cataract can be particularly disturbing in young patients, who are often the subjects that develop corticosteroid-induced glaucoma.

Canaloplasty is a non-perforating bleb-less technique, introduced some years ago, in which a 10-0 prolene suture is positioned and tensioned within Schlemm's canal, previously dilated with a viscoelastic agent, thus facilitating aqueous outflow through natural pathways [13,14].

The purpose of this study is to present the mid-term results of canaloplasty in a small cohort of patients with corticosteroid-induced glaucoma resistant to medical management.

## 2. Experimental Section

In this non-randomized prospective study, 9 eyes from 7 patients with uncontrolled corticosteroid-induced glaucoma under maximum tolerated medical therapy underwent canaloplasty under peribulbar anesthesia. Surgery was performed either at the Department of Ophthalmology at the Azienda Ospedaliero-Universitaria "Santa Maria della Misericordia" Hospital in Udine (Italy), or at the "Città di Udine" Health Center in Udine (Italy) by one surgeon (PB), with a 10-year experience with this type of surgery, from February 2008 to July 2016.

All patients provided written informed consent. The protocol was approved by the institutional review board or ethics committee.

Inclusion criteria included: (1) patients with ocular hypertension due to corticosteroid use; (2) IOP $\geq$ 24 mmHg with maximum tolerated medical therapy after stopping corticosteroid use (in the case of topical administration); (3) open irido-corneal angle; (4) age over 18 years. Patients with or without typical optic nerve alterations, and with or without glaucomatous visual field defects were considered.

Exclusion criteria included: (1) elapsed time after steroids stopping shorter than 3 months; (2) age under 18 years; (3) other possible causes of glaucoma (i.e., pseudoesfoliation, previous trauma, etc.); (4) previous ocular surgery, apart from cataract and intravitreal injections; (5) refusal to undergo surgery.

The patients' demographic data, causes of secondary glaucoma, preoperative IOP, number of drugs used, visual functions and length of the follow-up at the last visit and other clinical data are reported in Table 1.

Table 1. Patient data before surgery.

| Case | Sex | Age | Cause of OHT | | Pre-Op IOP | No. of Meds | VA | VF Stage (GSS 2) | Follow-Up Length (Months) |
|---|---|---|---|---|---|---|---|---|---|
| 1 | M | 49 | Dex IV | CRVO | 38 | 4 | 6/10 | NA | 31 |
| 2 | M | 45 | Triam IV | EM | 30 | 6 | 3/10 | NA | 16 |
| 3 | M | 48 | Dex drops | AC | 26 | 4 | 8/10 | 1 | 72 |
| 4 | M | 48 | Dex drops | AC | 24 | 4 | 9/10 | 1 | 60 |
| 5 | F | 18 | Dex drops | AC | 28 | 4 | 10/10 | 1 | 18 |
| 6 | F | 18 | Dex drops | AC | 30 | 4 | 10/10 | 1 | 23 |
| 7 | M | 69 | Dex IV | CRVO | 28 | 4 | 5/10 | 5 | 14 |
| 8 | F | 69 | Dex IV | EM | 45 | 5 | 2/0 | 0 | 19 |
| 9 | M | 34 | Dex drops | PK | 25 | 4 | CF | NA | 41 |
| Mean ($\pm$SD) | | 44.2 $\pm$ 10.6 | | | 30.4 $\pm$ 6.8 | 4.3 $\pm$ 0.7 | | | 32.7 $\pm$ 20.9 |

OHT = ocular hypertension; Pre-op IOP = preoperative intraocular pressure; Dex IV CRVO = Intravitreal dexametason for central retinal vein occlusion; Triam IV EM = Triamcinolone acetonide for exudative maculopathy; Dex drops AC = dexametason drops for allergic conjunctivitis; Dex drops PK = dexametason drops after perforating keratoplasty; VA = visual acuity; VF = visual field; GSS 2 = Glaucoma Staging System 2; NA = not applicable; CF = counting fingers; SD = standard deviation.

The canaloplasty surgical technique is well known and has been extensively reported in the literature [15–19]. Briefly, surgery starts with a fornix-based conjunctival flap, and a 3 × 4 mm superficial scleral flap, which is dissected forward into the clear cornea for 1.5 mm. A deep scleral flap is then created, in order to open the Schlemm's canal. The deep scleral flap is removed and the two openings of the canal are dilated with hyaluronic acid in order to cannulate the Schlemm's canal, by means of a special microcatheter (iTrack by iScience Interventional, Menlo Park, CA, USA), connected to a flickering red laser light source for easy identification of the distal tip through the sclera. The microcatheter is inserted and pushed forward within Schlemm's canal for the entire 360° until it comes out of the other end of the canal opening. A 10-0, prolene suture is then tied to the distal tip and the microcatheter is withdrawn back through the canal in the opposite direction. During this maneuver, a small amount of high-molecular weight viscoelastic agent (Healon GV, Abbot Medical Optics, Santa Ana, CA, USA) is delivered within the canal every two hours of circumference, using a special screw-driven syringe. The suture is then knotted under tension in order to inwardly distend the trabecular meshwork. The superficial scleral flap is sutured with seven 10-0 Polyglactin 910 stitches to ensure a watertight closure in order to prevent any bleb formation. The conjunctival flap is then sutured with two 10-0 sutures to complete the surgery.

All patients underwent a visit once a week for the first month in order to measure IOP and detect any possible postoperative complication, then went on to have a complete ophthalmic examination every six months, including slit-lamp examination, best corrected visual acuity (BCVA), IOP measurement with Goldmann applanation tonometer, fundus examination with a 78 D Volk lens, visual field testing (Humphrey Field Analyzer (Carl Zeiss Meditec Inc. Dublin, CA, USA) 30-2 SITA standard test), retinal nerve fiber layer assessment with spectral-domain OCT and gonioscopy. Moreover, the corneal astigmatism was measured after one week and one month by means of a keratometer of Javal and corneal topography. Visual field damage severity was assessed using the Glaucoma Staging System 2 (P. Brusini, Italy) [20]. The definition of success was based on two different criteria: post-operative IOP $\leq$ 21 mmHg and $\leq$ 16 mmHg. When this goal was obtained without any medical treatment, the success was defined as "complete". When the same IOP levels were obtained with or without medical treatment, the success was defined as "qualified". Moreover, the IOP reduction had to be $\geq$20% for defining a case as successful. The number of medications before and after canaloplasty was also taken into consideration.

Differences between test results were calculated using the paired $t$-test for variables that showed a normal distribution. The statistical analysis was performed using SPSS 11.0 (IBM Analytics, Chicago, IL, USA). Statistical significance was defined as $p < 0.05$.

## 3. Results

The entire standard procedure could be performed as planned in all of the nine eyes. Follow-up ranged from 14 to 72 months (mean: 32.7 $\pm$ 20.8). The mean pre-operative IOP was 30.4 $\pm$ 6.8 mmHg, ranging from 24 to 45 mmHg. The mean IOP after 6 and 12 months was 13.1 $\pm$ 2.6 mmHg, and 13.7 $\pm$ 1.9 mmHg, respectively, ranging 11 to 18 mmHg (paired $t$-test, $p = 0.0001$). The mean IOP reduction from baseline after 6 and 12 months was of 56.9% and 54.9%, respectively. The IOP values at various follow-up sessions within a period of 36 months are shown in Table 2. The scatter plot in Figure 1 shows the pre- and one-year post-operative IOP values. After the 6 and 12-month follow-up, a complete and qualified success, was obtained in all 9 eyes, using both the definitions of success (IOP $\leq$ 21 mmHg and $\leq$ 16 mmHg), with an IOP within normal limits during the entire follow-up period, except for one eye that showed an increase of IOP after two years, successfully controlled with medical therapy. The number of medications used pre- and at the 12-month follow-up was 4.3 $\pm$ 0.7, and 0.2 $\pm$ 1.0, respectively (difference statistically significant, $p < 0.001$). Only one patient (11%) was under IOP-lowering drops after one year, but medical treatment was needed in both the two patients which reached a five-year follow-up. No patient required adjunctive surgical procedures. Gonioscopy showed that the prolene suture remained correctly positioned within the Schlemm's canal for the entire follow-up period in all cases. At the last visit, visual acuity worsened of two lines in two eyes (case #1 and case #2), depending on retina conditions, and improved of three lines in one eye (case #7) due to the effects of corticosteroid treatment. A reliable visual field testing was not possible in three eyes due either to a poor visual acuity (case #9) or to artifacts related to retinal disease (case #1 and #2). Before surgery, visual field was normal in one case (#5), showed only slight defects in four cases, whereas only small islands of vision were present in another case (#9). All of these defects remained stable over time. Optic nerve appearance (normal in all eyes but one) and retinal nerve fiber layer did not show any significant change during the follow-up period.

Table 2. Mean post-operative intraocular pressure (IOP).

| Time Point | IOP, Mean ± SD (mmHg) | No. of Eyes |
| --- | --- | --- |
| Preoperative | 30.4 ± 6.8 | 9 |
| 1 month | 12.6 ± 1.9 * | 9 |
| 6 month | 13.2 ± 2.6 * | 9 |
| 12 month | 13.7 ± 1.9 * | 9 |
| 24 month | 16.8 ± 6.3 * | 5 |
| 30 month | 15.7 ± 2.5 * | 4 |
| 36 month | 15.7 ± 2.3 * | 3 |
| 42 month | 15.5 ± 2.1 * | 2 |
| 48 month | 17.0 ± 4.2 * | 2 |
| 54 month | 16.0 ± 1.4 * | 2 |
| 60 month | 14.5 ± 0.7 * | 2 |

* $p < 0.0001$ vs. preoperative values.

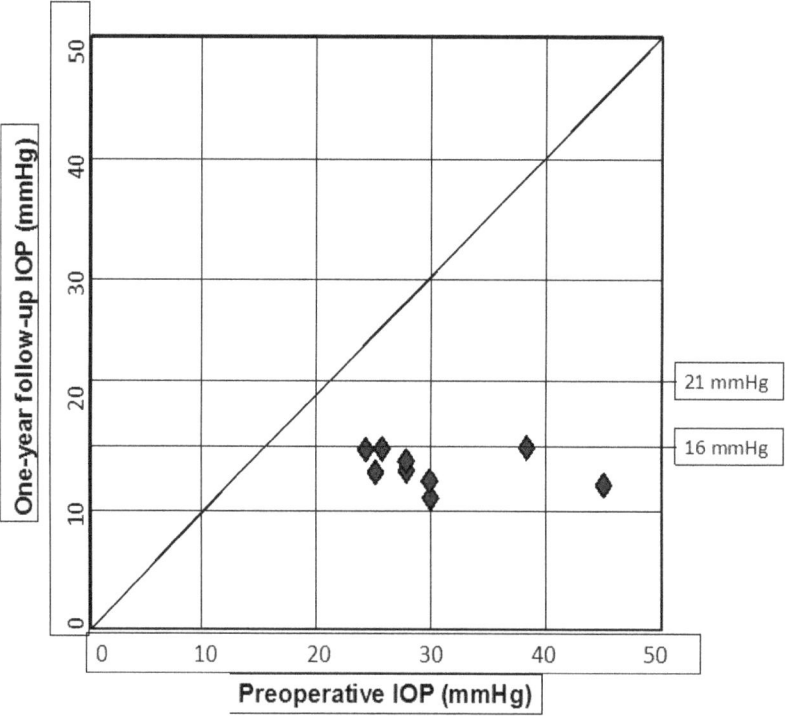

Figure 1. Pre- and one-year post-operative IOP values.

The early post-operative complications (within four weeks from surgery) included: microhyphema in two eyes (22.2%); hypotonus (IOP < 5 mm/Hg) in one eye (11.1%); and, IOP spikes > 10 mmHg in one case (11.1%). A transient decrease in visual acuity in the first weeks after canaloplasty was a rather common finding, which was due to an induced according to-the-rule astigmatism which can reach five diopters, but usually disappear within one month. No surgery-related complications were observed after two months.

## 4. Discussion

Surgery is sometimes needed to control ocular hypertension and delay damage progression in patients with corticosteroid-induced glaucoma, especially considering that visual field defect progression can be fast and severe if IOP is very high. However, unlike from patients with primary open-angle glaucoma or pseudoesfoliation glaucoma, which often show advanced visual field loss, patients with corticosteroid-induced glaucoma usually have normal optic nerves and visual fields at the beginning. For this reason, an IOP in the mid-teens is usually adequate in order to avoid any structural and/or functional damage. In this type of patient, even with very high pre-operative IOP levels, non-filtering surgical procedures, such as goniotomy [21], trabeculotomy [22–25], trabecular stents [26], viscocanalostomy [27] or deep sclerectomy [28] may be an interesting option, even if they are less effective than trabeculectomy in lowering IOP, considering the lower risk of complications. Nowadays, canaloplasty should be considered as a step ahead of these procedures with very interesting long-term outcomes in various forms of open-angle glaucoma [15–19].

Our mid-term results in a small cohort of patients with corticosteroid-induced glaucoma unresponsive to medical therapy appear to be particularly good in comparison with other types of glaucoma, where the mean IOP usually ranges between 15 and 17 mmHg, with a percentage of success after one year ranging between 60% and 95%, depending on the definition of success used [14–19]. In particular, if a cut-off of $\leq 16$ mmHg is taken in order to define successful cases, the percentage of qualified success reported in literature is about 50% in comparison with the 100% obtained in our nine cases.

The reasons for this favorable behavior are probably various and include: (1) histopatologic studies in corticosteroid-induced glaucoma demonstrated an increased density of the cribriform meshwork and thinning of the endothelial lining of Schlemm's canal [29,30]; in cases of elevated IOP, a collapse of aqueous plexus and collector channel ostia obstructed by herniation was observed in bovine eyes [31], resulting in a decrease in the effective filtration area. Canaloplasty is able to overcome this obstacle, allowing the restoration of the aqueous humor outflow; (2) patients with this type of glaucoma are usually relatively young with well-functioning aqueous humor pathways, which is a fundamental requirement to obtain satisfactory results after canaloplasty; (3) all of our patients were under medical therapy for a short period before the operation; it is well known that topical therapy for glaucoma has negative effects in all glaucoma surgeries.

It should be noted, however, that the percentage of patients which require a pharmacological therapy, even at a lower dosage, to maintain adequate IOP control seems to increase with time.

Even if the results we obtained are very promising, it should be remembered that this was a non-randomized study with a small sample of patients without a control group. Another limitation of our study is that both eyes of two patients have been considered. Even if this could be incorrect from a statistical point of view, considering the small number of patients treated, we decided to describe all cases we treated with this surgical procedure. The study is currently still underway. New patients with corticosteroid-induced glaucoma that fit the inclusion criteria are being added and follow-up data of existing patients are being constantly updated to provide long term results and a larger cohort for our future study. Regarding these patients, multicentric randomized studies with a larger population, where canaloplasty is compared to gold standard surgery (trabeculectomy), are needed to draw more definite and robust conclusions.

## 5. Conclusions

Canaloplasty is a very promising surgical technique in eyes with high IOP, which is usually the case in patients with corticosteroid-induced glaucoma. In our small cohort of patients, postoperative IOP was able to be maintained within physiological values, even if some medical therapy is occasionally still required. Considering that ocular hypertension is the main risk factor for structural and functional damage in corticosteroid-induced glaucoma, target IOP may not need to be very low to avoid the onset or the progression of the damage. Even if the sample taken into consideration in our study was limited, the good outcomes and the low rate of complications observed with this non-perforating procedure are very encouraging and could entice glaucoma specialists to consider early surgical treatment in the management of this kind of patient.

**Author Contributions:** P.B. and C.T. conceived and designed this research and analyzed data. C.T. visited the patients during the follow-up. P.B. wrote the paper. M.Z. checked patient's data e revised the manuscript.

**Conflicts of Interest:** The authors declare no conflict of interest.

## References

1. McDonnell, P.J.; Kerr Muir, M.G. Glaucoma associated with systemic corticosteroid therapy. *Lancet* **1985**, *17*, 386–387. [CrossRef]
2. Kersey, J.P.; Broadway, D.C. Corticosteroid-induced glaucoma: A review of the literature. *Eye (Lond.)* **2006**, *20*, 407–416. [CrossRef] [PubMed]
3. Kiddee, W.; Trope, G.E.; Sheng, L.; Beltran-Agullo, L.; Smith, M.; Strungaru, M.H.; Baath, J.; Buys, Y.M. Intraocular pressure monitoring post intravitreal steroids: A systematic review. *Surv. Ophthalmol.* **2013**, *58*, 291–310. [CrossRef] [PubMed]
4. Jain, S.; Thompson, J.R.; Foot, B.; Tatham, A.; Eke, T. Severe intraocular pressure rise following intravitreal triamcinolone: A national survey to estimate incidence and describe case profiles. *Eye (Lond.)* **2014**, *28*, 399–401. [CrossRef] [PubMed]
5. Mazzarella, S.; Mateo, C.; Freixes, S.; Burés-Jelstrup, A.; Rios, J.; Navarro, R.; García-Arumí, J.; Corcóstegui, B.; Arrondo, E. Effect of intravitreal injection of dexamethasone 0.7 mg (Ozurdex®) on intraocular pressure in patients with macular edema. *Ophthalmic Res.* **2015**, *54*, 143–149. [CrossRef] [PubMed]
6. Armaly, M. Effects of corticosteroids on intraocular pressure and fluid dynamics I. The effect of dexamethasone in normal subject. *Arch. Ophthalmol.* **1963**, *70*, 482–491. [CrossRef] [PubMed]
7. Becker, B. Intraocular pressure response to topic corticosteroids. *Investig. Ophthalmol. Vis. Sci.* **1965**, *4*, 198–205.
8. Pizzimenti, J.J.; Nickerson, M.M.; Pizzimenti, C.E.; Kasten-Aker, A.G. Selective laser trabeculoplasty for intraocular pressure elevation after intravitreal triamcinolone acetonide injection. *Optom. Vis. Sci.* **2006**, *83*, 421–425. [CrossRef] [PubMed]
9. Rubin, B.; Taglienti, A.; Rothman, R.F.; Marcus, C.H.; Serle, J.B. The effect of selective laser trabeculoplasty on intraocular pressure in patients with intravitreal steroid-induced elevated intraocular pressure. *J. Glaucoma* **2008**, *17*, 287–292. [CrossRef] [PubMed]
10. Tokuda, N.; Inoue, J.; Yamazaki, I.; Matsuzawa, A.; Munemasa, Y.; Kitaoka, Y.; Takagi, H.; Ueno, S. Effects of selective laser trabeculoplasty treatment in steroid-induced glaucoma. *Nippon Ganka Gakkai Zasshi* **2012**, *116*, 751–757. (In Japanese) [PubMed]
11. Ang, M.; Ho, C.L.; Tan, D.; Chan, C. Severe vernal keratoconjunctivitis requiring trabeculectomy with mitomycin C for corticosteroid-induced glaucoma. *Clin. Exp. Ophthalmol.* **2012**, *40*, e149–e155. [CrossRef] [PubMed]
12. Fitzgerald, J.T.; Saunders, L.; Ridge, B.; White, A.J.; Goldberg, I.; Clark, B.; Mills, R.A.; Craig, J.E. Severe intraocular pressure response to periocular or intravitreal steroid treatment in Australia and New Zealand: Data from the Australian and New Zealand Ophthalmic Surveillance Unit. *Clin. Exp. Ophthalmol.* **2015**, *43*, 234–238. [CrossRef] [PubMed]
13. Koerber, N. Canaloplasty—A new approach to nonpenetrating glaucoma surgery. *Tech. Ophthalmol.* **2007**, *5*, 102–106. [CrossRef]

14. Lewis, R.A.; von Wolff, K.; Tetz, M.; Korber, N.; Kearney, J.R.; Shingleton, B.; Samuelson, T.W. Canaloplasty: Circumferential viscodilation and tensioning of Schlemm's canal using a flexible microcatheter for the treatment of open-angle glaucoma in adults. Interim clinical study analysis. *J. Cataract. Refract. Surg.* **2007**, *33*, 1217–1226. [CrossRef] [PubMed]
15. Grieshaber, M.C.; Pienaar, A.; Olivier, J.; Stegmann, R. Canaloplasty for open-angle glaucoma: Long term outcome. *Br. J. Ophthalmol.* **2010**, *94*, 1478–1482. [CrossRef] [PubMed]
16. Lewis, R.A.; von Wolff, K.; Tetz, M.; Koerber, N.; Kearney, J.R.; Shingleton, B.J.; Samuelson, T.W. Canaloplasty: Three-year results of circumferential viscodilation and tensioning of Schlemm canal using a microcatheter to treat open-angle glaucoma. *J. Cataract. Refract. Surg.* **2011**, *37*, 682–690. [CrossRef] [PubMed]
17. Bull, H.; von Wolff, K.; Körber, N.; Tetz, M. Three-year canaloplasty outcomes for the treatment of open-angle glaucoma: European study results. *Graefe's Arch. Clin. Exp. Ophthalmol.* **2011**, *249*, 1537–1545. [CrossRef] [PubMed]
18. Brusini, P.; Caramello, G.; Benedetti, S.; Tosoni, C. Canaloplasty in open angle glaucoma. Mid-term results from a multicenter study. *J. Glaucoma* **2016**, *25*, 403–407. [CrossRef] [PubMed]
19. Brusini, P. Canaloplasty in open-angle glaucoma surgery: A four-year follow-up. *Sci. World J.* **2014**, *2014*, 469609. [CrossRef] [PubMed]
20. Brusini, P.; Filacorda, S. Enhanced glaucoma staging system (GSS 2) for classifying functional damage in glaucoma. *J. Glaucoma* **2006**, *15*, 40–46. [CrossRef] [PubMed]
21. Choi, E.Y.; Walton, D.S. Goniotomy for steroid-induced glaucoma: Clinical and tonographic evidence to support therapeutic goniotomy. *J. Pediatr. Ophthalmol. Strabismus* **2015**, *52*, 183–188. [CrossRef] [PubMed]
22. Kawamura, M.; Zako, M. Successful trabeculotomy in a patient with corticosteroid-induced glaucoma with anti-aquaporin 4 antibody-positive neuromyelitis optica: A case report. *J. Med. Case Rep.* **2013**, *7*, 101. [CrossRef] [PubMed]
23. Iwao, K.; Inatani, M.; Tanihara, H. Japanese Steroid-Induced Glaucoma Multicenter Study Group. Success rates of trabeculotomy for steroid-induced glaucoma: A comparative, multicenter, retrospective cohort study. *Am. J. Ophthalmol.* **2011**, *151*, 1047–1056. [CrossRef] [PubMed]
24. Dang, Y.; Kaplowitz, K.; Parikh, H.A.; Roy, P.; Loewen, R.T.; Francis, B.A.; Loewen, N.A. Steroid-induced glaucoma treated with trabecular ablation in a matched comparison with primary open-angle glaucoma. *Clin. Exp. Ophthalmol.* **2016**, *44*, 783–788. [CrossRef] [PubMed]
25. Ngai, P.; Kim, G.; Chak, G.; Lin, K.; Maeda, M.; Mosaed, S. Outcome of primary trabeculotomy ab interno (Trabectome) surgery in patients with steroid-induced glaucoma. *Medicine (Baltim.)* **2016**, *95*, e5383. [CrossRef] [PubMed]
26. Morales-Fernandez, L.; Martinez-De-La-Casa, J.M.; Garcia-Feijoo, J.; Diaz Valle, D.; Arriola-Villalobos, P.; Garcia-Sanchez, J. Glaukos® trabecular stent used to treat steroid-induced glaucoma. *Eur. J. Ophthalmol.* **2012**, *22*, 670–673. [CrossRef] [PubMed]
27. Krishnan, R.; Kumar, N.; Wishart, P.K. Viscocanalostomy for refractory glaucoma secondary to intravitreal triamcinolone acetonide injection. *Arch. Ophthalmol.* **2007**, *125*, 1284–1286. [CrossRef] [PubMed]
28. Detry-Morel, M.; Escarmelle, A.; Hermans, I. Refractory ocular hypertension secondary to intravitreal injection of triamcinolone acetonide. *Bull. Soc. Belg. Ophthalmol.* **2004**, *292*, 45–51.
29. Kayes, J.; Becker, B. The human trabecular meshwork in corticosteroid-induced glaucoma. *Trans. Am. Ophthalmol. Soc.* **1969**, *67*, 339–354. [PubMed]
30. Rohen, J.W.; Linner, E.; Witmer, R. Electron microscopic studies on the trabecular meshwork in two cases of corticosteroid glaucoma. *Exp. Eye Res.* **1973**, *17*, 19–31. [CrossRef]
31. Battista, S.A.; Lu, Z.; Hofmann, S.; Freddo, T.; Overby, D.R.; Gong, H. Reduction of the available area for aqueous humor outflow and increase in meshwork herniations into collector channels following acute IOP elevation in bovine eyes. *Investig. Ophthalmol. Vis. Sci.* **2008**, *49*, 5346–5352. [CrossRef] [PubMed]

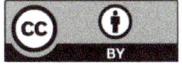 © 2018 by the authors. Licensee MDPI, Basel, Switzerland. This article is an open access article distributed under the terms and conditions of the Creative Commons Attribution (CC BY) license (http://creativecommons.org/licenses/by/4.0/).

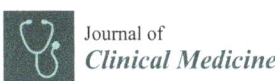 

*Communication*

# The Impact of the Brain-Derived Neurotrophic Factor Gene on Trauma and Spatial Processing

Jessica K. Miller [1,*], Siné McDougall [2], Sarah Thomas [3] and Jan Wiener [4]

1. Faculty of Human, Social & Political Science, University of Cambridge, Cambridge CB2 1TN, UK
2. Department of Psychology, Bournemouth University, Poole BH12 5BB, UK; smcdougall@bournemouth.ac.uk
3. Faculty of Health & Social Sciences, Clinical Research Unit, Bournemouth University, Poole BH12 5BB, UK; saraht@bournemouth.ac.uk
4. Department of Psychology, Ageing and Dementia Research Centre, Bournemouth University, Poole BH12 5BB, UK; jwiener@bournemouth.ac.uk
* Correspondence: jkm35@cam.ac.uk; Tel.: +44-1300-341-015

Academic Editor: Nuri B. Farber
Received: 15 September 2017; Accepted: 6 November 2017; Published: 27 November 2017

**Abstract:** The influence of genes and the environment on the development of Post-Traumatic Stress Disorder (PTSD) continues to motivate neuropsychological research, with one consistent focus being the Brain-Derived Neurotrophic Factor (BDNF) gene, given its impact on the integrity of the hippocampal memory system. Research into human navigation also considers the BDNF gene in relation to hippocampal dependent spatial processing. This speculative paper brings together trauma and spatial processing for the first time and presents exploratory research into their interactions with BDNF. We propose that quantifying the impact of BDNF on trauma and spatial processing is critical and may well explain individual differences in clinical trauma treatment outcomes and in navigation performance. Research has already shown that the BDNF gene influences PTSD severity and prevalence as well as navigation behaviour. However, more data are required to demonstrate the precise hippocampal dependent processing mechanisms behind these influences in different populations and environmental conditions. This paper provides insight from recent studies and calls for further research into the relationship between allocentric processing, trauma processing and BDNF. We argue that research into these neural mechanisms could transform PTSD clinical practice and professional support for individuals in trauma-exposing occupations such as emergency response, law enforcement and the military.

**Keywords:** BDNF; Brain-Derived Neurotrophic Factor; navigation; spatial processing; trauma; trauma processing; Post-Traumatic Stress Disorder; PSTD; allocentric; hippocampus

## 1. Introduction

Post-Traumatic Stress Disorder (PTSD) is an increasingly visible mental health issue that represents a considerable public health burden [1] across many civilian and professional populations. With mounting pressure on health, military and emergency response sectors (https://www.pdtrust.org/help/research/post-traumatic-stress/) to look after the psychological wellbeing of their staff in the face of unprecedented demand from major incidents and resource deficits, understanding PTSD has perhaps never been so critical. Fortuitously, neuropsychological research over recent years has also moved at a commensurate pace and in this paper, we seize the opportunity to reflect on the progress (and pitfalls) of that research. We review recent literature, present findings from exploratory research (provided in more detail in the Appendix A) and highlight design issues which may be key to understanding how genetic and environmental conditions interact to influence PTSD vulnerability, etiology and recovery. To do this, we look at another area of cognitive function—navigation—which may provide us with vital information about the resilience of a specific part of our brain (the hippocampus) on which we rely to process trauma exposure [2–6].

## 2. The Neural Basis of Post-Traumatic Stress Disorder (PTSD)

Contemporary theories of PTSD which have been developed from cognitive theories and clinical research [2–9] describe PTSD in the context of information processing. A predominant theory is that of dual representation [2,4,6–8]. Dual Representation Theory describes how trauma processing operates with two types of memory representations in the limbic system: those which are associative and those which are contextual [8]. Associative representations of trauma are typically involuntary, fear-based, and originate in the amygdala. Contextual representations, in contrast, are retrieved voluntarily and mediated by the hippocampus [10,11]. According to Dual Representation Theory, effective trauma processing involves applying context to the sensory and evocative experiences of trauma to consolidate them into long term memory and file them as "past". Trauma literature often refers to egocentric, associatively conditioned responses to stimuli as being typical in cases of post-traumatic stress, and these responses can be described by a signature symptom of PTSD, the "flashback" [9–13]. Hippocampal representations, on the other hand, provide episodic and spatial context for extreme experiences, which enables individuals to make sense of when and where traumatic incidents occurred [14–18]. However, when the hippocampus is down-regulated (e.g., by trauma or stress) it is less able to contextualise or anchor traumatic experiences in space and time, allowing them to intrude in the present, thus prolonging the stress response [4,19–24].

## 3. Brain-Derived Neurotrophic Factor (BDNF)

Stressful or traumatic incidents in the environment are not the only causes of down-regulation in the hippocampus; genetics also has a substantial impact [1,5,24–30]. Identifying genes which are relevant to the development of PTSD has been a relentless motivator for numerous genome-wide association studies, twin studies and candidate gene studies [1,5]. A recent review [31] identified 25 such studies, many of which highlighted the specific role of a gene called Brain-Derived Neurotrophic Factor (BDNF). BDNF is expressed in the limbic system, moderating fear responses and broadly regulating the stress response [5,20,22,23,30–32]. It is also expressed outside the limbic system, such as in the retina, kidneys and prostate [33], and has been considered integral to critical periods of human development [34]. The BDNF gene codes for the BDNF protein which is then expressed to promote the growth and survival of neurons, particularly those in the hippocampus [26,31,35]. BDNF-related neuroplasticity is considered an important component in maintaining the integrity of the hippocampus [5,25,34,35].

However, this operation is complicated by the fact that the BDNF gene has two variants, derived from carrying "met" and "val" alleles, which differ in their functionality [5,15,18,20,24,25,29,31,32,35]. At a genetic level, allelic variation occurs at codon 66 on chromosome 11, resulting in an amino acid switch from valine (val) to methionine (met) and producing a val66met polymorphism which is unique to humans [18,31,35,36]. In the Caucasian population, 30% carry the met allele, either as the metmet homozygotes or valmet heterozygotes [35]. Typically, met carriers show less activity-dependent release of the BDNF protein in the hippocampus than val homozygotes [5,24,25,29,35]. This means that in met carriers (rather than val homozygotes) sufficient BDNF protein may not be released into the hippocampus for it to respond appropriately to the demands that the environment may place on it, such as the demand for consolidating traumatic experiences into long term memory [20,22,26,30–32,37,38].

Given the compounding effect of the BDNF polymorphism on hippocampal function, we would anticipate that post-traumatic stress would be more prevalent and severe in met carriers, if other environmental conditions have been controlled for. This appears to be borne out by Zhang et al.'s (2014) finding that PTSD was more prevalent and severe in met allele carriers [32]. Specifically, the study revealed that the allelic frequency of BDNF met was twofold higher in those with probable PTSD. In support of this finding, it has recently been proposed that sufficient BDNF release may be involved in helping to prevent PTSD because its operation induces fear extinction and ensures successful trauma processing [5,20,22,30–32,37,38].

It is worth noting from BDNF and PTSD studies [32] the importance of controlling for environmental conditions. Indeed, a failure to consider the demand on the hippocampus that different environmental conditions can present may account for mixed findings to date in studies relating BDNF to PTSD [1,31,32,36]. Nonetheless, in 2014, Zhang and colleagues [32] successfully controlled for these conditions and reported a direct relationship between the BNDF gene and PTSD in a population of U.S. military Special Operations personnel.

## 4. Hippocampal Function, Navigation and BDNF

Next, we consider how navigation can be used to assay hippocampal function [10,11,39–41]. Our situational awareness and our ability to orient ourselves and navigate our way through the world rely on two forms of mental representations, those that are hippocampal independent (egocentric representations) and those that are hippocampal dependent (allocentric, see Figure 1).

(i) Egocentric processing is viewpoint dependent and associative, relying on local landmarks in line of sight. This form of processing is not dependent on hippocampal processing: egocentric spatial memory representations are independent of the hippocampus, relying on the striatal circuit, whereas allocentric representations are thought to rely heavily on the hippocampal circuit [2,6,8,10,11,39].

(ii) Allocentric processing enables individuals to construct a viewer-independent representation of the relationship between objects /landmarks/ places in an environment. A spatial "map" [11] is created in which key landmarks are represented in relation to one another rather than in relation to the viewer. This form of representation is particularly important in route planning and is vital for contextualising information during navigation [10,11,28,29]. Allocentric processing, in contrast to egocentric processing, relies heavily on the hippocampal circuit [10,11,39].

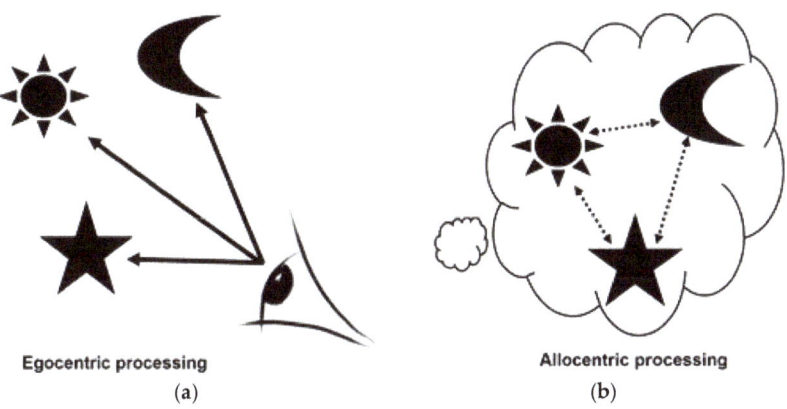

**Egocentric processing**
(a)

**Allocentric processing**
(b)

Figure 1. (a) Egocentric processing and (b) allocentric processing of spatial relationships.

So, given that the hippocampus facilitates (allocentric) spatial processing, individuals' navigation skills depend on effective hippocampal function and can therefore act as an index of hippocampal integrity [5,6,8,10,23,41]. There have been very few studies examining the effects of BDNF on navigation. However, there is evidence in recent neuropsychological literature for a relationship between the BDNF gene and hippocampal dependent (allocentric) spatial processing. A study from 2011 by Banner et al. [29] provides supportive evidence that met-carrying BDNF genotypes rely more on hippocampal independent (egocentric) spatial processing to complete a navigation task than valval homozygotes (see also Lövdén et al., 2011, for a similar proposal based on a study with a much smaller sample) [28]. To demonstrate this, Banner et al. assessed participants' spontaneous strategy use in a virtual maze. A higher proportion of BDNF metmet homozygotes spontaneously used egocentric strategies in comparison to valval homozygotes, whereas a higher proportion of valval homozygotes spontaneously used allocentric strategies. Both studies [28,29] made an explicit connection between less BDNF release in met carriers, lack of hippocampal engagement in spatial tasks and a bias toward implicit, associative spatial processing. In short, BDNF met carriers are generally considered to be more likely to engage in egocentric processing (which does not rely on the hippocampus) in comparison to valval homozygotes (see also [5,15,28,29,40]), who have greater access to effective allocentric processing via the hippocampus.

## 5. Bringing Together Allocentric Spatial Processing, the BDNF Gene and PTSD

This focused literature review shows that the relationship between BDNF and hippocampal dependent processing and trauma is complicated, as illustrated in Figure 2.

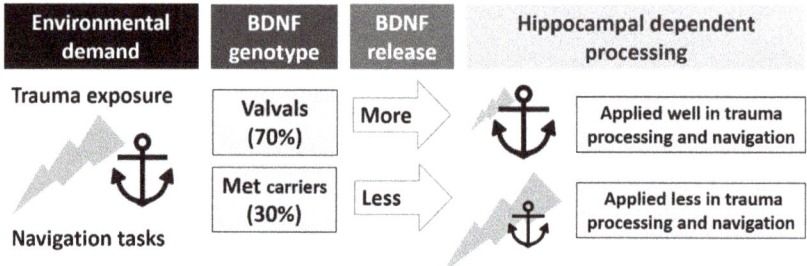

**Figure 2.** The relationship between Brain-Derived Neurotrophic Factor (BDNF) genotype, Post-Traumatic Stress Disorder (PTSD), hippocampal processing, and navigation skills (represented by the anchor). BDNF genotype influences activity-dependent release of the BDNF protein used in hippocampal processing of traumatic and spatial information, potentially placing some genotypes at a disadvantage for trauma resilience and navigation competence.

With regard to trauma processing, severity and prevalence of PTSD is positively related to carrying the BDNF met allele [5,20,30–32,36–38]. With regard to spatial processing, there is evidence of an egocentric bias in BDNF met carriers but no clear differences in allocentric performance between BDNF genotypes were reported in either study [28,29]. Interestingly, egocentric bias in navigation strategy use and allocentric performance deficits have also been recently demonstrated in cases of PTSD (and trauma exposure) [2,3,6,8,40]. Neuropsychology has yet to bring these findings about BDNF, hippocampal dependent processing and trauma (or PTSD) together into one human experiment. A rodent model in 2007 [41] went so far as to demonstrate impaired spatial learning in the Morris Water Maze and significantly reduced extinction of conditioned fear in BDNF "knockout" rats. Although based on deleting rodent genes rather than genotyping human populations, this cross-discipline study stresses the possibility that cognitive spatial processing deficits and impairment in managing trauma exposure may be directly related to BDNF gene expression in the hippocampus.

In 2012, we sought to investigate how spatial processing impairment and trauma exposure processing may be related to BDNF genotypes in an exploratory extension of a human study ($n = 150$) which assessed the impact of PTSD on navigation [6,40]. *Full details of and data from the exploratory study are provided in the Appendix A.* Our intention was to determine if any bias in BDNF met carriers toward hippocampal independent spatial processing:

(a) was evident in the virtual environment navigation task being used in the main study [6,28,29,40],
(b) remained, when controlling for hippocampal down-regulation from PTSD [2–4,6,8,40–42], and/or

(c) correlated with subjective measures of self-reported navigation competence [43–45].

In summary, in the diverse sample ($n = 150$) of civilian, police and military populations, PTSD severity and prevalence were similar across BDNF groups. In the sample population, 57 participants had probable levels of PTSD and of those without probable PTSD, 60 were trauma exposed and 33 were not. Participants' navigation performance was assessed using the Alternative Route paradigm [6,10,46]. When graphed (see Figure A1 in the Appendix A), the data showed a distinctly divergent pattern of egocentric performance between BDNF valval homozygotes and met carriers, resulting in significantly higher egocentric performance in met carriers at the end of the navigation task, echoing interpretations of egocentric bias in met carriers in the previous studies [28,29]. Using self-report navigation questionnaires (specific questions from which had been shown to "predict" allocentric spatial processing in earlier studies [43–45]), we were also able to show for the first time that only BDNF valval homozygotes (not met carriers) were accurate in judging their own competence at allocentric spatial processing (see Table A1 in the Appendix A). Overall, our exploratory data were indicative of BDNF-related differences in hippocampal dependent and independent navigation behaviour, irrespective of PTSD. While interesting, it is important to note that these findings were limited by several design features. These limitations provide valuable insights for further research, and it is to those insights that we now turn.

## 6. The Future of BDNF Research

For candidate gene (BDNF) research to shape the future of clinical trauma interventions or to influence professional practices in occupations requiring situational awareness, studies need to be able to deliver accurate and ecologically relevant data [1,3,47,48]. Our exploratory research [40] into the relationship between BDNF, PTSD and spatial processing was limited by several factors. If these factors could be addressed in replication studies, significant progress in our understanding of *gene* × *environment* interactions in trauma and navigation could be imminent. Here, we briefly critique the design limitations of recent studies (including our own) and offer suggestions for improving data quality in key areas: experimental groups, performance measurement, subjective measures of navigation, and collection of further neurological data.

Sample populations for BDNF studies can be a contentious issue, with some traditional academic disciplines [30] typically favouring large cohorts (of thousands) and genome-wide association studies over the much smaller designs and sample sizes seen in candidate gene studies [1,36,42,47,48]. While some candidate gene study sample sizes have simply been too small ($n < 20$) to adequately represent the three BDNF genotypes (see [1,28,46]), other moderate samples ($n > 100$) (see [24,26,29,32]) have been able to demonstrate the influence of the gene on PTSD when other environmental conditions within and between experimental groups have been adequately controlled. This was a lesson learnt by Zhang et al. in 2014 [32], in their replication of an earlier study from 2006 [42] which did not control for trauma exposure type or severity, time since exposure or treatment status. Another important factor to control for in studies of hippocampal function is age [2,5,6,10,25,46]. A primary recommendation is for future BDNF and PTSD research to control for: age, time since exposure, treatment status and trauma exposure type or severity (at least distinguishing between civilian exposure and occupational exposure, such as the military or blue light services).

Navigation performance as a measure or index of hippocampal integrity is also key to BDNF research design. Identifying navigation tasks which produce data that can discriminate between hippocampal dependent and independent performance is challenging [6,8,10,11,40,41,46], yet vital. In our own study, the purity of the egocentric performance measure [6,40,46] was somewhat compromised by the fact that egocentric trials in the route learning task could feasibly be solved allocentrically. Some theorists may challenge this concern on the basis that egocentric processing is generally considered more parsimonious and therefore more likely a universal default means of solving simple tasks [49,50]. Nonetheless, implementing spatial processing measures which can accurately distinguish between allocentric and egocentric processing should remain a priority for any future studies which intend to compare functionality of the two memory systems. Similarly, disparity between studies which assess performance in allocentric and egocentric strategy use as opposed to allocentric or egocentric spontaneous strategy choice, is also something to be mindful of when comparing participants' navigation behaviours [6,28,46,51]. Spontaneous navigation behaviour and navigation behaviour over the course of a learning paradigm likely measure different components of spatial processing and need to be clarified as such in research design. Asking participants directly how they think their behaviour may have changed over the course of a navigation task is a common approach and is it our recommendation that developing post-test self-report (i.e., think aloud) [28,29,43,46] measures may provide useful insights into how individuals think they navigate, even if this contradicts with their performance data.

Understanding individuals' self-awareness of their ability to apply hippocampal dependent processing when required is not only valuable to research into the declarative hippocampal dependent memory system [26,28,29] but could be highly valuable for clinical trauma processing and professional navigation training interventions that rely on that form of information processing [2,3,6,7,9,13,23,39,40]. Developing more ecologically relevant subjective measures of spatial processing would benefit future BDNF studies greatly. The navigation questionnaire literature shows that the Santa Barbara Sense of Direction questionnaire [43] and selected questions from the Questionnaire of Spatial Representation [44] and the Fragebogen Räumliche Strategien [45] can predict navigation performance, yet the validity of the questions could be enhanced by introducing terminology and frames of reference more aligned with the types of spatial processing that sample populations may be familiar with on a day-to-day basis. For example, a subjective navigation measure for a military population could refer to topographical (landscape) changes from conflict as a frame of reference for certain questions. Whereas for policing populations, references to using satellite navigation while driving a response vehicle may be a more meaningful context. Using terms participants can relate to, they may increase task engagement, and their more focused self-reflection could enhance the validity of the self-report measures.

Finally, we consider the use of supplementary neurological data to support future research into the influence of BDNF on hippocampal processing. While research to date has clearly suggested a relationship between BDNF, hippocampal dependent processing, PTSD and navigation, the precise neural mechanisms underlying this relationship are as yet undefined. BDNF research has looked at volumetric measurement in the hippocampus using magnetic resonance imaging (MRI) and fluorescent microscopy [51–53], but whether volume differences are the result of BDNF-related protein release, neurogenesis, neuronal survival or synaptic plasticity is not clear [50–54]. Investigating these neural mechanisms is further complicated by the possibility that BDNF is released in response to different environmental conditions over the life span, meaning that age (or critical periods of development) and time since trauma exposure may need to be controlled for when investigating levels of BDNF in plasma, blood or saliva (as opposed to BDNF genotypes) [5,25,33,34,36,54–58].

Implementing a solid framework for future research into the relationship between hippocampal integrity, PSTD and spatial processing is likely a daunting, but we argue, necessary task. Such a framework could comprise combining:

(a) ecologically valid behavioural and subjective tests of navigation, supported by
(b) functional MRI (fMRI) and MRI-assessing activity or volume, possibly pre- and post-trauma exposure, with
(c) adequate neurochemical assessment of activity-dependent hippocampal BDNF release (for example, using blood serum) between genotypes, and
(d) closely matching participants to control for numerous differentiating variables, which may influence hippocampal and broader neuro degradation syndromes, ranging from age and environmental conditions of trauma exposure to epigenetic history and even nutrition [59].

## 7. Conclusions

Understanding the *gene × environment* interaction in relation to both trauma exposure and spatial processing has far-reaching practical, clinical and academic implications. In practical terms, if research could accurately quantify the contribution that carrying the BDNF met allele makes to an individual being able to successfully adopt hippocampal dependent information processing techniques, this could transform how trauma management and navigation training interventions are delivered in clinical and occupational settings. If 30% of the Caucasian (and up to 50% of non-Caucasian) populations [31,35,36,60] (i.e., BDNF met carriers) could access interventions that either deliberately encouraged hippocampal dependent processing or provided workable alternatives to hippocampal dependent processing, this could equate to a substantial improvement in those intervention outcomes. The contribution that research on the hippocampus has made to 21st century neuropsychology (epitomized by the awarding of the Nobel Prize for Physiology or Medicine to Professor John O'Keefe in 2014 https://www.nobelprize.org/nobel_prizes/medicine/laureates/2014/okeefe-facts.html) is well recognised. Further research into the BDNF gene would reinforce the value of understanding how the human hippocampus shapes our emotional and professional lives. Perhaps above all, we believe that developing this research will enable science and society to take an important step toward protecting the wellbeing and mental integrity of the hundreds of thousands of men and women who put themselves in the face of trauma as part of their everyday public service, in defence, emergency response and law enforcement. To do this, we need to embrace lessons from earlier (sometimes exploratory) research across the disciplines of genetics, trauma and navigation to ensure that as we move forward, we can offer neuroscience the caliber of data it needs to meet some pressing public issues head on.

**Acknowledgments:** This work was financially supported by Army of Angels (registered charity 1143612). Recruitment to the research was supported by Combat Stress (registered charity 26002), Dorset Constabulary and Dorset University Healthcare Foundation Trust. Ethics clearance was secured with the support of Simon Wessely (King's Centre for Military Health Research) and Chris Brewin (University College London) who also kindly provided clinical supervision. Thanks goes to Olivier de Condappa for his technical support and to Kirsten Smith for her help with recruitment.

**Author Contributions:** Jessica K. Miller and Jan Wiener conceived and designed the experiments; Jessica K. Miller performed the experiments; Jessica K. Miller analysed the data; Sine McDougall and Sarah Thomas contributed analysis and advice; Jessica K. Miller wrote the paper, edited by Sine McDougall, Jan Wiener and Sarah Thomas.

**Conflicts of Interest:** The authors declare no conflict of interest. The founding sponsors had no role in the design of the study; in the collection, analyses, or interpretation of data; in the writing of the manuscript, and in the decision to publish the results.

## Appendix A. Exploratory Research Data

The appendix contains details and data from the exploratory research into the Brain-Derived Neurotrophic Factor (BDNF) gene, undertaken as part of a study into the impact of trauma and Post-Traumatic Stress Disorder (PTSD) on navigation behaviour [5,6,40,46].

*Appendix A.1. Participants*

The study sample population ($n = 150$) was diverse and was recruited from a university volunteer scheme ($n = 83$), two psychotherapy treatment centres (Traumatic Stress Clinic, Camden and Islington NHS) and the Intensive Psychotherapy Treatment Centre (Dorset Healthcare University NHS Foundation Trust) ($n = 10$), two police forces ($n = 26$) (Dorset and Cambridgeshire constabularies), and a military veteran treatment centre for PTSD (Combat Stress, Tyrwhitt House, Leatherhead, Surrey: registered charity #2060002) ($n = 25$ plus $n = 6$ staff). PTSD symptom severity and prevalence rates were measured using the PTSD Diagnostic Scale (PDS) [61]. Saliva samples for BDNF genotyping were collected using DNA *Genotek Orangene*™ self-test kits (DNA Genotek, Ottawa, ON, Canada). Participants were grouped according to whether they had been exposed to trauma or not, and if they had, whether or not they had clinical or probable levels of PTSD, using the PDS [46,61]. Sample sizes for PTSD were modest for the purpose of analysis by BDNF genotype. Of the 150 participants, 57 had probable levels of PTSD and of those who did not, 60 were trauma exposed and 33 were not trauma exposed. The frequency of the genotypes did not differ between experimental groups (*Trauma Unexposed, Trauma Exposed No PTSD,* and *PTSD*) for either the valval group, $\chi^2 = 0.24$, $p = 0.88$ or the "met carrying" group, $\chi^2 = 0.04$, $p = 0.98$. An independent samples *t*-test revealed no differences in PDS scores between BDNF groups, $t(54) = -1.23$, $p = 0.23$. This enabled the analysis of the influence of the BDNF gene to control for PTSD. The findings supported Zhang et al.'s conclusion in 2014 [32] that in order to demonstrate BDNF-related group differences in PTSD prevalence or severity, other environmental conditions may need to be controlled for (such as time since and severity of exposure, previous trauma and treatment access). It is important to note that this study could not assess the relationship between BDNF, spatial processing and PTSD, rather the relationship between BDNF and spatial processing.

*Appendix A.2. Methods*

DNA saliva samples were genotyped for one single nucleotide polymorphisms (SNP): rs6265 (Val66Met), using a Taqman® allele discrimination assay. The genotyping information acquired described which BDNF alleles were carried by the (anonymous) participant, i.e., whether they carried only the val allele (and were therefore valval homozygotes), both the val allele and the met allele (and were therefore valmet heterozygotes) or if they carried only the met allele (and were metmet homozygotes).

Allocentric and egocentric performance were assessed using a navigation paradigm, the Alternative Route (AR, [46]) which required participants to learn a route through a virtual environment. The task involved testing participants on their ability to re-join a route from the same direction and different directions from which they learned it. There were six blocks to the task. Mean performance on trials which involved joining the route from the same direction (same direction trials) provided a measure of egocentric performance. Mean performance on trials which involved joining the route from a different direction to the route as it was learned (different direction trials) provided a measure of allocentric performance. An ANOVA was used to assess BDNF group differences (met carriers vs. valval homozygotes) in egocentric and allocentric performance on a navigation task. Planned contrasts were then made at individual block level (1–11) using *t*-tests (see [6,40,46]).

Participants' self-reported navigation competence was assessed using validated questionnaires; the *Santa Barbara Sense of Direction* (SBSOD) [43] and two items from the *Questionnaire of Spatial Representation* (QSR) [44] that target allocentric processing. Correlation analysis was used to analyse the relationship between self-reported competence and navigation performance within the BDNF groups (met carriers and valval homozygotes).

*Appendix A.3. Results*

Appendix A.3.1. BDNF and Hippocampal Independent Performance

A repeated measures 2 × 6 ANOVA with the dependent variable egocentric performance, the between factor BDNF group (met carriers vs. valval homozygotes) and the within factor block (1 to 6) revealed no significant main effect of block, $F(4.49, 138) = 0.90$, $p = 0.48$, $\eta p^2 < 0.01$, nor BDNF group, $F(1, 138) = 0.99$, $p = 0.32$, $\eta p^2 < 0.01$, but a significant group × block interaction, $F(4.49, 138) = 2.48$, $p = 0.03$, $\eta p^2 = 0.02$, visible in the divergent pattern in performance in Figure A1.

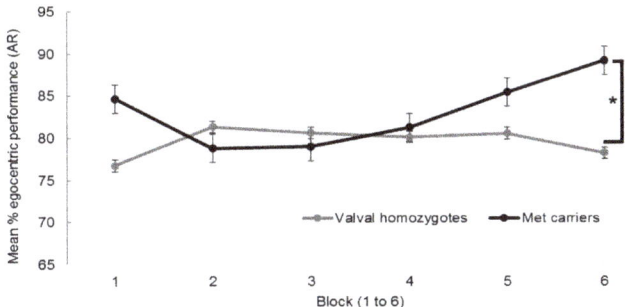

**Figure A1.** Mean egocentric performance on the Alternative Route (AR) paradigm between BDNF genotypes ($n = 140$, with $n = 96$ valval homozygotes and $n = 44$ met carriers) with standard error bars, showing significant performance differences in block 6, * $p < 0.05$.

Planned contrasts using independent samples $t$-tests revealed met carriers performed better than valval homozygotes in the final block 6 (89% SD ± 17% vs. 78% SD ± 28%), $t$ (138) = 5.65, $p = 0.006$ (equal variances not assumed). Applying Bonferroni's correction (0.05/6 blocks) would require a $p$ value of 0.008.

Despite the lack of significance in the overall BDNF group and egocentric performance interaction, closer examination of the data was undertaken to understand these final performance differences in block 6 and to look for any plausible explanation (other than chance) for the inverted curves in egocentric performance between the BDNF genotypes. The data showed there to be a statistically significant quadratic (rather than linear) effect of BDNF group, $F$ (1, 138) = 5.59, $p = 0.02$ which supports earlier hypotheses for met carrier status explaining differences in egocentric navigation strategy preference over the course of the task [28,29,62].

Allocentric performance was comparable between BDNF genotypes, as found by both Banner et al. and Lövdén et al. in 2011 [28,29] and as illustrated in Figure A2. A repeated measures 2 × 6 ANOVA with the dependent variable (DV) of allocentric performance, the between factor BDNF group and within factor block (1 to 6) revealed a significant main effect of block (with performance increasing by block), $F$ (4.07, 138) = 27.2, $p < 0.01$, $\eta p^2 = 0.17$, but no significant main effect of BDNF group, $F$ (1, 138) = 2.20, $p = 0.14$, $\eta p^2 = 0.02$, and no significant interaction $F$ (4.07, 138) = 1.71, $p = 0.14$, $\eta p^2 = 0.01$.

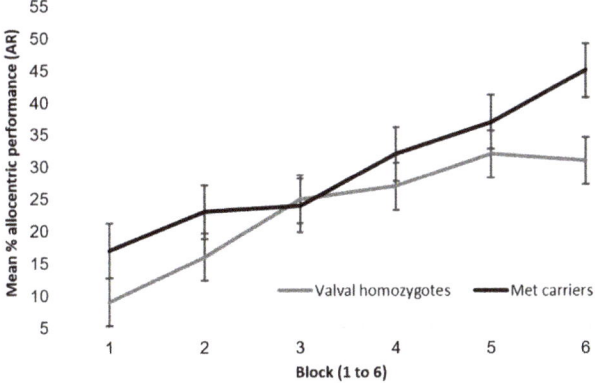

**Figure A2.** Mean allocentric performance on the AR paradigm between BDNF genotypes ($n = 140$, with $n = 96$ valval homozygotes and $n = 44$ met carriers) with standard error bars.

Appendix A.3.2. BDNF and Self-Reported Navigation Competence

The final part of the analysis was to assess the navigation questionnaire data in relation to BDNF genotype. Participants' scores for general self-reported competence in navigation (SBSOD) total score) and the allocentric targeted QSR questionnaire items were positively correlated with their performance in allocentric navigation in the AR task. As illustrated in Table A1, only valval homozygotes' self-reported competence positively correlated with their performance in allocentric navigation, suggesting that met carriers were less able than valval homozygotes to accurately describe their capacity for hippocampal dependent (allocentric) spatial processing.

**Table A1.** Pearson's correlations (r) between Questionnaire of Spatial Representation (QSR) allocentric items, the Santa Barbara Sense of Direction (SBSOD) and allocentric performance in the AR paradigm in BDNF valval homozygotes ($n = 102$) and met carriers ($n = 45$), $p < 0.01$ **, $p < 0.05$ *.

| Self-Reported Navigation Competence | Allocentric Performance in BDNF Valval Homozygotes ($n = 102$) | Allocentric Performance in BDNF Met Carriers ($n = 45$) |
|---|---|---|
| General competence (SBSOD) | 0.26 * | 0.05 |
| Allocentric competence (QSR) | 0.28 ** | 0.03 |

## References

1. Koenen, K.C.; Amstadter, A.B.; Nugent, N.R. Gene-environment interaction in post-traumatic stress disorder: An update. *J. Trauma. Stress* **2009**, *22*, 416–426. [CrossRef] [PubMed]
2. Smith, K.; Burgess, N.; Brewin, C.R.; King, J.A. Impaired allocentric spatial processing in posttraumatic stress disorder. *Neurobiol. Learn. Mem.* **2015**, *119*, 69–76. [CrossRef] [PubMed]
3. Kaur, M.; Murphy, D.; Smith, K.V. An adapted imaginal exposure approach to traditional methods used within trauma-focused cognitive behavioural therapy, trialled with a veteran population. *Cogn. Behav. Ther.* **2016**, *9*, 10. [CrossRef]
4. Bisby, J.A.; Horner, A.J.; Hørlyck, L.D.; Burgess, N. Opposing effects of negative emotion on amygdala and hippocampal memory for items and associations. *Soc. Cogn. Affect. Neurosci.* **2016**, *11*, 981–990. [CrossRef] [PubMed]
5. Miller, J.K.; Wiener, J.M. PTSD recovery, spatial processing, and the val66met polymorphism. *Front. Hum. Neurosci.* **2014**, *8*, 100. [CrossRef] [PubMed]
6. Miller, J.K.; McDougall, S.; Thomas, S.; Wiener, J.M. Impairment in active navigation from trauma and Post-Traumatic Stress Disorder. *Neurobiol. Learn. Mem.* **2017**, *140*, 114–123. [CrossRef] [PubMed]
7. Brewin, C.; Burgess, N. Contextualisation in the revised dual representation theory of PTSD: A response to Pearson and colleagues. *J. Behav. Ther. Exp. Psychiatry* **2014**, *45*, 217–219. [CrossRef] [PubMed]
8. Bisby, J.A.; King, J.A.; Brewin, C.R.; Burgess, N.; Curran, H.V. Acute effects of alcohol on intrusive memory development and viewpoint dependence in spatial memory support a dual representation model. *Biol. Psychiatry* **2010**, *68*, 280–286. [CrossRef] [PubMed]
9. Erwin, E. *The Freud Encyclopaedia*; Routledge: London, UK, 2003.
10. Wolbers, T.; Wiener, J.M. Challenges for identifying the neural mechanisms that support spatial navigation: The impact of spatial scale. *Front. Hum. Neurosci.* **2014**, *8*, 571. [CrossRef] [PubMed]
11. O'Keefe, J.; Nadel, L. *The Hippocampus as a Cognitive Map*; Oxford University Press: Oxford, UK, 1978.
12. Maren, S. Seeking a Spotless Mind: Extinction, Deconsolidation, and Erasure of Fear Memory. *Neuron* **2011**, *70*, 830–845. [CrossRef] [PubMed]
13. Lang, P.J. Imagery in therapy: An information-processing analysis of fear. *Behav. Ther.* **1977**, *8*, 862–886. [CrossRef]
14. Eichenmbaum, H. A corticol-hioppocampal system for declarative memory. *Nat. Rev. Neurosci.* **2000**, *1*, 41–50. [CrossRef] [PubMed]

15. Dennis, N.A.; Cabeza, R.; Need, A.C.; Waters-Metenier, S.; Goldstein, D.B.; LaBar, K.S. Brain-derived neurotrophic factor val66met polymorphism and hippocampal activation during episodic encoding and retrieval tasks. *Hippocampus* **2011**, *21*, 980–989. [CrossRef] [PubMed]
16. Byrne, P.; Becker, S.; Burgess, N. Remembering the past and imagining the future: A neural model of spatial memory and imagery. *Psychol. Rev.* **2007**, *114*, 340–375. [CrossRef] [PubMed]
17. Glazer, D.A.; Mason, O.; King, J.A.; Brewin, C.R. Contextual memory, psychosis-proneness, and the experience of intrusive imagery. *Cogn. Emot.* **2013**, *27*, 150–157. [CrossRef] [PubMed]
18. Hariri, A.R.; Goldberg, T.E.; Mattay, V.S.; Kolachana, B.S.; Callicott, J.H.; Egan, M.F.; Weinberger, D.R. Brain-derived neurotrophic factor val66met polymorphism affects human memory-related hippocampal activity and predicts memory performance. *J. Neurosci.* **2003**, *23*, 6690–6694. [PubMed]
19. Elzinga, B.M.; Bremner, J.D. Are the neural substrates of memory the final common pathway in posttraumatic stress disorder (PTSD)? *J. Affect. Disord.* **2002**, *70*, 1–17. [CrossRef]
20. Elzinga, B.M.; Molendijk, M.L.; Oude Voshaar, R.C.; Bus, B.A.; Prickaerts, J.; Spinhoven, P.; Penninx, B.J. The impact of childhood abuse and recent stress on serum brain-derived neurotrophic factor and the moderating role of BDNF Val66Met. *Psychopharmacology* **2011**, *214*, 319–328. [CrossRef] [PubMed]
21. Brewin, C.R.; Dalgleish, T.; Joseph, S. A dual representation theory of post-traumatic stress disorder. *Psychol. Rev.* **1996**, *103*, 670–686. [CrossRef] [PubMed]
22. Peters, J.; Dieppa-Perea, L.M.; Melendez, L.M.; Quirk, G.J. Induction of fear extinction with hippocampal-infralimbic BDNF. *Science* **2010**, *328*, 1288–1290. [CrossRef] [PubMed]
23. Holmes, E.A.; James, E.L.; Kilford, E.J.; Deeprose, C. Key Steps in Developing a Cognitive Vaccine against Traumatic Flashbacks: Visuospatial Tetris versus Verbal Pub Quiz. *PLoS ONE* **2010**, *5*, e13. [CrossRef] [PubMed]
24. Hashimoto, R.; Moriguchi, Y.; Yamashita, F.; Mori, T.; Nemoto, K.; Okada, T.; Hori, H.; Noguchi, H.; Kunugi, H.; Ohnishi, T. Dose-dependent effect of the Val66Met polymorphism of the brain-derived neurotrophic factor gene on memory-related hippocampal activity. *Neurosci. Res.* **2008**, *61*, 360–367. [CrossRef] [PubMed]
25. Sanchez, M.M.; Das, D.; Taylor, J.L.; Noda, A.; Yesavage, J.A.; Salehi, A. BDNF polymorphism predicts the rate of decline in skilled task performance and hippocampal volume in healthy individuals. *Transl. Psychiatry* **2011**, *1*, 10. [CrossRef] [PubMed]
26. Kambeitz, J.P.; Bhattacharyya, S.; Kambeitz-Ilankovic, L.M.; Valli, I.; Collier, D.A.; McGuire, P. Effect of BDNF val(66)met polymorphism on declarative memory and its neural substrate: A meta-analysis. *Neurosci. Biobehav. Rev.* **2012**, *36*, 2165–2177. [CrossRef] [PubMed]
27. Hajek, T.; Kopecek, M.; Hoschl, C. Reduced hippocampal volumes in healthy carriers of brain-derived neurotrophic factor Val66Met polymorphism: Meta-analysis. *World J. Biol. Psychiatry* **2012**, *13*, 178–187. [CrossRef] [PubMed]
28. Lövdén, M.; Schaefer, S.; Noack, H.; Kanowski, M.; Kaufmann, J.; Tempelmann, C.; Bodammer, N.C.; Kühn, S.; Heinze, H.J.; Lindenberger, U.; et al. Performance-related increases in hippocampal N-acetylaspartate (NAA) induced by spatial navigation training are restricted to BDNF Val homozygotes. *Cereb. Cortex* **2011**, *21*, 1435–1442. [CrossRef] [PubMed]
29. Banner, H.; Bhat, V.; Etchamendy, N.; Joober, R.; Bohbot, V.D. The brain-derived neurotrophic factor Val66Met polymorphism is associated with reduced functional magnetic resonance imaging activity in the hippocampus and increased use of caudate nucleus-dependent strategies in a human virtual navigation task. *Eur. J. Neurosci.* **2011**, *33*, 968–977. [CrossRef] [PubMed]
30. Rosas-Vidal, L.E.; Do-Monte, F.H.; Sotres-Bayon, F.; Quirk, G.J. Hippocampal—Prefrontal BDNF and Memory for Fear Extinction. *Neuropsychopharmacology* **2014**, *39*, 2161–2169. [CrossRef] [PubMed]
31. Notaras, M.; Hill, R.; van den Buuse, M. The BDNF gene Val66Met polymorphism as a modifier of psychiatric disorder susceptibility: Progress and controversy. *Mol. Psychiatry* **2015**, *20*, 916–930. [CrossRef] [PubMed]
32. Zhang, L.; Li, X.-X.; Hu, X.-Z. Post-traumatic stress disorder risk and brain-derived neurotrophic factor Val66Met. *World J. Psychiatry* **2014**, *6*, 1–6. [CrossRef] [PubMed]
33. Mandel, A.L.; Ozdener, H.; Utermohlen, V. Identification of pro- and mature brain-derived neurotrophic factor in human saliva. *Arch. Oral Biol.* **2009**, *54*, 689–695. [CrossRef] [PubMed]
34. Doidge, N. *The Brain That Changes Itself: Stories of Personal Triumph from the Frontiers of Brain Science*; James, H., Ed.; Silberman Books; Penguin: London, UK, 2007.

35. Egan, M.F.; Kojima, M.; Callicott, J.H.; Goldberg, T.E.; Kolachana, B.S.; Bertolino, A.; Zaitsev, E.; Gold, B.; Goldman, D.; Dean, M.; et al. The BDNF val66met polymorphism affects activity-dependent secretion of BDNF and human memory and hippocampal function. *Cell* **2003**, *112*, 257–269. [CrossRef]
36. Wang, T. Does BDNF Val66Met Polymorphism Confer Risk for Posttraumatic Stress Disorder. *Neuropsychobiology* **2015**, *71*, 149–153. [CrossRef] [PubMed]
37. Soliman, F.; Glatt, C.E.; Bath, K.G.; Levita, L.; Jones, R.M.; Pattwell, S.S.; Jing, D.; Tottenham, N.; Amso, D.; Somerville, L.H.; et al. A genetic variant BDNF polymorphism alters extinction learning in both mouse and human. *Science* **2010**, *327*, 863–866. [CrossRef] [PubMed]
38. Andero, R.; Ressler, K.J. Fear extinction and BDNF: Translating animal models of PTSD to the clinic. *Genes Brain Behav.* **2012**, *11*, 503–512. [CrossRef] [PubMed]
39. Dudchenko, P. *Why People Get Lost: The Psychology and Neuroscience of Spatial Cognition*; Oxford University Press: Oxford, UK, 2010.
40. Miller, J.K. Lost in Trauma: Post-Traumatic Stress Disorder, Spatial Processing and the Brain-Derived Neurotrophic Factor Gene. Ph.D. Thesis, Bournemouth University, Poole, UK, 2016. Available online: http://eprints.bournemouth.ac.uk/25012/ (accessed on 14 July 2016).
41. Heldt, S.A.; Stanek, L.; Chhatwal, J.P.; Ressler, K.J. Hippocampus-specific deletion of BDNF in adult mice impairs spatial memory and extinction of aversive memories. *Mol. Psychiatry* **2007**, *12*, 656–670. [CrossRef] [PubMed]
42. Zhang, H.; Ozbay, F.; Lappalainen, J.; Kranzler, H.R.; van Dyck, C.H.; Charney, D.S.; Price, L.H.; Southwick, S.; Yang, B.Z.; Rasmussen, A.; et al. Brain-Derived Neurotrophic Factor Gene (BDNF) Variants and Alzheimer's Disease, Affective Disorders, Posttraumatic Stress Disorder, Schizophrenia and Substance Dependence. *Am. J. Med. Genet.* **2006**, *141B*, 387–393. [CrossRef] [PubMed]
43. Hegarty, M.; Richardson, A.; Montello, D.; Lovelace, K.; Subbiah, I. Development of a self-report measure of environmental spatial ability. *Intelligence* **2002**, *30*, 425–447. [CrossRef]
44. Pazzaglia, F.; De Beni, R. Strategies of processing spatial information in survey and landmark-centred individuals. *Eur. J. Cogn. Psychol.* **2001**, *13*, 493–508. [CrossRef]
45. Münzer, S.; Hölscher, C. Entwicklung und Validierung eines Fragebogens zu räumlichen Strategien (Development and Validation of a Self-report Measure of Environmental Spatial Strategies). *Diagnostica* **2011**, *57*, 111–125. [CrossRef]
46. Wiener, J.M.; de Condappa, O.; Harris, M.A.; Wolbers, T. Maladaptive bias for extra hippocampal navigation strategies in aging humans. *J. Neurosci.* **2013**, *33*, 6012–6017. [CrossRef] [PubMed]
47. Zoladz, P.R.; Diamond, D.M. Current status on behavioral and biological markers of PTSD: A search for clarity in a conflicting literature. *Neurosci. Biobehav. Rev.* **2013**, *37*, 860–895. [CrossRef] [PubMed]
48. Bonne, O.; Gill, J.M.; Luckenbaugh, D.A.; Collins, C.; Owens, M.J.; Alesci, S.; Neumeister, A.; Yuan, P.; Kinkead, B.; Manji, H.K.; et al. Corticotropin-releasing factor, interleukin-6, brain-derived neurotrophic factor, insulin-like growth factor-1, and substance p in the cerebrospinal fluid of civilians with post-traumatic stress disorder before and after treatment with paroxetine. *J. Clin. Psychiatry* **2011**, *72*, 1124–1128. [CrossRef] [PubMed]
49. Furman, A.J.; Clements-Stephens, A.M.; Marchette, S.A.; Shelton, A.L. Persistent and stable biases in spatial learning mechanisms predict navigational style. *Cogn. Affect. Behav. Neurosci.* **2014**. [CrossRef] [PubMed]
50. Van Gerven, D.J.H.; Fergeson, T.; Skelton, R.W. Acute stress switches spatial navigation strategy from egocentric to allocentric in virtual Morris water maze. *Neurobiol. Learn. Mem.* **2016**, *132*, 29–39. [CrossRef] [PubMed]
51. Karnik, M.S.; Wang, L.; Barch, D.M.; Morris, J.; Csernansky, J.G. BDNF polymorphism rs6265, hippocampal structure and memory performance in healthy control subjects. *Psychiatry Res.* **2010**, *178*, 425–429. [CrossRef] [PubMed]
52. Bohbot, V.D.; Lerch, J.; Thorndycraft, B.; Iaria, G.; Zijdenbos, A.P. Gray matter differences correlate with spontaneous strategies in a human virtual navigation task. *J. Neurosci.* **2007**, *27*, 10078–10083. [CrossRef] [PubMed]
53. Joffe, R.T.; Gatt, J.M.; Kemp, A.H.; Grieve, S.; Dobson-Stone, C.; Kuan, S.A.; Schofield, P.R.; Gordon, E.; Williams, L.M. Brain derived neurotrophic factor Val66Met polymorphism, the five factor model of personality and hippocampal volume: Implications for depressive illness. *Hum. Brain Mapp.* **2009**, *30*, 1246–1256. [CrossRef] [PubMed]

54. Chaieb, L.; Antal, A.; Ambrus, G.G.; Paulus, W. Brain-derived neurotrophic factor: Its impact upon neuroplasticity and inducing transcranial brain stimulation protocols. *Neurogenetics* **2014**, *15*, 1–11. [CrossRef] [PubMed]
55. Van den Heuvel, L.; Suliman, S.; Malan-Müller, S.; Hemmings, S.; Seedat, S. Brain-derived neurotrophic factor (BDNF) Val66Met polymorphism and plasma levels in road traffic accident survivors. *Anxiety Stress Coping* **2016**. [CrossRef] [PubMed]
56. Hemmings, S.M.; Martin, L.I.; Klopper, M.; van der Merwe, L.; Aitken, L.; de Wit, E.; Black, G.F.; Hoal, E.G.; Walzl, G.; Seedat, S. BDNF val66met and drd2taq1a polymorphisms interact to influence PTSD symptom severity: A preliminary investigation in a South African population. *Progr. Neuropsychopharmacol. Biol. Psychiatry* **2012**, *40*, 273–280. [CrossRef] [PubMed]
57. Dror, I.E.; Schmitz-Williams, I.C.; Smith, W. Older adults use mental representations that reduce cognitive load: Mental rotation utilizes holistic representations and processing. *Exp. Aging Res.* **2005**, *31*, 409–420. [CrossRef] [PubMed]
58. Perroud, N.; Courtet, P.; Vincze, I.; Jaussent, I.; Jollant, F.; Bellivier, F.; Leboyer, M.; Baud, P.; Buresi, C.; Malafosse, A. Interaction between BDNF Val66Met and childhood trauma on adult's violent suicide attempt. *Genes Brain Behav.* **2008**, *7*, 314–322. [CrossRef] [PubMed]
59. Monti, J.M.; Baym, C.L.; Cohen, N.J. Identifying and Characterizing the Effects of Nutrition on Hippocampal Memory. *Adv. Nutr.* **2014**, *5*, 337S–343S. [CrossRef] [PubMed]
60. Bath, K.G.; Lee, F.S. Variant BDNF (Val66Met) impact on brain structure and function. *Cogn. Affect. Behav. Neurosci.* **2006**, *6*, 79–85. [CrossRef] [PubMed]
61. Foa, E.B.; Cashman, L.; Jaycox, L.H.; Perry, K. The validation of a self-report measure of PTSD: The PTSD Diagnostic Scale. *Psychol. Assess.* **1997**, *9*, 445–451. [CrossRef]
62. Iaria, G.; Petrides, M.; Dagher, A.; Pike, B.; Bohbot, V.D. Cognitive strategies dependent on the hippocampus and caudate nucleus in human navigation: Variability and change with practice. *J. Neurosci.* **2003**, *23*, 5945–5952. [PubMed]

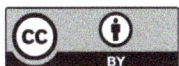

© 2017 by the authors. Licensee MDPI, Basel, Switzerland. This article is an open access article distributed under the terms and conditions of the Creative Commons Attribution (CC BY) license (http://creativecommons.org/licenses/by/4.0/).

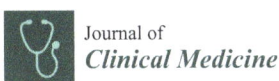 

*Review*

# A Review of HPV-Related Head and Neck Cancer

Kazuhiro Kobayashi [1], Kenji Hisamatsu [1], Natsuko Suzui [1], Akira Hara [1,2], Hiroyuki Tomita [2,*] and Tatsuhiko Miyazaki [1,*]

[1] Pathology Division, Gifu University Hospital, Gifu University Graduate School of Medicine, 1-1 Yanagido, Gifu 501-1194, Japan; hern@live.jp (K.K.); y3f3f84d72xsx@yahoo.co.jp (K.H.); nsuzui7@gifu-u.ac.jp (N.S.); ahara@gifu-u.ac.jp (A.H.)
[2] Department of Tumor Pathology, Gifu University Graduate School of Medicine, 1-1 Yanagido, Gifu 501-1194, Japan
* Correspondence: h_tomita@gifu-u.ac.jp (H.T.); tats@gifu-u.ac.jp (T.M.); Tel.: +81-58-230-7243 (H.T. & T.M.)

Received: 27 July 2018; Accepted: 22 August 2018; Published: 27 August 2018

**Abstract:** Head and neck squamous cell carcinomas (HNSCCs) arise in the mucosal lining of the upper aerodigestive tract. Tobacco and alcohol use have been reported to be associated with HNSCC. Infection with high-risk human papillomaviruses (HPVs) has recently been implicated in the pathogenesis of HNSCCs. It is now widely accepted that high-risk HPV is a cause of almost all cervical cancers as well as some forms of HNSCCs. HPV-related HNSCCs are increasing. HPV-related HNSCCs and HPV-unrelated HNSCCs differ with respect to the molecular mechanisms underlying their oncogenic processes. HPV-related HNSCCs are known to have a better prognosis response to treatment as compared with HPV-unrelated HNSCCs. Therefore, in recent years, it has been required to accurately discriminate between HPV-related and HPV-unrelated HNSCCs. To diagnose the HPV-related HNSCCs, various methods including *P16* immunohistochemistry, FISH, and genetic analyses of the HPV gene from histopathological and liquid biopsy specimens have been employed. Based on the results of the differential diagnosis, various treatments employing EGFR TKI and low-dose radiation have been employed. Here, we review the involvement of the HPV virus in HNSCCs as well as the molecular mechanism of carcinogenesis, classification, prognosis, diagnostic procedures, and therapy of the disease.

**Keywords:** human papillomavirus; human cancer; head and neck; reduction therapy

## 1. Introduction

The role of human papillomavirus (HPV) in carcinogenicity was confirmed in 1983 following the cloning of HPV 16 type from cervical carcinoma tissue by Durst and colleagues [1]. It has since become widely accepted that high-risk HPV is a cause of almost all cervical cancers. Many cases of HPV infection are asymptomatic and resolve spontaneously, but cervical cancer may arise in cases of persistent HPV infection of the cervical basal cells [1,2]. As reviewed by Kreimer et al. [3], HPV DNA has been detected by polymerase chain reaction (PCR) in head and neck squamous cell carcinoma arising from various anatomic sites. HPV16 is the predominant HPV type, accounting for 90% of HPV DNA-positive HNSCCs. Various studies involving mainly HPV 16 have shown that viral DNA is diffusely present in tumor cells of whole tumor, and exhibits clonality when detected by in situ hybridization (ISH) [4–6]. As shown in several oral and oropharyngeal carcinoma cell lines [7–9], the retention of viral DNA during the growth of tumor cells in culture provides further evidence suggestive of viral clonality.

Various studies have reported that oral and tonsillar epithelial cells can be immortalized by full-length HPV 16 or its E6/E7 oncogenes [10–14]. Additionally, transgenic mouse models have revealed that HPV 16 E6/E7 strongly increases susceptibility to oral and oropharyngeal carcinomas [15].

Although E7 was much more competent in inducing these tumors [15], a clear synergy between E6 and E7 in causing HNSCC was discovered [16]. In an analysis of paraffin-embedded biopsies of 116 cases of laryngeal squamous cell carcinomas by in situ DNA hybridization using 35S-labelled HPV (types 6, 11, 16 and 30) DNA probes, 15/116 (12.9%) tumors were shown to contain the DNA of at least 1 HPV type. HPV 11 was the most frequent DNA type, found in 9/116 (7.8%) of the lesions; HPV 16 was found in 5.2%, and HPV 6, in 4.3% [17]. HPV was recognized as a risk factor for oropharyngeal carcinogenesis by the International Agency for Research on Cancer (IARC) in 2007 [18].

A higher frequency of oral sex and a greater number of sex partners are thought to increase the risk of HPV-related cancer in the oropharynx [19,20].

The development of a vaccine for the primary prevention of HPV infection subsequently became an urgent worldwide priority. In 2017, Muranaka was awarded the John Maddox Prize for raising public awareness of the efficacy of the HPV vaccine for the prevention of cervical and other cancers (http://senseaboutscience.org/activities/2017-john-maddox-prize/). This review summarizes the involvement of HPV virus, molecular pathological implications, classification and prognosis, and prospects for future treatment in head and neck cancers.

## 2. Involvement of HPV Virus in Head and Neck Cancers

HPV is a DNA virus that infects the skin and mucous membranes. More than 100 types of HPV have been classified to date. Previous studies have examined the role of HPV-related carcinogenesis in uterine cervical cancer. HPV infecting the uterine cervix is divided into high- and low-risk groups. HPV 16, 18, 31, 33, 35, 39, 45, 51, 52, 56, 58, 68, 69, and 73 are classified as high-risk HPV [21], which is estimated to account for almost 100% of cases of cervical cancer, about 90% of cases of anal cancer, and 40% of vulva, vagina, and penile cancer. Additionally, at least 12% of pharyngeal cancer, 3% of oral cancer, and 30–60% of oropharyngeal carcinoma cases are caused by HPV infection [22]. An increase in squamous cell carcinoma of the head and neck has been reported and attracted global attention recently in the world [23]. It is now recognized that there are two types of squamous cell carcinoma of the head and neck. Classically, most oropharynx cancers are hyperdifferentiated and often show keratinization. Squamous cell carcinoma of the head and neck can be of the keratinized or nonkeratinized type. The former occurs most often in elderly males and is associated with smoking and alcohol consumption, but HPV is not involved. Conversely, nonkeratinizing squamous cell carcinoma occurs most commonly at age 40–55 years in men with little exposure to tobacco and alcohol, and HPV DNA is detected as the most characteristic feature [24–27]. Since the smoking rate in the USA is declining [28], the incidence of HPV-negative tobacco-related oropharyngeal cancer has decreased; however, that of HPV-positive oropharyngeal cancer is increasing [29]. According to repository data from the Surveillance, Epidemiology, and End Results (SEER) program, the prevalence of HPV-negative cancers decreased by 50% from 1988 to 2004, while HPV-positive oropharyngeal carcinoma increased by 225% [30]. In a study by Junor and associates involving patients at the Edinburgh Cancer Center, 41% of head and neck cancers were HPV-positive between 1999 and 2001 and 63% were HPV-positive between 2003 and 2005 [31]. HPV-positive oropharyngeal cancer is considered to be a separate disease with a causal relationship to HPV infection and a good prognosis. Several studies have shown that patients with HPV-positive oropharyngeal cancer, identified through PCR, in situ hybridization or *P16* immunohistochemistry on tumour tissues, have a significantly improved overall and disease-free survival compared with patients with HPV-negative oropharyngeal cancer patients [32–40]. In a prospective study involving 253 newly diagnosed or recurrent HNSCC patients, HPV was detected in 25% of patients. A low tumor grade and the oropharyngeal site increased the likelihood of the presence of HPV, respectively [5]. Oropharyngeal tumors are more likely to be positive for HPV (57%) compared with sites other than the tumor site and the oropharynx (14%) and the oral cavity (12%). HPV-positive oropharyngeal carcinoma occurs primarily in the tonsillar of the palatine or tonsils of the tongue. In the tonsils or tongue base, 62% of the tumors were HPV-positive, whereas in other parts of the oropharynx 25% were HPV-positive.

## 3. Pathological Molecular Mechanism in Carcinogenesis

HPV-unrelated HNSCC cigarette smoking and alcohol has p53 mutations [41]. Deletion of 9p21–22 is also observed early in the oncogenic process, and as a result, the function of the tumor suppressor gene *P16* is lost [42]. *P16*INK4a produced by the *P16* gene forms a complex with cyclin 1-cyclin-dependent kinase 4/cyclin-dependent kinase 6 (CDK4/CDK6), inhibits phosphorylation of Rb, and inhibits transcription factor E2F-related cell rotation (pRB pathway) [43]. In HPV-associated head and neck cancer, wild-type p53 is present and mutations occur at a rate of only 10% or less. However, HPVE6 inactivates p53 resulting in a decrease in function. Furthermore, there is no deletion of *P16* in these tumors. Since HPVE7 inactivates phosphorylated Rb, which controls cell cycling of host cells, control of E2F is inhibited [44] and *P16* is overexpressed. *P16* is a tumor suppressor gene encoding a CDK repressor, which inhibits the complex formation of cyclin D1 and cyclin-dependent kinase (CDK) 4/6. Cyclin D1 and CDK 4/6 complex promotes cell cycling through the release of E2F via phosphorylation of the Rb protein, whereas the Rb protein/E2F complex also suppress the transcription of *P16*, so that when HPV-E7 inactivates the Rb protein, *P16* is overexpressed (Figure 1) [45].

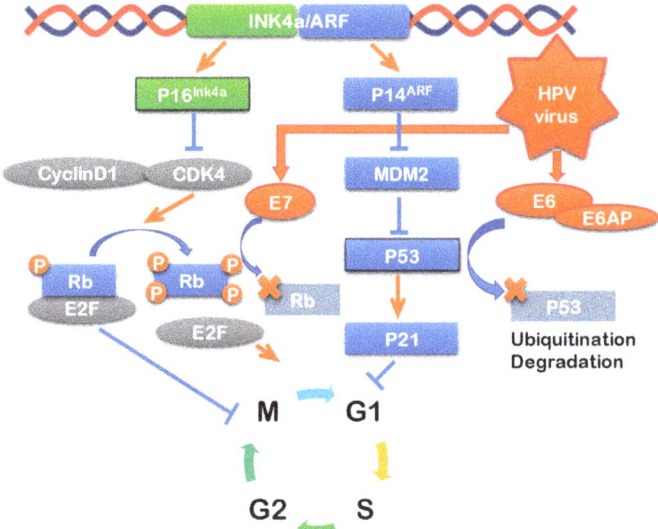

**Figure 1.** Signaling pathways of high-risk HPV oncogenes. High-risk HPVs encodes two known viral oncogenes. E6 protein inactivates tumor suppressor p53 mediated DNA damage and apoptosis pathway. E7 protein inactivates tumor suppressor pRb mediated cell cycle regulation pathway.

Thus, the phenotype at the molecular level is completely different between HPV-positive and HPV-negative cancer of the head and neck. Various methods have therefore been employed for the detection of HPV in head and neck cancer such as consensus primer or type-specific PCR, real-time PCR, in situ hybridization, and serum antibody assays. For cervical cancer screening, accepted international guidelines recommend using hybrid capture II (QIAGEN) and PCR (GP 5/GP 6).

*P16* immunohistochemistry is also useful as a surrogate maker for HPV infection detection, especially in head and neck cancers. *P16* immunohistochemistry has 100% sensitivity and 79% specificity; it is the gold standard for HPV detection, based on HPV 16 E6 and E7 mRNA, in head and neck cancer specimens and is useful as a surrogate maker for clinical HPV detection. *P16* is also a useful molecular marker for judging prognosis and is a component of the WHO classification scheme, described below. *P16*-positive and *P16*-negative HNSCCs could clearly be distinguished in our specimens (Figure 2).

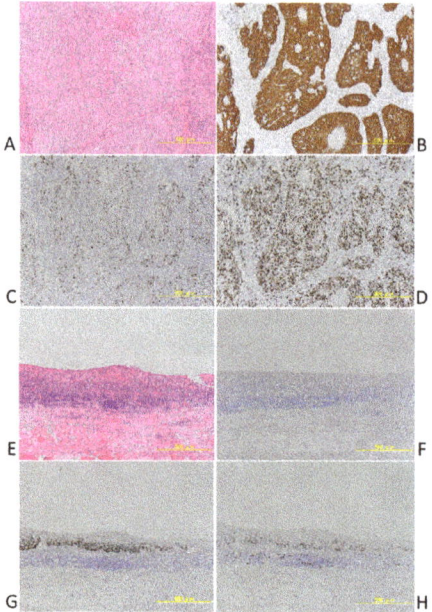

**Figure 2.** (**A–D**) A case of *P16* positive squamous cell carcinoma of Oropharynx. (**A**) HE, (**B**) *P16*, (**C**) p53, (**D**) MIB-1. (**E–H**) A case of *P16* positive squamous cell carcinoma of Oropharynx. (**E**) HE, (**F**) *P16*, (**G**) p53, (**H**) MIB-1.

A general consensus has been achieved for the definition of HPV associated tumors that require expression of the virus oncogenic proteins E6 and E7 that are involved in neoplastic transformation of infected cells. However, the integration of HPV-DNA into the host cell genome confirms the belief that it is an essential step for viral oncogene expression in oropharyngeal cancer, as in the case of cervical cancer. Regardless of the process leading to oncogene expression, HPV E6/E7 mRNA identification based on DNA or protein expression, for patient stratification and epidemiologic purposes, is considered a gold standard for HPV-related classification [46,47]. More accessible strategies are generally accepted. In the examination of the pathological specimen, the detection of HPV-DNA using PCR and ISH examination are typically used together with immunohistochemistry of *P16*. Various new methods have been examined for HPV testing in head and neck cancers [48]. When infected cells become malignant, HPV DNA remains in the nucleus, and viral oncoproteins, in particular against E6, are detected in virtually all cases of HPV-driven OPC cases [49,50]. There are reports that HPV-DNA and HPV16 E6 antibodies in oral and in body fluids can be used for detection of HPV-infected head and neck cancers and prediction of the risk of recurrence [51].

Studies using next-generation sequencing of HNSCCs have also been reported in recent years. Matthias Lechner did 20 HPV+ and 20 HPV-laser capture microdissection pharyngeal carcinoma studies. HPV-positive and HPV-negative oropharyngeal cancers are divided into two different subgroups. A TP53 mutation was detected in 100% of HPV-negative cases and invalidation of G1/S checkpoint by CDKN2A/B deficiency and/or CCND1 amplification was shown to occur in the majority of HPV tumors [52]. In a study that examined the somatic mutations of 279 HNSCCs performed in 2015, In HPV-positive oropharyngeal carcinoma, deletion of TRAF3, activation mutation of PIK3CA, and amplification of E2F1 were observed. In HPV-negative HNSCC, subsets recognizing simultaneous mutations of CASP8 with amplicons on 11q with CCND1, FADD, BIRC2, and YAP1, or with HRAS, were observed. Either type of tumor was abnormal with respect to target cell cycle, death, NF-κB and other oncogenic pathways [53]. In a study of 92 cases of HNSCC using the next generation sequencer, TPK 53was the most common mutation, occurring in 47 (51%) patients followed by CDKN 2A ($n = 23$, 25%), CCND 1 ($n = 22$, 24%), and PIK 3 CA ($n = 19$, 21%). Changes in TPV, CDKN2A, and CCND1 genes occurred more frequently in HPV-negative tumors, but the total amount of mutations was similar between HPV-negative and HPV-positive tumors. HPV-positive tumors were significantly associated with immune-related genes compared to HPV-negative tumors. Mutations in NOTCH1 ($p = 0.027$), CDKN2A ($p < 0.001$), and TP53 ($p = 0.038$) were significantly associated with decreased overall survival. FAT1 mutation was highly enriched in cisplatin responders and targetable alterations such as PIK3CA E545K and CDKN2A R58X were found in 14 patients (15%) [54].

As an emerging technology, liquid biopsies, involving the use of a small amount of DNA and mRNA collected from blood samples, have been used in recent cancer studies. Allen et al. [55] reported a novel in vitro diagnostic approach in which miRNA is examined from exposed cancer cells using sera from HNSCC patients. Of 377 miRNAs detected, 16 different miRNAs were found to be differentially expressed when comparing cells exposed to serum from HNSCC versus healthy individuals. Real-time PCR analysis revealed that serum from HNSCC patients downregulated the expression of 5 genes involved in carcinogenesis and 2 of these—P53 and SLC2A1—are direct targets for the detected miRNAs. This technique has potential for a new therapeutic approach using tumor-specific cell lines or single cell in vitro assays, and the possibility of more specific diagnosis could facilitate individual treatment and early detection of primary tumors or metastasis.

## 4. Classification and Prognosis of Head and Neck Cancers

In general, HPV-positive oropharyngeal carcinoma is highly susceptible to radiation and anticancer drugs and has a better prognosis compared with HPV-negative cancer. HPV-negative oropharyngeal carcinoma is caused by the disappearance of function due to p53 gene mutation [56–59]. In a prospective phase II clinical trial of pharyngeal and laryngeal cancer patients by the Eastern Cooperative Oncology Group, 63% of 60 cases were HPV 16 positive, and all of the HPV16-positive cases were also positive for *P16*. For HPV-positive and HPV-negative cancers the respective response rates were 84% versus 57%, the 2-year progression-free survival rates were 86% vs. 53%, the overall 2-year survival rates were 95% vs. 62%, and the prognosis for HPV-positive cancer was significantly better [37]. Previous reports have examined the prognosis of HPV in relation to *P16*, and the outcomes of oropharyngeal cancer in relation to tobacco exposure. In a phase III study involving 400 oropharyngeal carcinomas, the 2-year progression-free survival rates for HPV-positive and HPV-negative cancer were 72% vs. 51% and the 2-year overall survival rates were 88% vs. 67%. Due to differences in prognosis, squamous cell carcinoma of the head and neck was classified in the new WHO scheme as HPV-negative or HPV-positive. Classification by *P16* immunostaining or HPV testing is recommended. In addition, some recently proposed classification schemes are based on the EGFR status according to 2 categories: HPV-positive/*P16* positive squamous cell carcinoma and HPV-negative/*P16* negative squamous cell carcinoma [60]. Cetuximab, a monoclonal antibody that inhibits the function of EGFR, is known to have efficacy in colorectal cancer [61,62] and head and neck cancer [63,64], and it was also shown to be more specific and cost-effective for these types of cancers.

## 5. Prospects for Treatment

For the reasons outlined herein, HPV virus is expected to be a therapeutic target in the treatment of human cancer [65] We believe that the prognosis for cervical cancer can be greatly improved through the implementation of methods for early detection such as cytodiagnosis, HPV screening, and *P16* immunostaining, Furthermore, HPV vaccination may also be useful for preventing HPV-related cancers other than cervical cancer. For example, most cases of oropharyngeal carcinoma are caused by HPV 16 (about 90%) and HPV 18, and HPV vaccination for this condition can be expected to have a greater disease-suppressing effect than in cervical cancer. Randomized trials have provided strong evidence for high efficacy of the 2 FDA-approved VLP vaccines: the bivalent HPV16/18 vaccine

(Cervarix®, GlaxoSmithKline Biologicals, GlaxoSmithKline plc, Brentford, UK) and the quadrivalent HPV 6/11/16/18 vaccine (Gardasil™, Merck Sharp and Dohme, Merck & Co., Kenilworth, NJ, USA) against cervical, vaginal, and vulvar HPV16/18 infections and related diseases, and against anal HPV16/18 infections in women [66–70]. One of the methods proposed for prevention of HPV-related oropharyngeal cancer is vaccination. The US Centers for Disease Control Advisory Committee on Immunization Practices (ACIP) has recommended HPV vaccination for females and males between the ages of 11 and 12 years, starting as early as 9 years, with booster doses at up to 26 and 21 years for females and males, respectively. In order for the vaccination to be effective in preventing oropharyngeal cancer, the protective effect must last for at least 2 decades, and ongoing studies have shown no waning of systemic antibodies at 8 years after vaccination. However, in June 2013, the Ministry of Health, Labour and Welfare of Japan suspended proactive recommendation of the vaccine after unconfirmed reports of adverse events. To investigate any potential association between the vaccine and reported symptoms, the Nagoya City Council conducted a questionnaire-based survey. The anonymous postal questionnaire investigated the onset of 24 symptoms, associated hospital visits, frequency, and influence on school attendance. A total of 29,846 residents responded. No significant increase in occurrence of any of the 24 reported post-HPV vaccination symptoms was found. The results suggest no causal association between the HPV vaccines and reported symptoms [71].

Also, Reduction surgery or minimally invasive treatment should be considered in cases of HPV virus-related oropharyngeal carcinoma. Although limited to the T1 and T2 stages of oropharynx cancer, transoral robotic surgery approved by the FDA since 2009. In addition, many reduction surgeries and post-operative adjuvant therapies based on pathologic staging are being studied [72–74].

As mentioned above, it is known that EGFR is expressed in HNSCCs, and combination use of cetuximab and radiation is, therefore, being studied for treatment instead of standard cisplatin therapy [38,61,64,75–78]. Several researchers have hypothesized that radiation dose reduction is feasible and safe for some HPV-positive patients when induction chemotherapy (IC) is used for patient selection. Three points have been raised to support this assertion. First, HPV-positive HNSCCs are considered to be more radiosensitive than HPV-negative HNSCCs [79]. Second, doses comparable to the supplemental radiation dosage is sufficient for the treatment of patients with asymptomatic disease [80]. Finally, the response to chemotherapy can predict the future response to subsequent radiation therapy. Chen et al. [79] conducted an arm Phase II trial (NCT 01716195) in 44 patients with stage III/IV *P16*-positive OPCs treated 2 cycles of IC (paclitaxel and carboplatin was for 21 days), followed by radiation and paclitaxel. The radiation dose was also reduced in complete or partial responders (54 Gy, $n = 24$), and even in patients with partial or no response ($n = 20$, 60 Gy instead of standard 70 Gy). Except for 1patient, all patients completed the IC. Two years PFS and local region control were 92% (95% CI 77–97) and 95% (95% CI 80–99), respectively. The two-year degree of freedom for grade 3 or adverse events of worsening mucosa and esophagus was 85% (95% CI 80–90) in patients treated with 54 Gy. These results were achieved with doses reduced by 15–20% compared with these in the ECOG 2399 trial using the same protocol, except that a dose of 70 Gy, dose was used as a standard chemoradiotherapy regimen. Besides that, Removal of chemotherapy and Alternative to the "conventional" photon beam therapy are considered as new treatment methods [80].

Differences in the prognosis and etiologic mechanisms of HPV-related head and neck cancer from conventional head and neck cancers (mostly HPV-negative) suggest that the detection of HPV may significantly change the future diagnosis, treatment, and management [31]. HPV not only plays a role in the development of pharyngeal cancer but is also involved in 23.5% of oral cancer and 24% of laryngeal cancer cases, suggesting that indications for HPV vaccination could be expanded to also include oral and laryngeal cancer [37].

**Author Contributions:** K.K., K.H., N.S., A.H., H.T. and T.M. all contributed to the manuscript and have reviewed it.

**Funding:** This research was funded by the KAKENHI grant from the Ministry of Education, Culture, Sports, Science, and Technology of Japan: grant No. 26430111 (HT).

**Acknowledgments:** We thank all the members who work in the Division of Pathology.

**Conflicts of Interest:** The authors declare no conflicts of interest in this work.

## References

1. Durst, M.; Gissmann, L.; Ikenberg, H.; Zur Hausen, H. A papillomavirus DNA from a cervical carcinoma and its prevalence in cancer biopsy samples from different geographic regions. *Proc. Natl. Acad. Sci. USA* **1983**, *80*, 3812–3815. [CrossRef] [PubMed]
2. Walboomers, J.M.; Jacobs, M.V.; Manos, M.M.; Bosch, F.X.; Kummer, J.A.; Shah, K.V.; Snijders, P.J.H.; Peto, J.; Meijer, C.J.L.M.; Muñoz, N. Human papillomavirus is a necessary cause of invasive cervical cancer worldwide. *J. Pathol.* **1999**, *189*, 12–19. [CrossRef]
3. Kreimer, A.R.; Clifford, G.M.; Boyle, P.; Franceschi, S. Human papillomavirus types in head and neck squamous cell carcinomas worldwide: A systematic review. *Cancer Epidemiol. Biomark. Prev.* **2005**, *14*, 467–475. [CrossRef] [PubMed]
4. Niedobitek, G.; Pitteroff, S.; Herbst, H.; Shepherd, P.; Finn, T.; Anagnostopoulos, I.; Stein, H. Detection of human papillomavirus type 16 DNA in carcinomas of the palatine tonsil. *J. Clin. Pathol.* **1990**, *43*, 918–921. [CrossRef] [PubMed]
5. Gillison, M.L.; Koch, W.M.; Capone, R.B.; Spafford, M.; Westra, W.H.; Wu, L.; Zahurak, M.L.; Daniel, R.W.; Viglione, M.; Symer, D.E.; et al. Evidence for a causal association between human papillomavirus and a subset of head and neck cancers. *J. Natl. Cancer Inst.* **2000**, *92*, 709–720. [CrossRef] [PubMed]
6. Begum, S.; Cao, D.; Gillison, M.; Zahurak, M.; Westra, W.H. Tissue distribution of human papillomavirus 16 DNA integration in patients with tonsillar carcinoma. *Clin. Cancer Res.* **2005**, *11*, 5694–5699. [CrossRef] [PubMed]
7. Ferris, R.L.; Martinez, I.; Sirianni, N.; Wang, J.; Lopez-Albaitero, A.; Gollin, S.M.; Johnson, J.T.; Khan, S. Human papillomavirus-16 associated squamous cell carcinoma of the head and neck (SCCHN): A natural disease model provides insights into viral carcinogenesis. *Eur. J. Cancer* **2005**, *41*, 807–815. [CrossRef] [PubMed]
8. Steenbergen, R.D.; Hermsen, M.A.; Walboomers, J.M.; Joenje, H.; Arwert, F.; Meijer, C.J.; Snijders, P.J. Integrated human papillomavirus type 16 and loss of heterozygosity at 11q22 and 18q21 in an oral carcinoma and its derivative cell line. *Cancer Res.* **1995**, *55*, 546–55471.
9. Rampias, T.; Sasaki, C.; Weinberger, P.; Psyrri, A. E6 and e7 gene silencing and transformed phenotype of human papillomavirus 16-positive oropharyngeal cancer cells. *J. Natl. Cancer Inst.* **2009**, *101*, 412–423. [CrossRef] [PubMed]
10. Lace, M.J.; Anson, J.R.; Klussmann, J.P.; Wang, D.H.; Smith, E.M.; Haugen, T.H.; Turek, L.P. Human papillomavirus type 16 (HPV-16) genomes integrated in head and neck cancers and in HPV-16-immortalized human keratinocyte clones express chimeric virus-cell mRNAs similar to those found in cervical cancers. *J. Virol.* **2011**, *85*, 1645–1654. [CrossRef] [PubMed]
11. Sexton, C.J.; Proby, C.M.; Banks, L.; Stables, J.N.; Powell, K.; Navsaria, H.; Leigh, I.M. Characterization of factors involved in human papillomavirus type 16-mediated immortalization of oral keratinocytes. *J. Gen. Virol.* **1993**, *74*, 755–761. [CrossRef] [PubMed]
12. Park, N.H.; Min, B.M.; Li, S.L.; Huang, M.Z.; Cherick, H.M.; Doniger, J. Immortalization of normal human oral keratinocytes with type 16 human papillomavirus. *Carcinogenesis* **1991**, *12*, 1627–1631. [CrossRef] [PubMed]
13. Smeets, S.J.; van der Plas, M.; Schaaij-Visser, T.B.; van Veen, E.A.; van Meerloo, J.; Braakhuis, B.J.; Steenbergen, R.D.M.; Brakenhoff, R.H. Immortalization of oral keratinocytes by functional inactivation of the p53 and pRb pathways. *Int. J. Cancer* **2011**, *128*, 1596–1605. [CrossRef] [PubMed]
14. Chen, R.W.; Aalto, Y.; Teesalu, T.; Durst, M.; Knuutila, S.; Aaltonen, L.M.; Vaheri, A. Establishment and characterisation of human papillomavirus type 16 DNA immortalised human tonsillar epithelial cell lines. *Eur. J. Cancer* **2003**, *39*, 698–707. [CrossRef]
15. Strati, K.; Pitot, H.C.; Lambert, P.F. Identification of biomarkers that distinguish human papillomavirus (HPV)-positive versus HPV-negative head and neck cancers in a mouse model. *Proc. Natl. Acad. Sci. USA* **2006**, *103*, 14152–14157. [CrossRef] [PubMed]

16. Jabbar, S.; Strati, K.; Shin, M.K.; Pitot, H.C.; Lambert, P.F. Human papillomavirus type 16 E6 and E7 oncoproteins act synergistically to cause head and neck cancer in mice. *Virology* **2010**, *407*, 60–67. [CrossRef] [PubMed]
17. Syrjanen, S.; Syrjanen, K.; Mantyjarvi, R.; Collan, Y.; Karja, J. Human papillomavirus DNA in squamous cell carcinomas of the larynx demonstrated by in situ DNA hybridization. *ORL* **1987**, *49*, 175–186. [CrossRef] [PubMed]
18. Ragin, C.C.; Modugno, F.; Gollin, S.M. The epidemiology and risk factors of head and neck cancer: A focus on human papillomavirus. *J. Dent. Res.* **2007**, *86*, 104–114. [CrossRef] [PubMed]
19. Gillison, M.L.; D'Souza, G.; Westra, W.; Sugar, E.; Xiao, W.; Begum, S.; Viscidi, R. Distinct risk factor profiles for human papillomavirus type 16-positive and human papillomavirus type 16-negative head and neck cancers. *J. Natl. Cancer Inst.* **2008**, *100*, 407–420. [CrossRef] [PubMed]
20. D'Souza, G.; Agrawal, Y.; Halpern, J.; Bodison, S.; Gillison, M.L. Oral sexual behaviors associated with prevalent oral human papillomavirus infection. *J. Infect. Dis.* **2009**, *199*, 1263–1269. [CrossRef] [PubMed]
21. Munoz, N.; Bosch, F.X.; de Sanjose, S.; Herrero, R.; Castellsague, X.; Shah, K.V.; Snijders, P.J.F.; Meijer, C.J.L.M. Epidemiologic classification of human papillomavirus types associated with cervical cancer. *N. Engl. J. Med.* **2003**, *348*, 518–527. [CrossRef] [PubMed]
22. Parkin, D.M.; Bray, F. Chapter 2: The burden of HPV-related cancers. *Vaccine* **2006**, *24* (Suppl. 3), S11–S25. [CrossRef] [PubMed]
23. Chaturvedi, A.K.; Anderson, W.F.; Lortet-Tieulent, J.; Curado, M.P.; Ferlay, J.; Franceschi, S.; Rosenberg, P.S.; Bray, F.; Gillison, M.L. Worldwide trends in incidence rates for oral cavity and oropharyngeal cancers. *J. Clin. Oncol.* **2013**, *31*, 4550–4559. [CrossRef] [PubMed]
24. El-Mofty, S.K.; Lu, D.W. Prevalence of human papillomavirus type 16 DNA in squamous cell carcinoma of the palatine tonsil, and not the oral cavity, in young patients: A distinct clinicopathologic and molecular disease entity. *Am. J. Surg. Pathol.* **2003**, *27*, 1463–1470. [CrossRef] [PubMed]
25. Chernock, R.D.; El-Mofty, S.K.; Thorstad, W.L.; Parvin, C.A.; Lewis, J.S., Jr. HPV-related nonkeratinizing squamous cell carcinoma of the oropharynx: Utility of microscopic features in predicting patient outcome. *Head Neck Pathol.* **2009**, *3*, 186–194. [CrossRef] [PubMed]
26. Lewis, J.S., Jr.; Khan, R.A.; Masand, R.P.; Chernock, R.D.; Zhang, Q.; Al-Naief, N.S.; Muller, S.; McHugh, J.B.; Prasad, M.L.; Brandwein-Gensler, M.; et al. Recognition of nonkeratinizing morphology in oropharyngeal squamous cell carcinoma—A prospective cohort and interobserver variability study. *Histopathology* **2012**, *60*, 427–436. [CrossRef] [PubMed]
27. El-Mofty, S.K.; Zhang, M.Q.; Davila, R.M. Histologic identification of human papillomavirus (HPV)-related squamous cell carcinoma in cervical lymph nodes: A reliable predictor of the site of an occult head and neck primary carcinoma. *Head Neck Pathol.* **2008**, *2*, 163–168. [CrossRef] [PubMed]
28. Centers for Disease Control and Prevention, Chartbook on Long-term Trends in Heatlh, United States, 2016. Available online: https://www.cdc.gov/nchs/data/hus/hus16.pdf (accessed on 27 August 2018).
29. Chaturvedi, A.K.; Engels, E.A.; Anderson, W.F.; Gillison, M.L. Incidence trends for human papillomavirus-related and -unrelated oral squamous cell carcinomas in the United States. *J. Clin. Oncol.* **2008**, *26*, 612–619. [CrossRef] [PubMed]
30. Pytynia, K.B.; Dahlstrom, K.R.; Sturgis, E.M. Epidemiology of HPV-associated oropharyngeal cancer. *Oral Oncol.* **2014**, *50*, 380–386. [CrossRef] [PubMed]
31. Junor, E.; Kerr, G.; Oniscu, A.; Campbell, S.; Kouzeli, I.; Gourley, C.; et al. Benefit of chemotherapy as part of treatment for HPV DNA-positive but P16-negative squamous cell carcinoma of the oropharynx. *Br. J. Cancer* **2012**, *106*, 358–365. [CrossRef] [PubMed]
32. Elrefaey, S.; Massaro, M.A.; Chiocca, S.; Chiesa, F.; Ansarin, M. HPV in oropharyngeal cancer: The basics to know in clinical practice. *Acta Otorhinolaryngol. Italica* **2014**, *34*, 299–309.
33. Ang, K.K.; Harris, J.; Wheeler, R.; Weber, R.; Rosenthal, D.I.; Nguyen-Tan, P.F.; Westra, W.H.; Chung, C.H.; Jordan, R.C.; Lu, C.; et al. Human papillomavirus and survival of patients with oropharyngeal cancer. *N. Engl. J. Med.* **2010**, *363*, 24–35. [CrossRef] [PubMed]
34. Olshan, A.F. *Epidemiology, Pathogenesis, and Prevention of Head and Neck Cancer*; Springer: New York, NY, USA, 2010.
35. Marur, S.; D'Souza, G.; Westra, W.H.; Forastiere, A.A. HPV-associated head and neck cancer: A virus-related cancer epidemic. *Lancet Oncol.* **2010**, *11*, 781–789. [CrossRef]

36. Chung, C.H.; Gillison, M.L. Human papillomavirus in head and neck cancer: Its role in pathogenesis and clinical implications. *Clin. Cancer Res.* **2009**, *15*, 6758–6762. [CrossRef] [PubMed]
37. Fakhry, C.; Westra, W.H.; Li, S.; Cmelak, A.; Ridge, J.A.; Pinto, H.; Forastiere, A.; Gillison, M.L. Improved survival of patients with human papillomavirus-positive head and neck squamous cell carcinoma in a prospective clinical trial. *J. Natl. Cancer Inst.* **2008**, *100*, 261–269. [CrossRef] [PubMed]
38. Rischin, D.; Young, R.J.; Fisher, R.; Fox, S.B.; Le, Q.T.; Peters, L.J.; Solomon, B.; Choi, J.; O'Sullivan, B.; Kenny, L.M.; et al. Prognostic significance of *P16*INK4A and human papillomavirus in patients with oropharyngeal cancer treated on TROG 02.02 phase III trial. *J. Clin. Oncol.* **2010**, *28*, 4142–4148. [CrossRef] [PubMed]
39. Lassen, P.; Eriksen, J.G.; Krogdahl, A.; Therkildsen, M.H.; Ulhoi, B.P.; Overgaard, M.; Specht, L.; Andersen, E.; Johansen, J.; Grau, C.; et al. The influence of HPV-associated *P16*-expression on accelerated fractionated radiotherapy in head and neck cancer: Evaluation of the randomised DAHANCA 6&7 trial. *Radiother. Oncol.* **2011**, *100*, 49–55. [PubMed]
40. Posner, M.R.; Lorch, J.H.; Goloubeva, O.; Tan, M.; Schumaker, L.M.; Sarlis, N.J.; Haddad, R.I.; Cullen, K.J. Survival and human papillomavirus in oropharynx cancer in TAX 324: A subset analysis from an international phase III trial. *Ann. Oncol.* **2011**, *22*, 1071–1077. [CrossRef] [PubMed]
41. Carlos de Vicente, J.; Junquera Gutierrez, L.M.; Zapatero, A.H.; Fresno Forcelledo, M.F.; Hernandez-Vallejo, G.; Lopez Arranz, J.S. Prognostic significance of p53 expression in oral squamous cell carcinoma without neck node metastases. *Head Neck* **2004**, *26*, 22–30. [CrossRef] [PubMed]
42. Reed, A.L.; Califano, J.; Cairns, P.; Westra, W.H.; Jones, R.M.; Koch, W.; Ahrendt, S.; Eby, Y.; Sewell, D.; Nawroz, H.; et al. High frequency of *P16* (CDKN2/MTS-1/INK4A) inactivation in head and neck squamous cell carcinoma. *Cancer Res.* **1996**, *56*, 3630–3633. [PubMed]
43. Satyanarayana, A.; Rudolph, K.L. *P16* and ARF: Activation of teenage proteins in old age. *J. Clin. Investig.* **2004**, *114*, 1237–1240. [CrossRef] [PubMed]
44. Perrone, F.; Suardi, S.; Pastore, E.; Casieri, P.; Orsenigo, M.; Caramuta, S.; Dagrada, G.; Losa, M.; Licitra, L.; Bossi, P.; et al. Molecular and cytogenetic subgroups of oropharyngeal squamous cell carcinoma. *Clin. Cancer Res.* **2006**, *12*, 6643–6651. [CrossRef] [PubMed]
45. Romagosa, C.; Simonetti, S.; Lopez-Vicente, L.; Mazo, A.; Lleonart, M.E.; Castellvi, J.; y Cajal, S.R. *P16*(Ink4a) overexpression in cancer: A tumor suppressor gene associated with senescence and high-grade tumors. *Oncogene* **2011**, *30*, 2087–2097. [CrossRef] [PubMed]
46. Gao, G.; Johnson, S.H.; Kasperbauer, J.L.; Eckloff, B.W.; Tombers, N.M.; Vasmatzis, G.; Smith, D.I. Mate pair sequencing of oropharyngeal squamous cell carcinomas reveals that HPV integration occurs much less frequently than in cervical cancer. *J. Clin. Virol.* **2014**, *59*, 195–200. [CrossRef] [PubMed]
47. Snijders, P.J.; Meijer, C.J.; van den Brule, A.J.; Schrijnemakers, H.F.; Snow, G.B.; Walboomers, J.M. Human papillomavirus (HPV) type 16 and 33 E6/E7 region transcripts in tonsillar carcinomas can originate from integrated and episomal HPV DNA. *J. Gen. Virol.* **1992**, *73*, 2059–2066. [CrossRef] [PubMed]
48. Morbini, P.; Benazzo, M. Human papillomavirus and head and neck carcinomas: Focus on evidence in the babel of published data. *Acta Otorhinolaryngol. Italica* **2016**, *36*, 249–258.
49. Holzinger, D.; Wichmann, G.; Baboci, L.; Michel, A.; Hofler, D.; Wiesenfarth, M.; Sehroeder, L.; Boscolo-Rizzo, P.; Herold-Mende, C.; Dyckhoff, G.; et al. Sensitivity and specificity of antibodies against HPV16 E6 and other early proteins for the detection of HPV16-driven oropharyngeal squamous cell carcinoma. *Int. J. Cancer* **2017**, *140*, 2748–2757. [CrossRef] [PubMed]
50. Lang Kuhs, K.A.; Pawlita, M.; Gibson, S.P.; Schmitt, N.C.; Trivedi, S.; Argiris, A.; Kreimer, A.; Ferris, R.L.; Waterboer, T. Characterization of human papillomavirus antibodies in individuals with head and neck cancer. *Cancer Epidemiol.* **2016**, *42*, 46–52. [CrossRef] [PubMed]
51. Mirghani, H.; Lang Kuhs, K.A.; Waterboer, T. Biomarkers for early identification of recurrences in HPV-driven oropharyngeal cancer. *Oral Oncol.* **2018**, *82*, 108–114. [CrossRef] [PubMed]
52. Lechner, M.; Frampton, G.M.; Fenton, T.; Feber, A.; Palmer, G.; Jay, A.; Pillay, N.; Forster, M.; Cronin, M.T.; Lipson, D.; et al. Targeted next-generation sequencing of head and neck squamous cell carcinoma identifies novel genetic alterations in HPV+ and HPV- tumors. *Genome Med.* **2013**, *5*, 49. [CrossRef] [PubMed]
53. The Cancer Genome Atlas Network. Comprehensive genomic characterization of head and neck squamous cell carcinomas. *Nature* **2015**, *517*, 576–582. [CrossRef] [PubMed]

54. Lim, S.M.; Cho, S.H.; Hwang, I.G.; Choi, J.W.; Chang, H.; Ahn, M.J.; Park, K.U.; Kim, J.-W.; Ko, Y.H.; Ahn, H.K.; et al. Investigating the Feasibility of Targeted Next-Generation Sequencing to Guide the Treatment of Head and Neck Squamous Cell Carcinoma. *Cancer Res. Treat.* **2018**. [CrossRef] [PubMed]
55. Allen, B.; Schneider, A.; Victoria, B.; Nunez Lopez, Y.O.; Muller, M.; Szewczyk, M.; Pazdrowski, J.; Majchrzak, E.; Barcazk, W.; Golusinski, W.; et al. Blood Serum From Head and Neck Squamous Cell Carcinoma Patients Induces Altered MicroRNA and Target Gene Expression Profile in Treated Cells. *Front. Oncol.* **2018**, *8*, 217. [CrossRef] [PubMed]
56. Lindel, K.; Beer, K.T.; Laissue, J.; Greiner, R.H.; Aebersold, D.M. Human papillomavirus positive squamous cell carcinoma of the oropharynx: A radiosensitive subgroup of head and neck carcinoma. *Cancer* **2001**, *92*, 805–813. [CrossRef]
57. Butz, K.; Geisen, C.; Ullmann, A.; Spitkovsky, D.; Hoppe-Seyler, F. Cellular responses of HPV-positive cancer cells to genotoxic anti-cancer agents: Repression of E6/E7-oncogene expression and induction of apoptosis. *Int. J. Cancer* **1996**, *68*, 506–513. [CrossRef]
58. Bristow, R.G.; Benchimol, S.; Hill, R.P. The p53 gene as a modifier of intrinsic radiosensitivity: Implications for radiotherapy. *Radiother. Oncol.* **1996**, *40*, 197–223. [CrossRef]
59. Lindquist, D.; Romanitan, M.; Hammarstedt, L.; Nasman, A.; Dahlstrand, H.; Lindholm, J.; Onelöv, L.; Ramqvist, T.; Ye, W.; Munck-Wikland, E.; et al. Human papillomavirus is a favourable prognostic factor in tonsillar cancer and its oncogenic role is supported by the expression of E6 and E7. *Mol. Oncol.* **2007**, *1*, 350–355. [CrossRef] [PubMed]
60. Barnes, L.; Eveson, J.; Reichart, P.; Sidransky, D. World Health Organization classification of tumours. Pathology and genetics of head and neck tumours. *Int. Agency Res. Cancer* **2005**, *85*, 75–81.
61. Mirghani, H.; Amen, F.; Moreau, F.; Guigay, J.; Hartl, D.M.; Lacau St Guily, J. Oropharyngeal cancers: Relationship between epidermal growth factor receptor alterations and human papillomavirus status. *Eur. J. Cancer* **2014**, *50*, 1100–1111. [CrossRef] [PubMed]
62. Saltz, L.B.; Meropol, N.J.; Loehrer, P.J., Sr.; Needle, M.N.; Kopit, J.; Mayer, R.J. Phase II trial of cetuximab in patients with refractory colorectal cancer that expresses the epidermal growth factor receptor. *J. Clin. Oncol.* **2004**, *22*, 1201–1208. [CrossRef] [PubMed]
63. Cunningham, D.; Humblet, Y.; Siena, S.; Khayat, D.; Bleiberg, H.; Santoro, A.; Bets, D.; Mueser, M.; Harstrick, A.; Verslype, C.; et al. Cetuximab monotherapy and cetuximab plus irinotecan in irinotecan-refractory metastatic colorectal cancer. *N. Engl. J. Med.* **2004**, *351*, 337–345. [CrossRef] [PubMed]
64. Bonner, J.A.; Harari, P.M.; Giralt, J.; Azarnia, N.; Shin, D.M.; Cohen, R.B.; Jones, C.U.; Sur, R.; Raben, D.; Jassem, J.; et al. Radiotherapy plus cetuximab for squamous-cell carcinoma of the head and neck. *N. Engl. J. Med.* **2006**, *354*, 567–578. [CrossRef] [PubMed]
65. Hellner, K.; Munger, K. Human papillomaviruses as therapeutic targets in human cancer. *J. Clin. Oncol.* **2011**, *29*, 1785–1794. [CrossRef] [PubMed]
66. Kreimer, A.R. Prospects for prevention of HPV-driven oropharynx cancer. *Oral Oncol.* **2014**, *50*, 555–559. [CrossRef] [PubMed]
67. Kreimer, A.R.; Gonzalez, P.; Katki, H.A.; Porras, C.; Schiffman, M.; Rodriguez, A.C.; Solomon, D.; Jiménez, S.; Schiller, J.T.; Lowy, D.R.; et al. Efficacy of a bivalent HPV 16/18 vaccine against anal HPV 16/18 infection among young women: A nested analysis within the Costa Rica Vaccine Trial. *Lancet Oncol.* **2011**, *12*, 862–870. [CrossRef]
68. Schiller, J.T.; Castellsague, X.; Garland, S.M. A review of clinical trials of human papillomavirus prophylactic vaccines. *Vaccine* **2012**, *30* (Suppl. 5), F123–F138. [CrossRef] [PubMed]
69. Munoz, N.; Kjaer, S.K.; Sigurdsson, K.; Iversen, O.E.; Hernandez-Avila, M.; Wheeler, C.M.; Perez, G.; Brown, D.R.; Koutsky, L.A.; Tay, E.H.; et al. Impact of human papillomavirus (HPV)-6/11/16/18 vaccine on all HPV-associated genital diseases in young women. *J. Natl. Cancer Inst.* **2010**, *102*, 325–339. [CrossRef] [PubMed]
70. Lehtinen, M.; Paavonen, J.; Wheeler, C.M.; Jaisamrarn, U.; Garland, S.M.; Castellsague, X.; Skinner, S.R.; Apter, D.; Naud, P.; Salmerón, J.; et al. Overall efficacy of HPV-16/18 AS04-adjuvanted vaccine against grade 3 or greater cervical intraepithelial neoplasia: 4-year end-of-study analysis of the randomised, double-blind PATRICIA trial. *Lancet Oncol.* **2012**, *13*, 89–99. [CrossRef]

71. Suzuki, S.; Hosono, A. No Association between HPV Vaccine and Reported Post-Vaccination Symptoms in Japanese Young Women: Results of the Nagoya Study. *Papillomavirus Res.* **2018**, *5*, 96–103. [CrossRef] [PubMed]
72. Weinstein, G.S.; O'Malley, B.W., Jr.; Magnuson, J.S.; Carroll, W.R.; Olsen, K.D.; Daio, L.; Moore, E.J.; Holsinger, F.C. Transoral robotic surgery: A multicenter study to assess feasibility, safety, and surgical margins. *Laryngoscope* **2012**, *122*, 1701–1707. [CrossRef] [PubMed]
73. de Almeida, J.R.; Genden, E.M. Robotic surgery for oropharynx cancer: Promise, challenges, and future directions. *Curr. Oncol. Rep.* **2012**, *14*, 148–157. [CrossRef] [PubMed]
74. Dowthwaite, S.A.; Franklin, J.H.; Palma, D.A.; Fung, K.; Yoo, J.; Nichols, A.C. The role of transoral robotic surgery in the management of oropharyngeal cancer: A review of the literature. *ISRN Oncol.* **2012**, *2012*, 945162. [CrossRef] [PubMed]
75. Buglione, M.; Maddalo, M.; Corvo, R.; Pirtoli, L.; Paiar, F.; Lastrucci, L.; Stefanacci, M.; Belgioia, L.; Crociani, M.; Vecchio, S.; et al. Subgroup Analysis According to Human Papillomavirus Status and Tumor Site of a Randomized Phase II Trial Comparing Cetuximab and Cisplatin Combined With Radiation Therapy for Locally Advanced Head and Neck Cancer. *Int. J. Radiat. Oncol. Biol. Phys.* **2017**, *97*, 462–472. [CrossRef] [PubMed]
76. Roesler, R.; Schwartsmann, G. Failure of anti-EGFR therapy in *P16*-positive head and neck cancer. *Lancet Oncol.* **2013**, *14*, e436–e437. [CrossRef]
77. Keck, M.K.; Zuo, Z.; Khattri, A.; Stricker, T.P.; Brown, C.D.; Imanguli, M.; Rieke, D.; Endhardt, K.; Bragelmann, J.; DeBoer, R.; et al. Integrative analysis of head and neck cancer identifies two biologically distinct HPV and three non-HPV subtypes. *Clin. Cancer Res.* **2015**, *21*, 870–881. [CrossRef] [PubMed]
78. Hu, Z.; Muller, S.; Qian, G.; Xu, J.; Kim, S.; Chen, Z.; Jiang, N.; Wang, D.; Zhang, H.; Saba, N.F.; et al. Human papillomavirus 16 oncoprotein regulates the translocation of beta-catenin via the activation of epidermal growth factor receptor. *Cancer* **2015**, *121*, 214–225. [CrossRef] [PubMed]
79. Chen, A.M.; Felix, C.; Wang, P.C.; Hsu, S.; Basehart, V.; Garst, J.; Beron, P.; Wong, D.; Rosove, R.H.; Rao, S.; et al. Reduced-dose radiotherapy for human papillomavirus-associated squamous-cell carcinoma of the oropharynx: A single-arm, phase 2 study. *Lancet Oncol.* **2017**, *18*, 803–811. [CrossRef]
80. Mirghani, H.; Amen, F.; Tao, Y.; Deutsch, E.; Levy, A. Increased radiosensitivity of HPV-positive head and neck cancers: Molecular basis and therapeutic perspectives. *Cancer Treat. Rev.* **2015**, *41*, 844–852. [CrossRef] [PubMed]

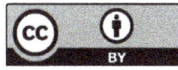

© 2018 by the authors. Licensee MDPI, Basel, Switzerland. This article is an open access article distributed under the terms and conditions of the Creative Commons Attribution (CC BY) license (http://creativecommons.org/licenses/by/4.0/).

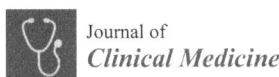 

*Review*

# The Role of Procalcitonin in the Diagnosis of Meningitis: A Literature Review

Dimitrios Velissaris [1], Martina Pintea [2], Nikolaos Pantzaris [3], Eirini Spatha [3], Vassilios Karamouzos [4], Charalampos Pierrakos [5] and Menelaos Karanikolas [6,*]

1. Department of Medicine, University of Patras, 26504 Patras, Greece; dimitrisvelissaris@yahoo.com
2. University of Medicine and Pharmacy, 400337 Cluj-Napoca, România; martina.pintea@yahoo.com
3. School of Medicine University of Patras, 26500 Patras, Greece; npantzaris@gmail.com (N.P.); eirini.spatha@outlook.com (E.S.)
4. Intensive Care Unit, University Hospital of Patras, Rion 26500, Greece; karamouzos@hotmail.com
5. Intensive Care Department, Brugmann University Hospital, 1020 Brussels, Belgium; charalampos.pierrakos@chu-brugmann.be
6. Department of Anesthesiology, Washington University School of Medicine, St. Louis, MO 63144, USA
* Correspondence: menelaos.karanikolas@wustl.edu; Tel.: +1-314-362-2330

Received: 4 June 2018; Accepted: 8 June 2018; Published: 11 June 2018

**Abstract:** Objective: To review the current published literature on the use of procalcitonin as a diagnostic and prognostic marker in adult patients with meningitis. Methods: We conducted a PubMed search to identify all relevant publications regarding the diagnostic and prognostic value of serum procalcitonin in patients with a known or suspected central nervous system infection. We also reviewed the bibliographies of all identified manuscripts in an attempt to identify additional relevant references. Results: A significant body of evidence suggests that serum procalcitonin has a promising role and can be a useful biomarker in the assessment of patients with meningitis. Conclusions: Our literature review suggests that data on the role of Cerebrospinal Fluid (CSF) procalcitonin are limited, whereas serum procalcitonin (S–PCT) is probably a useful tool in the evaluation of patients with a known or suspected central nervous system infection and can help distinguish between bacterial and viral meningitis.

**Keywords:** procalcitonin; bacterial meningitis; viral meningitis; antibiotic therapy; biomarker; differential diagnosis

---

## 1. Introduction

Meningitis is a serious medical condition and can be a major cause of morbidity and mortality. Early diagnosis and timely initiation of appropriate antibiotic therapy is crucial for reducing mortality from bacterial meningitis.

The term "biomarker", as used in daily clinical practice, refers to molecules and biological products used as markers for the assessment of disease progression or as indicators for the presence of an abnormal clinical state. Biomarkers can be specific cells or genes, gene products, enzymes or hormones, have characteristic defined biological properties, and can be detected and measured in biological fluids (plasma, serum, cerebrospinal fluid, bronchoalveolar lavage) or body tissues. More than 178 biomarkers have been identified in the field of sepsis, but none seem to have sufficient specificity or sensitivity for routine use in daily clinical practice [1] and some require considerable time, effort, and costs to measure. In addition, the reliability and validity of certain proposed biomarkers have not been thoroughly tested [2]. Procalcitonin (PCT) and C-reactive Protein (CRP) are the biomarkers most commonly used, but have a limited ability to distinguish sepsis from other inflammatory and non-inflammatory states or to predict outcomes.

Serum procalcitonin (S–PCT) has been used as biomarker in sepsis because S–PCT levels are elevated in bacterial, parasitic, or fungal infections, while they remain normal or only slightly elevated in viral infections. Because early recognition of viral versus bacterial meningitis is critical for the prompt initiation of treatment to improve prognosis, a reliable method distinguishing bacterial from viral meningitis could help clinicians limit inappropriate antibiotic treatment. This review was conducted to evaluate the current knowledge on the use of S–PCT as a tool for the diagnosis of meningitis and for distinguishing bacterial meningitis (BM) from viral meningitis (VM).

## 2. Methods

To identify relevant publications of interest, we conducted a PubMed search on 24 May 2018 using the terms 'procalcitonin and meningitis' as "Title/Abstract" or as "MeSH Terms". Because "Procalcitonin" is not a "Mesh Term" in PubMed, we also used the term "Calcitonin" in "Mesh Terms" during the search. The structure of the search in the "Search details" window of the PubMed website was (procalcitonin [Title/Abstract] OR "calcitonin" [MeSH Terms]) AND (meningitis [Title/Abstract] OR "meningitis" [MeSH Terms]). For the purposes of this review, we then limited the search to "Humans" and only considered manuscripts presenting data on adults. We also reviewed the bibliographies of all identified manuscripts to identify additional relevant publications. For the purposes of this review, we included all types of publications, including case reports, case series, and review articles, regardless of publication date. Publications in languages other than English were included only if they had a meaningful detailed abstract in English.

## 3. Results

The PubMed literature search generated 157 references, but the number of references was reduced to 125 after limiting the search to "Humans". After further evaluation, 38 publications were included in this review.

In a prospective study published in 1999, Viallon et al. evaluated 105 emergency department patients admitted with suspected meningitis. Based on clinical findings, gram staining, cultures, and Cerebrospinal Fluid (CSF) chemical analysis, 23 patients had bacterial meningitis, 57 had viral meningitis, and meningitis was ruled out in 25 patients. Although two patients with previous antibiotic therapy had S–PCT levels of <0.5, S–PCT was the best marker for differentiating between bacterial and viral meningitis: Using S–PCT of >0.2 ng/mL as the threshold, S–PCT sensitivity and specificity approaches 100% for the diagnosis of acute bacterial meningitis [3].

A prospective study published by Schwarz in 2000 included 30 patients with meningitis (16 with acute bacterial and 14 with abacterial meningitis) and assessed whether S–PCT levels were elevated in patients with bacterial meningitis. Results of the study showed that, although false negative results can occur, S–PCT is a useful variable for distinguishing bacterial from non-bacterial meningitis: Because S–PCT levels do not increase in cases of viral meningitis, even with viral sepsis, increased S–PCT levels indicated bacterial origins of an infection with high specificity [4].

In 2000, Viallon et al. published the results of a prospective study on 179 patients admitted to the emergency department on suspicion of meningitis. Of those, 32 patients had bacterial meningitis and 90 had viral meningitis, whereas 57 patients did not have meningitis. The authors assessed the role of CSF parameters (cytology, protein, glucose, lactate) and serum parameters (CRP, S–PCT) for differentiating between bacterial and viral meningitis, and demonstrated that S–PCT was the most discriminant variable, using a threshold value of 0.93 ng/mL in their population [5].

Shimetani et al. reported extremely high CSF CRP levels in patients with bacterial meningitis, but only in 10% of patients with viral meningitis. Among patients with bacterial meningitis, S–PCT levels were more elevated in those with a more serious infection. PCT levels in CSF did not differ significantly between patients with bacterial, viral, or mycotic meningitis. However, S–PCT levels were very high in all bacterial meningitis patients, especially in the most serious cases [6].

A report by Hoffmann et al., published in 2001, assessed S–PCT levels in 12 adult patients with meningitis and suggested that S–PCT has limited diagnostic value in adults with bacterial meningitis, especially in cases with unusual agents or nosocomial origin. Increased S–PCT levels in bacterial meningitis may indicate the presence of bacterial inflammation outside the Central Nervous System (CNS) [7].

A review by O'Connor published in 2001 included manuscripts published from 1990–2001 to assess the diagnostic usefulness of S–PCT in critical illness. This publication concluded that, although there is debate regarding the superiority of S–PCT as a sepsis biomarker compared to other biomarkers, a number of studies support the usefulness of S–PCT in differentiating between bacterial and viral meningitis [8].

A prospective study on 45 adult patients with CNS infection (20 with bacterial meningitis and 25 with tick-borne encephalitis), published in 2001, evaluated the role of S–PCT and CSF procalcitonin in differentiating acute bacterial vs. viral meningitis. Median S–PCT level was 6.45 ng/mL (0.25–43.76 ng/mL) in patients with bacterial meningitis vs. 0.27 ng/mL (0.05–0.44 ng/mL) in patients with viral meningitis, and the authors concluded that S–PCT and CSF PCT concentrations >0.5 ng/mL seem to be reliable indicator of bacterial CNS infection [9].

A study by Martinez et al. in 2002 attempted to evaluate the role of S–PCT monitoring in the differential diagnosis of ventriculitis in adult Intensive Care Unit (ICU) patients. The study included 15 consecutive ICU patients with ventriculitis and a ventricular catheter in place, and compared these data with 10 patients with community-acquired bacterial meningitis. The authors concluded that, in contrast to bacterial meningitis, monitoring of S–PCT alone is not helpful for the diagnosis of ventriculitis [10].

A case report published in 2004 presented the case of a 73-year-old woman with progressively worsening headaches, nausea, vomiting, and neck stiffness. As her clinical condition deteriorated, she developed diffuse brain edema and hydrocephalus, requiring external ventricular drainage (EVD) and admission to a neurologic ICU, with a subsequent diagnosis of severe post-myelographic chemical meningitis. The authors compared CSF and serum inflammatory markers of this patient versus seven patients with proven bacterial meningitis and concluded that S–PCT may be useful in differentiating between bacterial and chemical causes of CNS inflammation [11].

A study by Kepa et al. assessed the role of CSF PCT and S–PCT levels in the differential diagnosis of adults with CNS infections. The study included 17 patients with bacterial meningoencephalitis and 16 patients with lymphocytic meningitis and showed that CSF and plasma PCT levels were significantly different between these two patient groups. These results supported the usefulness of measuring plasma PCT levels in the differential diagnosis of CNS infections in adults. With regards to the role of CSF PCT, the authors concluded that CSF PCT levels are less important for differential diagnosis, but correlate with the severity of bacterial meningoencephalitis and can be taken into consideration when predicting prognosis and outcomes [12].

In 2005, a study by Viallon et al. described the change in S–PCT levels during the treatment of 48 patients with community-acquired acute bacterial meningitis. Bacterial infection was documented in 45 patients and initial antibiotic treatment was effective in all patients. Serum PCT levels were measured on admission and on day two, and showed that S–PCT levels decline rapidly with appropriate antibiotic therapy. The authors concluded that the rapid decline of S–PCT levels reduces the value of performing lumbar puncture 48 to 72 h after admission to assess the effectiveness of antibiotic therapy [13].

Ernst and colleagues evaluated serum and CSF procalcitonin levels in patients with dementia disorders and neuro-inflammation. The study included 40 patients with probable Alzheimer's disease, 12 patients with frontotemporal dementia (FTD), 8 patients with dementia with Lewy bodies (DLB), 12 patients with vascular dementia (VD), 16 patients with acute neuroinflammation, and 50 non-dementia control patients (18 surgery patients and 32 patients with other neurologic diseases)and showed that, compared to non-dementia controls, CSF procalcitonin levels were increased in patients with dementia diseases and acute neuro-inflammation. In addition, in matched serum samples, S–PCT levels were elevated in meningitis patients, but not in dementia patients [14].

An observational cohort study by Knudsen et al. included 55 patients with suspected meningitis and compared the diagnostic value of serum sCD163 levels, CRP, and procalcitonin in bacterial infection and meningitis and showed that, although elevated serum sCD163 levels seem to be the most specific biomarker for differentiating between bacterial and non-bacterial disease (specificity 0.91; sensitivity 0.47), the overall diagnostic accuracy of CRP (Area Under the Curve (AUC) = 0.91) and PCT (AUC = 0.87) were superior compared to sCD163. The authors concluded that, although PCT and CRP had very high accuracy for distinguishing between bacterial and viral infection, none of them were useful as an independent tool for diagnosis in patients presenting with purulent meningitis [15].

A prospective multicenter study, published in 2007, included 151 patients with bacterial or nonbacterial meningitis and negative initial Gram stains from three teaching hospitals in France and reported laboratory data, including results of CSF analysis (CSF leukocyte count, percentage of CSF leukocyte, CSF/blood glucose ratio, CSF protein), serum CRP, and serum PCT, together with clinical findings and outcomes. The study evaluated the accuracy of laboratory results in differentiating between bacterial and non-bacterial meningitis in patients with meningitis and a negative gram stain, and concluded that CSF laboratory results have some role in distinguishing bacterial from non-bacterial meningitis, whereas serum CRP (AUC 0.81 (95% CI 0.58–0.92) and S–PCT levels (AUC 0.98, 95% CI, 0.83–1.00) are excellent predictors of bacterial meningitis, with S CPT being clearly superior ($p < 0.05$) [16].

A prospective study from the Saint-Etienne University Hospital in France collected data from all patients admitted to the emergency unit with suspected meningitis between 1997 and 2009. Data were collected on 97 patients with bacterial meningitis and 218 patients with viral meningitis, but, after 62 patients with Bacterial Meningitis (BM) were excluded for various reasons, the study only included data from 35 patients with BM and negative direct CSF examination. The aim of the study was to determine the ability of several parameters used for the diagnosis of acute meningitis in differentiating between bacterial and viral meningitis in adult patients with a negative CSF examination. In this study, S–PCT had a 95% sensitivity, 100% specificity, and 100% negative predictive value, as well as a 97% positive predictive value for distinguishing BM versus Viral Meningitis (VM) when using a diagnostic cut-off level of 0.28 ng/mL (AUC, 0.99; 95% CI, 0.99 to 1) [17].

A prospective study on 36 adult patients with acute meningitis was published in 2012. The aim of the study was to evaluate the role of serum procalcitonin levels over time during treatment for central nervous system infections. Serum procalcitonin levels were measured before the initiation of treatment and 24 and 72 h after treatment started. Results showed that mean PCT levels were higher in patients who did not improve and that the reduction of serum PCT levels were more significant after 72 h in patients who improved. The authors emphasized the role of serum PCT levels as a marker for follow up in treating patients with bacterial meningitis [18].

A study by Choi assessed the value of serum procalcitonin in differentiating post-operative bacterial meningitis (PBM) versus postoperative aseptic meningitis (PAM) after neurological surgery and included patients who had cerebrospinal fluid pleocytosis within 14 days of surgery. The study compared PCT in 14 patients with PBM against 64 patients with PAM and showed that serum PCT had limited value for diagnosing PBM and serum PCT levels of $\geq 0.15$ ng/mL had 80% specificity. However, CPT combined with other biomarkers can be a useful adjunct for increasing diagnostic sensitivity [19].

An observational study by Tian et al., from Guadong, China and published in 2014, investigated the value of procalcitonin in the discrimination between sepsis and systemic inflammatory response syndrome (SIRS). The study included patients treated in a neurological intensive care unit and serum levels of C-reactive protein and S–PCT were evaluated on admission day, on the day of diagnosis of SIRS or sepsis, and on days three and seven after the diagnosis. Results of the study showed significant differences in S–PCT levels between groups at all stages of sepsis. The authors concluded that S–PCT has significant value as an index for discriminating sepsis from SIRS and in determining sepsis severity [20].

A study by Abdelkader et al. published in 2014 evaluated 40 patients with suspected acute meningitis and negative gram stains compared to 10 healthy controls. The goal of the study was to evaluate the role of S–PCT in differentiating bacterial from aseptic meningitis in patients with negative cerebrospinal fluid (CSF) examination on admission and after three days of treatment, and to assess the role of PCT and other inflammatory markers in relation to treatment efficacy. In this study, patients in the bacterial group had significantly higher serum PCT on admission compared to the aseptic group ($2.49 \pm 2.54$ vs. $0.89 \pm 0.69$, $p < 0.001$), and there was a significant difference in bacterial versus. aseptic meningitis, even after three days of treatment ($1.70 \pm 1.58$ vs. $0.64 \pm 0.51$, $p < 0.001$) [21].

A prospective observational study, published by Shen et al. in 2015, assessed the diagnostic value of serum and CSF PCT levels in 120 patients with meningitis-like symptoms and showed that both S–PCT and CSF PCT levels were increased in patients with bacterial meningitis (BM). The area under the Receiver Operator Characteristic (ROC) curve was 0.96 (CI 0.93–1.00) for S–PCT versus 0.9 (CI 0.83–0.96) for CSF PCT in the diagnosis of BM. When using 0.88 ng/mL as a threshold, S–PCT had an 87% sensitivity and 100% specificity for the diagnosis of BM. The study concluded that both S–PCT and CSF PCT have value for the diagnosis of BM, but the diagnostic value of S–PCT is superior [22].

In another prospective observational study, Omar et al. collected data on CRP, S–PCT, and CSF cultures every other day in 36 adult patients with severe head trauma and ventriculostomy, and observed elevated S–PCT concentration in all five patients who developed ventriculostomy-related infections. Mean serum PCT was <2.0 ng/mL in patients with negative CSF cultures versus 4.18 ng/mL in patients with positive cultures. The study concluded that an early increase of S–PCT levels is a valid indicator of bacterial CNS infection in patients with head trauma and External Ventricular Drainage (EVD) [23].

A retrospective clinical study by Li et al. assessed the diagnostic value of CSF procalcitonin combined with CSF lactate levels in distinguishing post-neurosurgical bacterial meningitis (PNBM) from aseptic meningitis in 178 hospitalized patients with suspected PNMB (50 patients with PNBM vs. 128 patients without PNBM). Median (min, max) CSF procalcitonin levels were 0.2 (0–3.1) in patients with PNBM versus 0 (0–0.5) in patients with non-PNBM ($p < 0.001$), and ROC analysis revealed a cut-off value of 0.075 ng/mL (AUC = 0.746, sensitivity 68.0%; specificity 72.7%, $p < 0.001$) for CSF procalcitonin. Similarly, median (min, max) CSF lactate levels were 5.3 (2.2–10.6) in patients with PNBM versus 2.3 (1.2–5.4) in patients with non-PNBM ($p < 0.001$), and ROC analysis revealed a cut-off value of 3.45 mmol/L (AUC = 0.943, sensitivity 90.0%; specificity 84.4%, $p < 0.001$) for CSF lactate. The study showed that PNBM patients have significantly higher CSF procalcitonin and CSF lactate levels compared with non-PNBM patients and concluded that CSF lactate and PCT levels have significant diagnostic value for PNBM, and could be useful in differentiating PNBM from non-PNBM [24].

A publication by Konstantinidis et al. in 2015 evaluated CSF procalcitonin levels and compared CSF procalcitonin levels with CSF levels of other established markers of infection, such as CRP, high-sensitivity CRP, and White Blood Cells (WBC) in 30 ICU, Medicine, Neurology, Hematology, and Pediatric patients with bacterial ($n = 19$) or viral ($n = 11$) meningitis, and in 28 patients with non-infectious diseases. In this study, CSF PCT levels were $4.714 \pm 1.59$ ng/mL in bacterial meningitis versus $0.1327 \pm 0.03$ ng/mL in patients with viral meningitis versus <0.1 ng/mL in patients with non-infectious diseases, with the authors concluding that S–PCT can be helpful in distinguishing bacterial meningitis from viral meningitis and other noninfectious CNS diseases [25].

A meta-analysis published in 2015 by Vikse et al. included nine studies with a total of 725 patients and concluded that serum procalcitonin had a pooled sensitivity of 0.90 (95% CI 0.84–0.94), a specificity of 0.98 (0.97–0.99), a positive likelihood ratio of 27.3 (8.2–91.1), a negative likelihood ratio of 0.13 (0.07–0.26), a diagnostic odds ratio of 287.0 (58.5–1409.0), and, thus, is far superior to CRP for rapid differentiation between bacterial and viral meningitis [26].

Kim et al. compared S–PCT levels in 26 patients with tuberculosis meningitis versus 70 patients with BM and 49 patients with VM in a retrospective study and showed that low S–PCT levels ($\leq 1.27$ ng/mL) independently distinguished tuberculosis meningitis from bacterial meningitis, with a 96.2% sensitivity and a 62.9% specificity. However, S–PCT levels were not significantly different in patients with tuberculosis versus viral meningitis. Logistic regression showed that an S–PCT level of >0.4 ng/mL was an independent predictor of a poor prognosis in patients with tuberculosis meningitis and had a negative correlation with Glasgow Coma Scale (GCS) scores at discharge ($r = 0.437, p = 0.026$) [27].

A prospective observational study published by Morales-Casado et al. in 2016 assessed the role of 32 clinical and epidemiological variables as predictors of bacterial meningitis in 154 patients aged over 15 years who presented in the Emergency Department with symptoms of acute meningitis. Multivariate logistic regression showed that four variables (S–PCT, CSF lactate $\geq 33$ mg/dL, CSF glucose <60% of blood value, and CSF polymorphonuclears $\geq 50$%) were excellent tools for the prediction of bacterial meningitis; the model using S–PCT $\geq 0.8$ ng/mL and CSF lactate $\geq 33$ mg/dL had an AUC of 0.992, with a 99% sensitivity and a 98% specificity for predicting bacterial meningitis (95% CI: 0.979–1; $p < 001$) [28].

Another prospective observational study by Morales-Casado et al. evaluated the usefulness of inflammatory markers for the diagnosis of bacterial meningitis in 220 patients and showed that S–PCT had the highest AUC (0.972; 95% CI, 0.946–0.998; $p < 001$) for the diagnosis of BM. Using 0.52 ng/mL as a cutoff, S–PCT had 93% sensitivity and 86% specificity for the diagnosis of BM overall, but sensitivity was 96% and specificity was 75% in patients >75 years old [29].

In 2016, Wei and colleagues published a systematic review and meta-analysis on the role of procalcitonin in the diagnosis of bacterial versus non-bacterial meningitis. The review included twenty-two studies with a total of 2058 patients; diagnostic accuracy of S–PCT and CSF PCT was assessed using the bivariate model and analysis showed that PCT is a useful biomarker for the diagnosis of bacterial meningitis: CSF PCT had 0.86 specificity and 0.8 sensitivity, whereas S–PCT had 0.97 specificity and 0.95 sensitivity [30].

A prospective, observational study published in 2016 by Morales Casado et al. evaluated serum PCT and C-reactive protein as markers for detection of bacterial meningitis in 98 patients diagnosed with acute meningitis in the emergency department (38 pts with BM, 33 with VM, 15 with probable VM, and 12 with presumptively diagnosed, partially treated acute meningitis). Data analysis showed that S–PCT levels were significantly higher in patients with BM (11.47 $\pm$ 7.76 ng/mL vs. 0.10 $\pm$ 0.15 ng/mL in viral meningitis, $p < 0.001$). Using 1.1 ng/mL as cutoff, S–PCT as diagnostic tool achieved 94.6% sensitivity, 72.4% specificity, 95.4% NPV, and 69.2% PPV, and AUC was 0.965 (95% CI, 0.921–1; $p < 0.001$). Based on these results, the authors concluded that S–PCT performs better than CRP in the detection of bacterial meningitis [31].

In a prospective observational study published in 2017, Zhang et al. measured S–PCT and CSF PCT, high-sensitivity C-reactive proteins (Hs-CRP), proteins, chloride, and glucose in three patient groups: 24 patients with suppurative meningitis, 20 with VM, and 22 with tuberculous meningitis (TBM). S–PCT values were significantly higher in the suppurative meningitis group, but declined significantly in suppurative meningitis patients after 72 h and seven days of treatment. In addition, admission CSF PCT levels were significantly lower in VM compared to TBM and suppurative meningitis patients, but CSF PCT values did not change significantly with treatment. The authors concluded that S–PCT changes over time can be useful in evaluating disease progression and response to treatment in patients with suppurative meningitis [32].

A retrospective clinical study on 80 patients with BM and 58 with VM, published by Park in 2017, showed that S–PCT >0.12 ng/mL is a significant marker for differentiating BM from VM, and also that

S–PCT levels >7.26 ng/mL are associated with higher risk of death (OR = 9.09, 95% CI: 1.74–47.12, $p$ = 0.016) [33].

Last, a prospective observational study published by Li et al. in 2017 included 143 ICU patients (49 with BM, 25 with TBM, 34 with viral meningitis/encephalitis (VM/E), 15 with autoimmune encephalitis (AIE), and 20 with non-inflammatory nervous system diseases (NINSD) to assess the value of CSF PCT, S–PCT and other biomarkers in the diagnosis of BM. In this study, CSF PCT levels (median, range) were significantly ($P$ < 0.01) higher in BM patients (0.22, 0.13–0.54 ng/mL) compared to TBM (0.12, 0.07–0.16 ng/mL), VM/E (0.09, 0.07–0.11 ng/mL), AIE (0.06, 0.05–0.10 ng/mL), or NINSD (0.07, 0.06–0.08 ng/mL) patients. Furthermore, CSF PCT had the highest area under the receiver operating characteristic curve (AUROC) (0.881; 95% CI 0.810–0.932; cutoff 0.15 ng/mL; sensitivity 69.39%; specificity 91.49%), whereas S–PCT was less useful (AUROC 0.759, 95% CI 0.669–0.849, cutoff 0.19 ng/mL, with sensitivity 67.35% and specificity 75.53% for the diagnosis of BM [34]. Findings of clinical studies evaluating the role of PCT in patients with known or suspected meningitis are summarized in Table 1. Quantitative measures, including AUC, sensitivity, specificity, and cut-off points, reported in clinical studies included in this review are summarized in Table 2.

**Table 1.** Clinical studies evaluating the role of procalcitonin (PCT) in patients with known or suspected meningitis.

| Reference | Origin | Study Design | Patient Population | Findings |
|---|---|---|---|---|
| [3] | St. Etienne, France | Prospective study | 105 pts (23 with BM, 57 with VM, 25 controls), 54 women, 51 men, mean age 42 years (range 16–82 years) | S–PCT was the best marker for differentiating BM vs. VM. with S–PCT > 0.2 ng/mL as the cutoff, S–PCT sensitivity and specificity approaches 100% for diagnosing acute BM |
| [4] | Heidelberg, Germany | Prospective case series | 30 pts (13 men, 17 women), mean age 52 (range, 16–87 years) | S–PCT is useful for distinguishing BM from VM. Increased S–PCT levels have a high specificity for bacterial infection |
| [5] | St. Etienne, France | Prospective study | 179 patients with suspected meningitis: 32 patients with BM, 90 patients with VM, 57 patients did not have meningitis | S–PCT is the most discriminant variable for differentiating BM vs. VM, with a threshold value 0.93 ng/mL |
| [6] | Saitama, Japan | Prospective study | 42 patients requiring CSF examination, 12 patients with non-inflammatory CNS disease as controls, 22 men, mean age 37.8 years; 20 women, mean age 38.1 years | CSF PCT levels not significantly different in BM, VM, or mycotic meningitis. S–PCT > 0.1 mcg/L in all BM patients. AUC and cut-off values were not reported |
| [7] | Berlin, Germany | Case series, 12 adults with meningitis | 12 pts: 7 men, 5 women, mean age 48.6 years | S–PCT has a limited diagnostic value for BM in adults |
| [9] | Ljubljana, Slovenia | Prospective study, 45 adults with CNS infection | 20 BM patients: 11 men, 9 women, mean age 55 years; 25 TBE patients: 13 men, 12 women, mean age 49 years | Median S–PCT 6.45 ng/mL (0.25–43.76) in patients with BM vs. 0.27 ng/mL (0.05–0.44) in patients with TBE. S–PCT and CSF PCT > 0.5 ng/mL is a reliable indicator of BM |
| [10] | Dresden, Germany | Prospective ICU study | 11 ventriculitis patients with negative CSF (6 men, 5 women, mean age 44.3 years), 4 ventriculitis patients with positive CSF (2 men, 2 women, mean age 56.2 years), 10 community BM (7 men, 3 women, mean age 49.4 years) | S–PCT alone is not helpful for diagnosis of ventriculitis |
| [11] | Munich, Germany | Case report: 73 year old woman, post-myelogram chemical meningitis | 7 ICU BM patients (4 men, 3 women, mean age 55 years), and one woman with aseptic, chemical meningitis | S–PCT is useful in differentiating bacterial vs. chemical CNS inflammation |
| [12] | Poland | Observational study, 33 adult patients | 17 bacterial meningoencephalitis patients vs. 16 lymphocytic meningitis patients | CSF PCT and S–PCT significantly higher in BM vs. lymphocytic meningitis (CSF PCT 0.63 ng/mL vs. 0.23 ng/mL, $p$ < 0.05, S–PCT 9.97 ng/mL vs. 0.27 ng/mL, $p$ < 0.01 |
| [13] | St. Etienne, France | Prospective study, 48 BM patients with S–PCT > 0.5 ng/mL on admission | 48 BM patients: 21 men, 27 women, mean age 55 years | S–PCT levels declined rapidly with antibiotic therapy |
| [14] | Borgsdorf, Germany | Prospective Study | 40 patients with AD, 12 with FTD, 8 with DLB, 12 with VD, 16 with acute neuroinflammation, 50 controls | Measured S–PCT, CSF PCT. S–PCT elevated in meningitis, CSF PCT helpful in diagnosing dementia |

Table 1. Cont.

| Reference | Origin | Study Design | Patient Population | Findings |
|---|---|---|---|---|
| [15] | Hvidovre, Denmark | Observational cohort study | 52 patients (25 men, 27 women) with suspected meningitis, median age 36 (range, 13–92 years) | S–PCT has a moderate overall accuracy for differentiating BM vs. non-bacterial disease |
| [16] | Paris, France | Prospective multicenter study, 151 meningitis patients | 133 NBM patients: 66 men, 67 women, mean age 33 years vs. 18 BM patients: 9 men, 9 women, mean age 52 years | Serum CRP and S–PCT are excellent predictors of BM |
| [17] | St. Etienne, France | Prospective study, patients with negative CSF exam | 35 patients (17 men, 18 women, mean age 55 years) with BM, 218 patients (116 men, 102 women, mean age 35 years) with VM | S–PCT had very high diagnostic value for distinguishing BM vs. VM |
| [18] | Ahvaz, Iran | Prospective study, 36 patients with acute meningitis | 36 acute meningitis patients: 26 men, 10 women, mean age 38.4 years | S–PCT levels were reduced after 72 h in patients who improved, but remained higher in patients who did not improve |
| [19] | Seoul, Korea | Prospective study, 78 postoperative meningitis patients | 14 patients with BM: 4 men, 10 women, median age 52 (range 44–63) vs. 64 aseptic meningitis patients: 35 men, 29 women, median age 47.5 (range 35–61 years) | S–PCT has limited value for diagnosing BM (50% sensitivity, 80% specificity for S–PCT $\geq$ 0.15 ng/mL). |
| [20] | Guangzhou, China | Retrospective study, NICU pts | 22 sepsis patients (16 men, 6 women, mean age 58 years), 22 severe sepsis patients (17 men, 5 women, mean age 55.4 years), 12 septic shock patients (5 men, 6 women, mean age 51.9 years), and 48 SIRS patients (28 men, 20 women, mean age 51.8 years) | Assessed S–PCT for discrimination between sepsis and SIRS. S–PCT levels were significantly different between groups at all stages of sepsis. S–PCT has value for discriminating sepsis from SIRS and for determining sepsis severity |
| [21] | Cairo, Egypt | Prospective study, 40 patients with suspected acute meningitis | 16 ABM patients (9 men, 7 women, mean age 39 years) and 24 patients with acute ASM (21 men, 3 women, mean age 29 years), 10 controls (7 men, 3 women, mean age 40 years) | S–PCT significantly higher in BM compared to ASM patients (2.49 $\pm$ 2.54 vs. 0.89 $\pm$ 0.69, $p < 0.001$). Difference in BM vs. ASM persisted after 3 days of therapy |
| [22] | Nanjing, China | Prospective observational study, 120 patients | 45 BM patients (30 men, 15 women, mean age 50) vs. 75 non-BM patients (55 men, 20 women, mean age 47 years) | S–PCT and CSF PCT levels increase in patients with BM |
| [23] | Abu Dhabi, UAE | Prospective, observational study | 36 head trauma patients with EVD (30 men, 6 women, mean age 32.8 years) | High S–PCT in patients with ventriculostomy-related infections. Early S–PCT increase is a valid indicator of bacterial CNS infection |
| [24] | Beijing, China | Retrospective study, 178 post-neurosurgical patients | 50 with PNBM (23 men, 27 women, median age 42 years) vs. 128 without PNBM 49 men, 79 women, median age 42 years) | CSF lactate and PCT have significant diagnostic value for PNBM and could be useful in differentiating PNBM from non-PNBM |
| [25] | Alexandroupolis, Greece | Prospective, observational study, 58 patients | 19 BM patients (12 men, 7 women, mean age 41 years) vs. 11 VM patients (8 men, 3 women, mean age 24 years) vs. 28 controls (20 men, 8 women, mean age 30 years) | CSF–PCT is helpful in distinguishing BM from VM and other noninfectious CNS diseases |
| [27] | Busan, Korea | Retrospective study of patients with TBM who had S–PCT measured | 26 TBM patients (13 men, 13 women, mean age 57 years) vs. 70 BM patients (42 men, 28 women, mean age 64 years) vs. 49 VM patients (24 men, 25 women, mean age 40 years) | S–PCT levels not significantly different in TBM vs. VM, but S–PCT > 0.4 ng/mL was a predictor of poor prognosis in TBM |
| [29] | Toledo, Spain | Prospective, observational study | 220 meningitis patients (136 men, 84 women, mean age 30 years) | PCT has high diagnostic powers and outperforms CRP and leukocytes for the detection of bacterial meningitis |
| [28] | Toledo, Spain | Prospective observational study | 154 ED patients over age 15 | Logistic regression shows that S–PCT $\geq$ 0.8 ng/mL + CSF lactate $\geq$ 33 mg/dL are strong predictors of BM ($p < 0.001$) |
| [31] | Toledo, Spain | Prospective, observational study | 98 ED patients (66 men, 32 women, mean age 44 years), 38 BM patients (mean age 61.5 years), 33 VM patients (mean age 36 years) 15 with probable VM, but negative cultures, 12 with antibiotic treatment and negative cultures | S–PCT higher in BM vs. VM (11.47 $\pm$ 7.76 vs. 0.10 $\pm$ 0.15 ng/mL, $p < 0.001$). S–PCT is superior to S-CRP for BM detection |
| [32] | Jilin, China | Prospective observational study | 66 meningitis patients: 37 men, 29 women, mean age 40.21 years (24 suppurative meningitis, 20 VM, 22 TBM), 20 controls: 11 men, 9 women, mean age 43.05 years | S–PCT is significantly higher in suppurative meningitis, declined significantly after 72 h and 7 days of treatment. CSF PCT is significantly lower in VM compared to TBM and suppurative meningitis. |

**Table 1.** Cont.

| Reference | Origin | Study Design | Patient Population | Findings |
|---|---|---|---|---|
| [33] | Busan, Korea | Retrospective study, suspected meningitis patients | 80 patients with BM (49 patients, 31 women, median age 66 years) vs. 58 VM patients (30 men, 28 women, median age 37 years) | S–PCT levels >0.12 ng/mL are significant marker for differentiating BM vs. VM |
| [34] | Xi'an, China | Prospective observational study, 143 ICU patients with CNS disease | 49 BM patients (36 men, 13 women, median age 43 years) vs. 25 TBM patients (15 men, 10 women, median age 42 years) vs. 34 VM patients (25 men, 9 women, median age 39.5 years) vs. 15 AIE patients (6 men, 9 women, median age 27 years) vs. 20 NINSD (11 men, 9 women, median age 43 years) | CSF PCT levels were significantly higher in BM compared to TBM, VM, AIE, or NINSD |

ABM = Acute Bacterial Meningitis, AD = Alzheimer's disease, AIE = Autoimmune Encephalitis, ASM = Aseptic Meningitis, AUC = Area Under the Curve, AUROC = Area Under The Receiver Operating Characteristic Curve, BM = Bacterial Meningitis, CI = Confidence Interval, CRP = C-reactive protein, CSF = cerebrospinal fluid, DLB = Dementia with Lewy bodies, ED = Emergency Department, EVD = External Ventricular Drainage, FTD = Frontotemporal dementia, LP = Lumbar Puncture, NBM = Nonbacterial Meningitis, NICU = Neurological Intensive Care Unit, NINSD = Non-Inflammatory Nervous System Disease, NPV = Negative Predictive Value, PMN = Polymorphonuclear, PNBM = Post-Neurosurgical Bacterial Meningitis, PPV = Positive Predictive Value, Pts = patients, S–PCT = Serum Procalcitonin, SIRS = Systemic Inflammatory Response Syndrome, Tb = Tuberculosis, TBE = Tick-Borne Encephalitis, TBM = Tuberculous Meningitis, VD = Vascular Dementia, VM/E = Viral Meningitis/Encephalitis, VM = Viral Meningitis.

**Table 2.** Area under the Curve (AUC), sensitivity, specificity, and cut-off points reported in clinical studies evaluating Serum Procalcitonin (S–PCT) or Cerebrospinal Fluid Procalcitonin (CSF PCT) in patients with known or suspected meningitis.

| Reference | Biomarker | AUC (95% CI) $p$ Value | Cut-off Point | Sensitivity | Specificity | Comments |
|---|---|---|---|---|---|---|
| [3] | S–PCT | Not reported | 0.2 ng/mL | 100% | 100% | CSF PCT found only in two patients with hemorrhage. S–PCT sensitivity and specificity approach 100% for diagnosing acute BM |
| [4] | S–PCT | Not reported | 0.5 ng/mL | 69% (41–89%) | 100% (79–100%) | S–PCT is a useful variable for distinguishing BM from VM. Increased S–PCT levels have a high specificity for bacterial infection |
| [5] | S–PCT | Not reported | 0.93 ng/mL | Not reported | 100% | S–PCT is the most discriminant variable for differentiating BM vs. VM |
| [7] | S–PCT | Not reported | 1 ng/mL | 58.3% | Not reported | S–PCT has limited diagnostic value in adults with BM |
| [9] | CSF PCT / S–PCT | Not reported | 0.5 ng/mL / 0.5 ng/mL | 55% / 90% | 100% / 100% | Median S–PCT is significantly higher in BM (6.45 ng/mL range 0.25–43.76) vs. TBE (0.27 ng/mL, 0.05–0.44). S–PCT, CSF PCT > 0.5 ng/mL is a reliable indicator of BM |
| [10] | S–PCT | Not reported | 1.0 ng/mL | 100% | 83% | S–PCT is not helpful for diagnosis of ventriculitis, but is highly diagnostic for BM |
| [11] | S–PCT | Not reported | 1.0 ng/mL | Not reported | Not reported | S–PCT is useful in differentiating bacterial vs. chemical causes of CNS inflammation |
| [12] | CSF-PCT / S–PCT | Not reported | Not reported | Not reported | Not reported | CSF PCT and S–PCT are significantly higher in bacterial meningoencephalitis vs. lymphocytic meningitis |
| [13] | S–PCT | Not reported | Not reported | Not reported | Not reported | Rapid S–PCT decline with antibiotic therapy reduces the value of repeating LP to assess antibiotic therapy effectiveness |
| [14] | CSF-PCT | 0.83 (0.76–0.91), $p < 0.0001$ | 57 pg/mL / 65 pg/mL | 75% / 63.9% | 80% / 90% | S–PCT levels are elevated in meningitis, but not in dementia |
| [15] | S–PCT | 0.93 (0.64–0.99) | 0.25 ng/mL | 0.90 (0.55–1.0) | 0.92 (0.62–1.0) | S–PCT is helpful for differentiating BM vs. VM, with an overall moderate accuracy (AUC 0.75, 0.50–0.89) |
| [16] | S-CRP / S–PCT | 0.81 (0.58–0.92) / 0.98 (0.83–1.00) | 22 mg/L / 2.13 ng/mL | 78% / 87% | 74% / 100% | S-CRP and S–PCT are excellent predictors of BM |
| [17] | S–PCT | 0.99 (0.99–1.00) | 0.28 ng/mL | 97% | 100% | S–PCT: High diagnostic value for distinguishing BM vs. VM |
| [18] | S–PCT | Not reported | Not reported | Not reported | Not reported | S–PCT can be a useful marker for the follow up of BM patients |

**Table 2.** Cont.

| Reference | Biomarker | AUC (95% CI) p Value | Cut-off Point | Sensitivity | Specificity | Comments |
|---|---|---|---|---|---|---|
| [19] | S–PCT | 0.617 | 0.15 ng/mL | 50% | 80% | S–PCT is of limited value for diagnosing BM |
| [20] | S–PCT | 0.799 (0.711–0.887) | 2 ng/mL | 75% | 83.3% | S–PCT has value for discriminating sepsis vs. SIRS and determining sepsis severity |
| [21] | S–PCT | AUC shown, but value not reported | 1.2 ng/mL | 68.8% | 83.3% | Admission S–PCT is higher in BM patients compared to ASM patients (2.49 ± 2.54 vs. 0.89 ± 0.69, $p < 0.001$). The difference in BM vs. ASM persisted after 3 days of therapy (1.70 ± 1.58 vs. 0.64 ± 0.51, $p < 0.001$) |
| [22] | S–PCT | 0.96 (0.93–1.00) | 0.88 ng/mL | 87% | 100% | S–PCT and CSF PCT increased in BM patients. |
| [23] | S–PCT | Not reported | Not reported | Not reported | Not reported | Mean S–PCT < 2.0 ng/mL in patients with negative vs. 4.18 ng/mL in patients with positive CSF cultures |
| [24] | CSF PCT / CSF lactate | 0.746 $p < 0.001$ / 0.943 $p < 0.001$ | 0.075 ng/mL / 3.45 mmoL/L | 68.0% / 90% | 72.7% / 84.4% | CSF lactate and CSF PCT have significant diagnostic value for PNBM |
| [25] | CSF PCT | Not reported | Not reported | 100% | 96.4% | CSF PCT 4.71 ± 1.59 ng/mL in BM, 0.13 ± 0.03 ng/mL in VM, <0.1 in patients with non-infectious disease |
| [27] | S–PCT | 0.876 (0.688–0.972) | 1.27 ng/mL | 96.2% (80.4–99.9) | 62.9% (50.5–74.1) | S–PCT useful for distinguishing TBM from BM. S–PCT > 0.4 ng/mL is predictor of poor outcome in TBM |
| [29] | S–PCT | 0.972 (0.946–0.998) | 0.52 ng/mL | 93% | 86% | Sensitivity 96%, Specificity 75% for ages >75 years |
| [28] | S–PCT + CSF lactate | 0.992 (0.979–1.000, $p < 0.001$) | S–PCT ≥ 0.8 ng/mL + CSF lactate ≥33mg/dL | 99% | 98% | The combination of S–PCT ≥ 0.8 ng/mL + CSF lactate ≥ 33 mg/dL has excellent diagnostic value for predicting BM |
| [31] | S–PCT | 0.965 (0.921–1), $p < 0.001$ | 1.1 ng/mL | 94.6% | 72.4% | S–PCT significantly higher in BM vs. VM (11.47 ± 7.76 vs. 0.10 ± 0.15 ng/mL, $p < 0.001$). Concluded that S–PCT is superior to serum CRP for detecting BM |
| [32] | S–PCT | Not reported | Not reported | Not reported | Not reported | S–PCT is significantly higher in suppurative meningitis and declined 72 h and 7 days after treatment |
| [33] | S–PCT | Not reported | 0.12 ng/mL | 88.75% | 74.14% | S–PCT > 0.12 ng/mL is useful for differentiating BM vs. VM. S–PCT > 7.26 ng/mL associated with higher mortality (OR = 9.09, 95% CI: 1.74–47.12, $p = 0.016$) |
| [34] | CSF PCT | 0.881 (0.810–0.932) | 0.15 ng/mL | 69.39 | 91.49% | CSF PCT levels are the most useful biomarker for the diagnosis of BM |
| [34] | S–PCT | 0.759 (0.669–0.849) | 0.19 ng/mL | 67.35% | 75.53% | S–PCT is less useful than CSF PCT for the diagnosis of BM |

## 4. Discussion

Procalcitonin, a precursor of calcitonin, is a 116 amino acid peptide and a member of the calcitonin superfamily of peptides, with a molecular weight of 14.5 kDa. PCT is synthesized by the parafollicular C cells of the thyroid gland and is involved in calcium homeostasis. In addition, PCT is also produced by the neuroendocrine cells of the lung and the intestine. In the CNS, cells likely to be sources of CSF PCT include the neurons, astrocytes, and microglia in the parenchyma and meningeal cells. Normal S–PCT concentration is <0.05 ng/mL, with a reported half-life of 25–30 h [35]. Procalcitonin is considered a sensitive and specific marker of certain bacterial infections, such as pneumonia, meningitis, and pyelonephritis, and has been used as tool for the assessment of disease severity. In addition to bacterial infections, increased PCT levels have been identified in other clinical conditions, including severe fungal infections, trauma, burns, major surgery, and medical therapy that stimulates cytokine production. In these cases, S–PCT levels are less elevated and rarely exceed 0.5 ng/mL [36]. There are several hypotheses regarding the pathophysiology of PCT; most suggesting that procalcitonin may be involved in calcium metabolism, cytokine network, and the modulation of nitric oxide (NO) synthesis [37]. In sepsis, PCT hypersecretion emanates from multiple tissues throughout the body, which are not traditionally viewed as endocrine tissues. It is likely that PCT in sepsis potentiates the inflammation cascade by increasing leukocyte-derived cytokines and augmenting reactive oxygen species [38]. PCT secretion is stimulated in bacterial infections by various cytokines, such as IL–1, IL–6, and tumor necrosis factor-alpha. In contrast, PCT production is down-regulated in viral infections, probably due to increased interferon gamma production. Consequently, PCT is considered a useful tool for diagnosing sepsis and repeat S–PCT measurements over time can be used to monitor response to therapy. Most currently used inflammatory markers do not reliably differentiate between a systemic inflammatory response and sepsis. However, because PCT is, generally, not induced by severe viral infections or non-infectious inflammatory reactions, PCT can help distinguish bacterial from viral infections and differentiate between infectious and non-infectious origins of systemic inflammatory response syndrome (SIRS), acute respiratory distress syndrome (ARDS), pancreatitis, cardiogenic shock, and acute rejection of transplanted organs [39].

In CNS infections, disruption of the blood brain barrier (BBB) has been documented in patients with bacterial infections and in experimental models [40,41]. Elevated CSF PCT levels in bacterial meningitis patients seem to be the result of this mechanism and some studies have shown higher CSF PCT levels in patients with Gram-negative bacteria compared to patients with Gram-positive bacteria [42]. In CNS infection cases, microglia and meningeal cells express the responding receptors (Toll-like receptors [TLRs]) to the invading bacteria [43]. Several questions regarding PCT synthesis and secretion by brain cells during bacterial meningitis have not been resolved and need further investigation.

Prompt diagnosis and appropriate antimicrobial treatment are of paramount importance and can contribute to a reduced morbidity and mortality in sepsis. Procalcitonin is an acute-phase protein with faster kinetics than C-reactive protein (CRP) and erythrocyte sedimentation rate (ESR), and is detectable in serum within 4–6 h after the onset of a bacterial infection. PCT serum levels peak within 24 h and start to decline by approximately 50% daily with effective treatment [44–46]. Although there is no "gold standard" for the diagnosis of most infections, several biomarkers have been used as tools to monitor disease progression. An ideal marker should help with early diagnosis and therapeutic decision-making in bacterial infections and should also help clinicians assess the course and prognosis and, in that regard, PCT seems to be superior compared to other commonly used biomarkers.

Despite advances in diagnosis and treatment, bacterial meningitis is a neurological emergency, requires treatment in a high acuity care unit, and remains an important cause of mortality. The diagnosis and management of bacterial meningitis requires various biological tests and a multidisciplinary approach. Empiric antimicrobial and adjunctive therapy should start as soon as there is clinical suspicion of meningitis. Regarding laboratory findings, a left shift in peripheral white blood cell count, elevated serum PCT and C-reactive protein, CSF pleocytosis with predominance of polymorphonuclear leukocytes, and decreased glucose concentration are predictive of bacterial meningitis. CSF analysis is a gold standard for the diagnosis of meningitis: CSF gram staining reveals bacteria in 50% to 80% of cases and cultures are positive in 80% of cases, at best. However, the sensitivity of both tests is <50% in patients already receiving antibiotics. CSF leukocyte count, protein, glucose and lactate concentration, and a latex agglutination test adapted for the rapid direct detection of soluble bacterial antigens in CSF lack the specificity and sensitivity for the diagnosis of meningitis and can only define a clinical probability. In fact, the relatively imprecise nature of the cutoff values for these markers can make their interpretation difficult. Furthermore, in the early phases of acute bacterial and viral meningitis, differential diagnosis is difficult because signs and symptoms are often non-specific and, therefore, differentiation between bacterial and viral meningitis remains a difficult problem for clinicians. Biomarkers, like CRP, procalcitonin, or sTREM–1, may be useful for diagnosis and can help differentiate between viral and bacterial meningitis [47,48]. Serum and CSF PCT levels can be more useful in the diagnosis of bacterial meningitis and in distinguishing bacterial from viral meningitis. A systematic review published by Markanday in 2015 compared serum PCT versus CRP as markers for bacterial infection and showed that, compared to CRP, S–PCT had a higher sensitivity and specificity for differentiating bacterial from noninfectious causes of inflammation [49].

Diagnosis of meningitis requires a detailed history and physical examination combined with high clinical suspicion and appropriate cultures. Prognosis of meningitis depends on rapid diagnosis, identification of the cause, and prompt implementation of appropriate antibiotic treatment. Because clinical and laboratory data available within a few hours after hospital admission are not reliable (except for when bacteria are found in CSF under the microscope), use of biological markers has been proposed as a tool to improve the accuracy of initial diagnosis and, in this setting, serum and CSF procalcitonin measurements seem to be of great value. Because of its high specificity and positive predictive value, elevated S–PCT concentrations (>0.5 ng/mL) indicates ongoing and, potentially, severe systemic infection. Because C-reactive protein is the inflammatory marker most widely used in emergency departments to discriminate bacterial from viral infections, Gerdes et al. published a meta-analysis in 1998 from 35 studies aiming to assess the usefulness of CRP in discriminating bacterial from viral meningitis. The meta-analysis showed that, although the majority of authors propose using CRP as an additional tool for discriminating bacterial from viral meningitis, only negative CRP tests are highly informative in most clinical settings [50]. However, procalcitonin seems to be a valuable tool for discriminating the causative factor of meningitis as, since 1997 and 1998, two French studies showed that, using a cut-off range of 0.5–2 ng/mL, S–PCT had 100% sensitivity and specificity in discriminating bacterial from viral meningitis [51]. Similarly, a more recent meta-analysis published by Vikse et al. in 2015 showed that procalcitonin has a 90% sensitivity and a 98% specificity in the discrimination between bacterial and viral meningitis [26].

This review aims to provide clinicians with an overview of the role of S–PCT and CSF-PCT as diagnostic markers in CNS infections. Several publications assessing the role of PCT as a guide for antibiotic therapy in adult meningitis patients suggest that S–PCT is a sensitive, specific, and prognostic marker of bacterial infections, therefore, S–PCT and CSF PCT measurement can help differentiate bacterial from viral meningitis. Interpretation of PCT levels must take into consideration the clinical presentation of the CNS infection. In addition, knowledge of assay characteristics is important for setting specific cut-off values and functional assay sensitivities. Most clinical studies presented in this review have limitations, including small sample sizes and inconsistent reporting of laboratory findings: In some, AUC values and cut-off values were not reported, while a few were published in languages other than English and, therefore, we only included in the review data reported in the Abstract. Therefore, even though S–PCT seems to be a useful biomarker for the diagnosis and possible prognosis in patients with BM, additional data from larger, well-designed studies are needed to better evaluate the role of procalcitonin in the differentiation between viral and bacterial meningitis and as tool to improve the overall management of patients with meningitis.

## 5. Conclusions

Serum PCT is a biomarker with high sensitivity and specificity in identifying patients with sepsis and can be useful for the diagnosis of bacterial infections. This literature review identified several studies evaluating the role of S–PCT in the assessment of patients with central nervous system infections. Published data suggests that, compared to other acute phase biomarkers, S–PCT is superior as a sepsis biomarker in acute meningitis and can help differentiate bacterial from viral meningitis. Combined with good clinical judgment and appropriate use of antimicrobial agents, S–PCT could be a valuable adjunct in the timely diagnosis and management of sepsis in patients with CNS infection.

**Author Contributions:** D.V. did literature search, wrote and edited manuscript; M.P. did literature search and wrote manuscript; N.P. did literature search; E.S. did literature search; V.K. did literature search; C.P. did literature search, M.K. did literature search, edited, revised and submitted the manuscript.

**Acknowledgments:** This work, including the costs to publish in open access was supported in its entirety by Department funds, without financial support by industry or by any external grants.

**Conflicts of Interest:** The authors declare no conflict of interest.

## References

1. Pierrakos, C.; Vincent, J.L. Sepsis biomarkers: A review. *Crit Care* **2010**, *14*, R15. [CrossRef] [PubMed]
2. Marshall, J.C.; Reinhart, K. Biomarkers of sepsis. *Crit. Care Med.* **2009**, *37*, 2290–2298. [CrossRef] [PubMed]
3. Viallon, A.; Zeni, F.; Lambert, C.; Pozzetto, B.; Tardy, B.; Venet, C.; Bertrand, J.C. High sensitivity and specificity of serum procalcitonin levels in adults with bacterial meningitis. *Clin. Infect. Dis.* **1999**, *28*, 1313–1316. [CrossRef] [PubMed]
4. Schwarz, S.; Bertram, M.; Schwab, S.; Andrassy, K.; Hacke, W. Serum procalcitonin levels in bacterial and abacterial meningitis. *Crit. Care Med.* **2000**, *28*, 1828–1832. [CrossRef] [PubMed]
5. Viallon, A.; Pouzet, V.; Zeni, F.; Tardy, B.; Guyomarc'h, S.; Lambert, C.; Page, Y.; Bertrand, J.C. Rapid diagnosis of the type of meningitis (bacterial or viral) by the assay of serum procalcitonin. *Presse Med.* **2000**, *29*, 584–588. [PubMed]
6. Shimetani, N.; Shimetani, K.; Mori, M. Levels of three inflammation markers, C-reactive protein, serum amyloid A protein and procalcitonin, in the serum and cerebrospinal fluid of patients with meningitis. *Scand. J. Clin. Lab. Investig.* **2001**, *61*, 567–574. [CrossRef]
7. Hoffmann, O.; Reuter, U.; Masuhr, F.; Holtkamp, M.; Kassim, N.; Weber, J.R. Low sensitivity of serum procalcitonin in bacterial meningitis in adults. *Scand. J. Infect. Dis.* **2001**, *33*, 215–218. [PubMed]
8. O'Connor, E.; Venkatesh, B.; Lipman, J.; Mashongonyika, C.; Hall, J. Procalcitonin in critical illness. *Crit. Care Resusc.* **2001**, *3*, 236–243. [PubMed]
9. Jereb, M.; Muzlovic, I.; Hojker, S.; Strle, F. Predictive value of serum and cerebrospinal fluid procalcitonin levels for the diagnosis of bacterial meningitis. *Infection* **2001**, *29*, 209–212. [CrossRef] [PubMed]
10. Martinez, R.; Gaul, C.; Buchfelder, M.; Erbguth, F.; Tschaikowsky, K. Serum procalcitonin monitoring for differential diagnosis of ventriculitis in adult intensive care patients. *Intensive Care Med.* **2002**, *28*, 208–210. [CrossRef] [PubMed]
11. Bender, A.; Elstner, M.; Paul, R.; Straube, A. Severe symptomatic aseptic chemical meningitis following myelography: The role of procalcitonin. *Neurology* **2004**, *63*, 1311–1313. [CrossRef] [PubMed]
12. Kepa, L.; Oczko-Grzesik, B.; Bledowski, D. Procalcitonin (PCT) concentration in cerebrospinal fluid and plasma of patients with purulent and lymphocytic meningoencephalitis—Own observations. *Przegl. Epidemiol.* **2005**, *59*, 703–709. [PubMed]
13. Viallon, A.; Guyomarc'h, P.; Guyomarc'h, S.; Tardy, B.; Robert, F.; Marjollet, O.; Caricajo, A.; Lambert, C.; Zéni, F.; Bertrand, J.C. Decrease in serum procalcitonin levels over time during treatment of acute bacterial meningitis. *Crit. Care* **2005**, *9*, R344–R350. [CrossRef] [PubMed]
14. Ernst, A.; Morgenthaler, N.G.; Buerger, K.; Dodel, R.; Noelker, C.; Sommer, N.; Schwarz, M.; Koehrle, J.; Bergmann, A.; Hampel, H. Procalcitonin is elevated in the cerebrospinal fluid of patients with dementia and acute neuroinflammation. *J. Neuroimmunol.* **2007**, *189*, 169–174. [CrossRef] [PubMed]
15. Knudsen, T.B.; Larsen, K.; Kristiansen, T.B.; Møller, H.J.; Tvede, M.; Eugen-Olsen, J.; Kronborg, G. Diagnostic value of soluble CD163 serum levels in patients suspected of meningitis: Comparison with CRP and procalcitonin. *Scand. J. Infect. Dis.* **2007**, *39*, 542–553. [CrossRef] [PubMed]
16. Ray, P.; Badarou-Acossi, G.; Viallon, A.; Boutoille, D.; Arthaud, M.; Trystram, D.; Riou, B. Accuracy of the cerebrospinal fluid results to differentiate bacterial from non bacterial meningitis, in case of negative gram-stained smear. *Am. J. Emerg. Med.* **2007**, *25*, 179–184. [CrossRef] [PubMed]
17. Viallon, A.; Desseigne, N.; Marjollet, O.; Birynczyk, A.; Belin, M.; Guyomarch, S.; Borg, J.; Pozetto, B.; Bertrand, J.C.; Zeni, F. Meningitis in adult patients with a negative direct cerebrospinal fluid examination: Value of cytochemical markers for differential diagnosis. *Crit. Care* **2011**, *15*, R136. [CrossRef] [PubMed]
18. Alavi, S.M.; Shokri, S. Can serum procalcitonin measurement help monitor the treatment of acute bacterial meningitis? A prospective study. *Caspian J. Intern. Med.* **2012**, *3*, 382–385. [PubMed]
19. Choi, Se.-H.; Choi, Sa.-H. Predictive performance of serum procalcitonin for the diagnosis of bacterial meningitis after neurosurgery. *Infect. Chemother.* **2013**, *45*, 308–314. [CrossRef] [PubMed]
20. Tian, G.; Pan, S.Y.; Ma, G.; Liao, W.; Su, Q.G.; Gu, B.C.; Qin, K. Serum levels of procalcitonin as a biomarker for differentiating between sepsis and systemic inflammatory response syndrome in the neurological intensive care unit. *J. Clin. Neurosci.* **2014**, *21*, 1153–1158. [CrossRef] [PubMed]

21. Abdelkader, N.A.; Mahmoud, W.A.; Saber, S.M. Serum procalcitonin in Egyptian patients with acute meningitis and a negative direct cerebrospinal fluid examination. *J. Infect. Public Health* **2014**, *7*, 106–113. [CrossRef] [PubMed]
22. Shen, H.Y.; Gao, W.; Cheng, J.J.; Zhao, S.D.; Sun, Y.; Han, Z.J.; Hua, J. Direct comparison of the diagnostic accuracy between blood and cerebrospinal fluid procalcitonin levels in patients with meningitis. *Clin. Biochem.* **2015**, *48*, 1079–1082. [CrossRef] [PubMed]
23. Omar, A.S.; ElShawarby, A.; Singh, R. Early monitoring of ventriculostomy-related infections with procalcitonin in patients with ventricular drains. *J. Clin. Monit. Comput.* **2015**, *29*, 759–765. [CrossRef] [PubMed]
24. Li, Y.; Zhang, G.; Ma, R.; Du, Y.; Zhang, L.; Li, F.; Fang, F.; Lv, H.; Wang, Q.; Zhang, Y.; et al. The diagnostic value of cerebrospinal fluids procalcitonin and lactate for the differential diagnosis of post-neurosurgical bacterial meningitis and aseptic meningitis. *Clin. Biochem.* **2015**, *48*, 50–54. [CrossRef] [PubMed]
25. Konstantinidis, T.; Cassimos, D.; Gioka, T.; Tsigalou, C.; Parasidis, T.; Alexandropoulou, I.; Nikolaidis, C.; Kampouromiti, G.; Constantinidis, T.; Chatzimichael, A.; et al. Can procalcitonin in cerebrospinal fluid be a diagnostic tool for meningitis? *J. Clin. Lab. Anal.* **2015**, *29*, 169–174. [CrossRef] [PubMed]
26. Vikse, J.; Henry, B.M.; Roy, J.; Ramakrishnan, P.K.; Tomaszewski, K.A.; Walocha, J.A. The role of serum procalcitonin in the diagnosis of bacterial meningitis in adults: A systematic review and meta-analysis. *Int. J. Infect. Dis.* **2015**, *38*, 68–76. [CrossRef] [PubMed]
27. Kim, J.; Kim, S.E.; Park, B.S.; Shin, K.J.; Ha, S.Y.; Park, J.; Kim, S.E.; Park, K.M. Procalcitonin as a diagnostic and prognostic factor for tuberculosis meningitis. *J. Clin. Neurol.* **2016**, *12*, 332–339. [CrossRef] [PubMed]
28. Morales-Casado, M.I.; Julian-Jimenez, A.; Lobato-Casado, P.; Cámara-Marín, B.; Pérez-Matos, J.A.; Martínez-Maroto, T. Predictive factors of bacterial meningitis in the patients seen in emergency departments. *Enferm. Infecc. Microbiol. Clin.* **2017**, *35*, 220–228. [CrossRef] [PubMed]
29. Morales-Casado, M.I.; Julian-Jimenez, A.; Moreno-Alonso, F.; Valente-Rodríguez, E.; López-Muñoz, D.; Saura-Montalbán, J.; Cuena-Boy, R. Diagnostic usefulness of procalcitonin and C-reactive protein in the Emergency Department for predicting bacterial meningitis in the elderly. *Enferm. Infecc. Microbiol. Clin.* **2016**, *34*, 8–16. [CrossRef] [PubMed]
30. Wei, T.T.; Hu, Z.D.; Qin, B.D.; Ma, N.; Tang, Q.Q.; Wang, L.L.; Zhou, L.; Zhong, R.Q. Diagnostic accuracy of procalcitonin in bacterial meningitis versus nonbacterial meningitis: A systematic review and meta-analysis. *Medicine* **2016**, *95*, e3079. [CrossRef] [PubMed]
31. Morales Casado, M.I.; Moreno, A.F.; Juarez Belaunde, A.L.; Heredero Gálvez, E.; Talavera Encinas, O.; Julián-Jiménez, A. Ability of procalcitonin to predict bacterial meningitis in the emergency department. *Neurologia* **2016**, *31*, 9–17. [CrossRef] [PubMed]
32. Zhang, X.F.; Zhang, X.Q.; Wu, C.C.; Wu, H.W.; Wei, D. Application value of procalcitonin in patients with central nervous system infection. *Eur. Rev. Med. Pharmacol. Sci.* **2017**, *21*, 3944–3949. [PubMed]
33. Park, B.S.; Kim, S.E.; Park, S.H.; Kim, J.; Shin, K.J.; Ha, S.Y.; Park, J.; Kim, S.E.; Lee, B.I.; Park, K.M. Procalcitonin as a potential predicting factor for prognosis in bacterial meningitis. *J. Clin. Neurosci.* **2017**, *36*, 129–133. [CrossRef] [PubMed]
34. Li, W.; Sun, X.; Yuan, F.; Gao, Q.; Ma, Y.; Jiang, Y.; Yang, X.; Yang, F.; Ma, L.; Jiang, W. Diagnostic accuracy of cerebrospinal fluid procalcitonin in bacterial meningitis patients with empiric antibiotic pretreatment. *J. Clin. Microbiol.* **2017**, *55*, 1193–1204. [CrossRef] [PubMed]
35. Dandona, P.; Nix, D.; Wilson, M.F.; Aljada, A.; Love, J.; Assicot, M.; Bohuon, C. Procalcitonin increase after endotoxin injection in normal subjects. *J. Clin. Endocrinol. Metab.* **1994**, *79*, 1605–1608. [PubMed]
36. Ryu, J.A.; Yang, J.H.; Lee, D.; Park, C.M.; Suh, G.Y.; Jeon, K.; Cho, J.; Baek, S.Y.; Carriere, K.C.; Chung, C.R. Clinical usefulness of procalcitonin and c-reactive protein as outcome predictors in critically ill patients with severe sepsis and septic shock. *PLoS ONE* **2015**, *10*, e0138150. [CrossRef] [PubMed]
37. Maruna, P.; Nedelnikova, K.; Gurlich, R. Physiology and genetics of procalcitonin. *Physiol. Res.* **2000**, *49* (Suppl. 1), S57–S61. [PubMed]
38. Becker, K.L.; Snider, R.; Nylen, E.S. Procalcitonin in sepsis and systemic inflammation: A harmful biomarker and a therapeutic target. *Br. J. Pharmacol.* **2010**, *159*, 253–264. [CrossRef] [PubMed]
39. Ferriere, F. Procalcitonin, a new marker for bacterial infections. *Ann. Biol. Clin.* **2000**, *58*, 49–59.

40. Leppert, D.; Leib, S.L.; Grygar, C.; Miller, KM.; Schaad, U.B.; Holländer, G.A. Matrix metalloproteinase (MMP)-8 and MMP-9 in cerebrospinal fluid during bacterial meningitis: Association with blood-brain barrier damage and neurological sequelae. *Clin. Infect. Dis.* **2000**, *31*, 80–84. [CrossRef] [PubMed]
41. Ricci, S.; Grandgirard, D.; Wenzel, M.; Braccini, T.; Salvatore, P.; Oggioni, M.R.; Leib, SL.; Koedel, U. Inhibition of matrix metalloproteinases attenuates brain damage in experimental meningococcal meningitis. *BMC Infect. Dis.* **2014**, *14*, 726. [CrossRef] [PubMed]
42. Charles, P.E.; Ladoire, S.; Aho, S.; Quenot, J.P.; Doise, J.M.; Prin, S.; Olsson, N.O.; Blettery, B. Serum procalcitonin elevation in critically ill patients at the onset of bacteremia caused by either Gram negative or Gram positive bacteria. *BMC Infect. Dis.* **2008**, *8*, 38. [CrossRef] [PubMed]
43. Gerber, J.; Nau, R. Mechanisms of injury in bacterial meningitis. *Curr. Opin. Neurol.* **2010**, *23*, 312–318. [CrossRef] [PubMed]
44. Schuetz, P.; Christ-Crain, M.; Muller, B. Procalcitonin and other biomarkers to improve assessment and antibiotic stewardship in infections—Hope for hype? *Swiss Med. Wkly.* **2009**, *139*, 318–326. [PubMed]
45. Schneider, H.G.; Lam, Q.T. Procalcitonin for the clinical laboratory: A review. *Pathology* **2007**, *39*, 383–390. [CrossRef] [PubMed]
46. Hausfater, P.; Juillien, G.; Madonna-Py, B.; Haroche, J.; Bernard, M.; Riou, B. Serum procalcitonin measurement as diagnostic and prognostic marker in febrile adult patients presenting to the emergency department. *Crit. Care* **2007**, *11*, R60. [CrossRef] [PubMed]
47. Carbonnelle, E. Laboratory diagnosis of bacterial meningitis: Usefulness of various tests for the determination of the etiological agent. *Med. Mal. Infect.* **2009**, *39*, 581–605. [CrossRef] [PubMed]
48. Viallon, A.; Botelho-Nevers, E.; Zeni, F. Clinical decision rules for acute bacterial meningitis: Current insights. *Open Access Emerg. Med.* **2016**, *8*, 7–16. [CrossRef] [PubMed]
49. Markanday, A. Acute phase reactants in infections: Evidence-based review and a guide for clinicians. *Open Forum Infect. Dis.* **2015**, *2*, ofv098. [CrossRef] [PubMed]
50. Gerdes, L.U.; Jorgensen, P.E.; Nexo, E.; Wang, P. C-reactive protein and bacterial meningitis: A meta-analysis. *Scand. J. Clin. Lab. Investig.* **1998**, *58*, 383–393. [CrossRef]
51. Mary, R.; Veinberg, F.; Couderc, R. Acute meningitidis, acute phase proteins and procalcitonin. *Ann. Biol. Clin.* **2003**, *61*, 127–137.

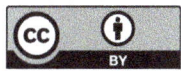

© 2018 by the authors. Licensee MDPI, Basel, Switzerland. This article is an open access article distributed under the terms and conditions of the Creative Commons Attribution (CC BY) license (http://creativecommons.org/licenses/by/4.0/).

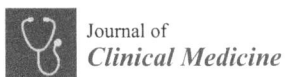 

*Review*

# Imaging Characteristics of Malignant Sinonasal Tumors

Masaya Kawaguchi [1,2], Hiroki Kato [1,*], Hiroyuki Tomita [2,*], Keisuke Mizuta [3], Mitsuhiro Aoki [3], Akira Hara [2] and Masayuki Matsuo [1]

1. Department of Radiology, Gifu University School of Medicine, 1-1 Yanagido, Gifu 501-1194, Japan; kawamasaya0713@yahoo.co.jp (M.K.); matsuo_m@gifu-u.ac.jp (M.M.)
2. Department of Tumor Pathology, Gifu University School of Medicine, Gifu 501-1194, Japan; ahara@gifu-u.ac.jp
3. Department of Otolaryngology, Gifu University School of Medicine, Gifu 501-1194, Japan; kmizuta@gifu-u.ac.jp (K.M.); aoki@gifu-u.ac.jp (M.A.)
* Correspondence: hkato@gifu-u.ac.jp (H.K.); h_tomita@gifu-u.ac.jp (H.T.); Tel.: +81-58-230-6439 (H.K.); +81-58-230-6225 (H.T.); Fax: +81-58-230-6440 (H.K.); +81-58-230-6226 (H.T.)

Received: 30 October 2017; Accepted: 4 December 2017; Published: 6 December 2017

**Abstract:** Malignancies of the nasal cavity and paranasal sinuses account for 1% of all malignancies and 3% of malignancies of the upper aerodigestive tract. In the sinonasal tract, nearly half of all malignancies arise in the nasal cavity, whereas most of the remaining malignancies arise in the maxillary or ethmoid sinus. Squamous cell carcinoma is the most common histological subtype of malignant tumors occurring in this area, followed by other epithelial carcinomas, lymphomas, and malignant soft tissue tumors. Although many of these tumors present with nonspecific symptoms, each tumor exhibits characteristic imaging features. Although complex anatomy and various normal variants of the sinonasal tract cause difficulty in identifying the origin and extension of large sinonasal tumors, the invasion of vital structures such as the brain, optic nerves, and internal carotid artery affects patients' prognosis. Thus, diagnostic imaging plays a key role in predicting the histological subtype and in evaluating a tumor extension into adjacent structures. This article describes the computed tomography and magnetic resonance imaging findings for malignant sinonasal tumors.

**Keywords:** sinonasal tract; malignant tumor; CT; MRI

## 1. Introduction

Sinonasal neoplasms are relatively rare and malignant sinonasal neoplasms are more common than their benign counterparts. Sinonasal malignancies comprise only 3% of all head and neck cancers and 1% of all malignancies [1–3]. The complex anatomy of the region and the rare occurrence of these tumors pose diagnostic and therapeutic challenges. Of the various histological subtypes of malignant sinonasal tumors, squamous cell carcinoma (SCC) is the most common subtype, whereas the other subtypes, such as adenocarcinoma, minor salivary gland carcinoma, undifferentiated carcinoma, neuroendocrine carcinoma, and nonepithelial malignancies (such as sarcoma, lymphoma, plasmacytoma, olfactory neuroblastoma, and melanoma) are considerably less common. The treatment modalities vary depending on the tumor histological subtype, location, and extent of the disease and include surgery, radiation, chemotherapy, or a combination of two or more of these modalities. The prognosis of the patients largely depends on tumor histology, location, and stage.

## 2. Anatomy

The sinonasal tract comprises the nasal cavity, maxillary sinus, ethmoid sinus, frontal sinus, and sphenoid sinus. It includes various tissue types such as epithelium, mucosal epithelium, vessel, nerve, cartilage, bone, and lymphatic tissue. The maxillary, ethmoid, nasal, frontal, palatine, sphenoid, and lacrimal bones are also included. This area comprises bone and cartilage lined with ciliated respiratory epithelium and is located between the orbit and the oral cavity. This area is also close to the frontal cortex through the cribriform plate of the ethmoid bone and is connected with the cerebrum by vessels, lymph channels, and nerves.

The nasal cavity is divided by the nasal septum in the midline. Bilateral nasal cavities include the superior, middle, and inferior turbinates; in addition, the nasal meatus is located under each of them. The common nasal meatus lies between the nasal turbinate and the nasal septum, and the olfactory cleft is located superior to the lower border of the middle turbinate. The paranasal sinuses are connected to the nasal cavity and categorized according to the location of the ostium. The middle meatus drains the maxillary, frontal, and anterior ethmoid sinuses, whereas the superior meatus drains the posterior ethmoid and sphenoidal sinuses. These are located close to important structures, such as the cavernous sinus, the internal carotid artery, the pituitary gland, and the optic nerve.

The upper third of the nasal cavity, the frontal sinus, and parts of the ethmoid and sphenoid sinuses are supplied by the ophthalmic artery, whereas most of the remaining sinonasal tracts are supplied by facial and maxillary arteries. The olfactory mucosa in the upper part of the nasal cavity is innervated by the olfactory nerve. The ophthalmic nerve (V1) provides sensory innervation to the ethmoid sinus, sphenoid sinus, lateral wall of the nasal cavity, and the anterior part of the nasal septum. The maxillary nerve (V2) provides sensory innervation to the maxillary sinus. Submandibular lymph nodes drain the anterior components of the sinonasal tract (anterior drainage pathway), whereas the retropharyngeal lymph nodes drain the posterior components of the sinonasal tract (posterior drainage pathway). These routes of lymphatic drainage finally reach the superior deep cervical lymph nodes.

## 3. Clinical Presentation

The clinical presentations of sinonasal malignancies are nonspecific and identical to those of inflammatory sinus disease, such as nasal obstruction, rhinorrhea, epistaxis, headache, and facial pain. In addition, these malignancies are often asymptomatic until they erode and invade the adjacent structures. Therefore, sinonasal malignancies are usually diagnosed in advanced stages, and the survival rate and prognosis of these patients remain poor. Sinonasal malignancies should be considered in patients with unilateral nasal obstruction or recurrent epistaxis. Progressive sinonasal malignancies that often invade the adjacent structures produce characteristic symptoms, such as cranial neuropathies due to intracranial extension, facial subcutaneous soft tissue swelling, exophthalmos, diplopia, visual disturbances, eye movement disorders, olfactory dysfunction, and respiratory symptoms. Early detection and adequate treatment are required to improve the survival and mortality rates.

## 4. Imaging

Computed tomography (CT) and magnetic resonance imaging (MRI) are very useful tools for the assessment of tumor size, nature, extent, and invasion. The evaluation of the potential extension into adjacent regions impacts the surgical or therapeutic planning, particularly in cases with the involvement of the anterior and middle cranial fossa, orbit, pterygopalatine fossa, palate, or infratemporal fossa (masticator and parapharyngeal space). CT is the most commonly used imaging modality because of its wider availability, easy access, lower cost, and potential to offer greater anatomic detail. In comparison to MRI, CT is particularly effective in delineating calcification and evaluating the pattern of bone invasion. Intralesional calcifications are observed in some sinonasal disorders, such as adenocarcinoma, olfactory neuroblastoma, inverted papilloma, fibrous dysplasia, osteoma, osteosarcoma, cartilaginous tumor, fungal sinusitis, and dentigerous tumor. Characteristic patterns of bone invasion help predict the tumor histology. High grade malignancies show extensive bony destruction, whereas small round cell tumors show permeative invasion and lack of bony destruction. Benign lesions and low grade malignancies may cause bony expansion due to their slow and expansile growth. Contrast-enhanced CT is invaluable for the identification of the feeding artery (because of its high spatial resolution) and for the diagnosis of hypervascular tumors. In contrast, MRI provides higher contrast resolution and affords an excellent characterization of the soft tissue components of the tumor. The signal intensity within a tumor varies according to the tissue components. Malignant tumors usually exhibit nonspecific hyperintensity on T2-weighted images (T2WI) and hypo- to isointensity on T1-weighted images (T1WI). On T2WI, mucinous or cartilaginous tumors show marked hyperintensity, hypercellular tumors show slight hyperintensity, and tumors with fibrosis, calcification, or flow void show hypointensity. On T1WI, hyperintensity within a tumor is indicative of the presence of methemoglobin, melanin, lipid, protein, and mineral elements. Diffusion-weighted image (DWI) with measurement of apparent diffusion coefficient (ADC) captures the degree of Brownian movement of the water molecules in tissues, which serves as a useful imaging biomarker. Low-ADC lesions with strong diffusion restriction indicate hypercellularity, abscess, or hemorrhage, whereas high-ADC lesions indicate hypocellularity, mucus, cartilage, or fluid. Therefore, DWI with ADC measurement is usually useful to differentiate between benign and malignant tumors. The ADC values of malignant sinonasal tumors ($0.87$–$1.10 \times 10^{-3}$ mm$^2$/s) have been shown to be significantly lower than those of benign sinonasal lesions ($1.35$–$1.78 \times 10^{-3}$ mm$^2$/s) [4–6]. Contrast-enhanced MRI is a useful method in detecting perineural spread and dural invasion. Perineural spread can be diagnosed as nerve thickening, widening of the neural foramen, loss of perineural fat, and enhancement of the nerve. Linear enhancement alone is not a conclusive sign of dural invasion; however, dural thickening > 5 mm, pial enhancement, or the presence of focal dural nodules are indicative of dural invasion.

## 5. Sinonasal Malignancies

### 5.1. Squamous Cell Carcinoma

Squamous cell carcinoma (SCC) is the most common histological subtype and accounts for more than half of all sinonasal malignant tumors. It most commonly affects patients in the sixth and seventh decade of life with male predominance. The maxillary sinus is the most frequently affected site, followed by the nasal cavity and the ethmoid sinus. Primary SCCs of the sphenoid sinus and frontal sinus are rare. In the past, sinonasal SCC has been linked to cigarette smoking and occupational exposures [7]. However, in recent years, the generational changes in sexual behavior may have led to an increased positivity rate for human papillomavirus (HPV) among patients with sinonasal SCC; consequently, HPV has been identified in 32–62% of all sinonasal SCCs [8,9]. HPV positivity is more common in SCCs of the nasal cavity than in paranasal SCCs [9]. As with oropharyngeal SCCs, patients with a HPV-positive sinonasal SCC have a better prognosis than patients with a HPV-negative sinonasal SCC [8,9].

Sinonasal SCCs are characterized by aggressive bony destruction of the adjacent sinus walls (Figure 1). Because sinonasal SCCs are often detected at an advanced stage, the invasion of the contralateral sinonasal area, orbital wall, infratemporal fossa, and skull base is sometimes observed. Hypoxia is a common feature in most cases of SCC, and prolonged oxygen deprivation often leads to chronic hypoxic stress and consequent tumor necrosis [10]. Thus, intratumoral necrosis is also one of the characteristic findings in SCCs. On MRI, isointensity on T1WI, slight hyperintensity on T2WI, and moderate enhancement on contrast-enhanced T1WI are typical and nonspecific imaging findings for SCCs. Smaller lesions are typically homogeneous, whereas larger tumors are usually more heterogeneous and exhibit areas of necrosis and hemorrhage [11]. In the maxillary sinus, the ADC values of SCC ($0.95 \times 10^{-3}$ mm$^2$/s) were higher than those of non-Hodgkin's lymphoma (NHL) ($0.61 \times 10^{-3}$ mm$^2$/s) [12].

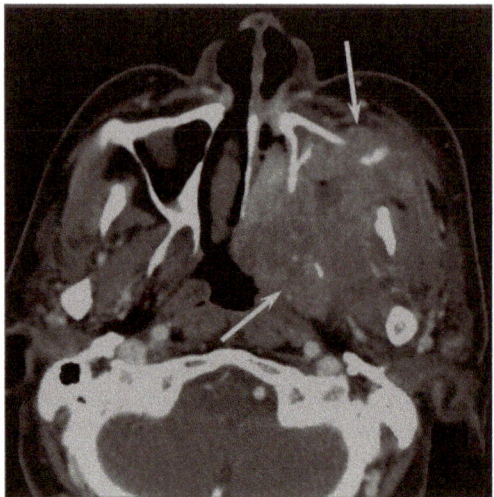

**Figure 1.** Squamous cell carcinoma of the left maxillary sinus. Contrast-enhanced CT image showing an ill-demarcated, heterogeneously enhanced bulky mass with extensive bony destruction (arrows).

*5.2. Adenocarcinoma*

Adenocarcinomas account for 10–20% of all sinonasal malignancies. Sinonasal adenocarcinomas are categorized into salivary type adenocarcinomas and non-salivary type adenocarcinomas [13]. The latter are further classified into intestinal-type adenocarcinomas (ITAC) and nonintestinal-type adenocarcinomas (non-ITAC) [13]. Sinonasal ITACs, which histopathologically resemble colorectal adenocarcinoma, can occur sporadically or are associated with occupational exposure to hardwood and leather dust. Sinonasal non-ITACs do not exhibit the histopathological features of sinonasal ITACs or of salivary type adenocarcinomas; they are categorized into high-grade type and low-grade type. Most sinonasal non-ITACs are of the low-grade type, whereas high-grade non-ITACs are rare. Although the age of the patients with sinonasal ITAC and non-ITAC may vary widely, patients in the sixth decade of life are most commonly affected. The nasal cavity is the most common site for ITAC and non-ITAC, whereas the paranasal sinuses are less commonly affected [14].

On CT, sinonasal adenocarcinomas appear as a soft-tissue mass and occasionally exhibit areas of calcification, which reflect the mucin content. In unilateral olfactory cleft adenocarcinomas, the bulging of the nasal septum across the midline and widening of the olfactory cleft are observed [15]. High-grade adenocarcinomas often show bone destruction. Adenocarcinomas arising from the ethmoid sinus may potentially extend to the skull base and intracranially to the frontal lobes [16]. On MRI, the signal intensity of the adenocarcinomas varies according to their mucin content, cellularity and the presence of hemorrhage. Mucin-producing adenocarcinomas usually show hyperintensity on T2WI and exhibit gradual enhancement on contrast-enhanced T1WI, whereas adenocarcinomas without mucin production show iso- to hypointensity on T2WI. The imaging characteristics of adenocarcinomas are often indistinguishable from those of SCCs (Figure 2).

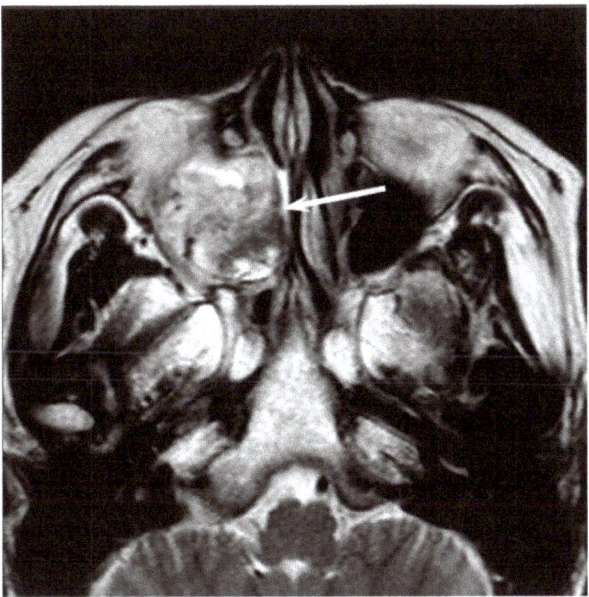

**Figure 2.** Non-intestinal type adenocarcinomas of the right maxillary sinus. T2-weighted image showing a heterogeneously hyperintense lesion (arrow).

## 5.3. Adenoid Cystic Carcinoma

Adenoid cystic carcinomaa (ACC) are slow-growing and relentless salivary gland tumors comprising epithelial and myoepithelial neoplastic cells. ACCs are the most common malignant salivary gland tumors of the sinonasal tract; sinonasal ACCs account for 10–25% of all head and neck ACCs. The average age at presentation is the fifth to sixth decade of life. The maxillary sinus is the most commonly affected primary site, followed by the nasal cavity, ethmoid sinus, and sphenoid sinus [17]. There are three distinct histopathological subtypes of ACC: tubular, cribriform, and solid subtype. ACCs are characterized by wide local infiltration, perineural spread, a propensity for local recurrence, and late distant metastasis. Bone invasion (41%), perineural invasion (40%), and angioinvasion (3.8%) are observed in the surgical specimens of sinonasal ACCs [17]. Lymph node and distant metastases are uncommon at presentation, but the reported overall recurrence rate is 56.2% [17]. The most common sites of distant metastases are the lungs, followed by the liver and bone.

Low-grade sinonasal ACCs may present as polypoid lesions that remodel the bone and mimic a simple polyp, whereas high-grade sinonasal ACCs may present as large irregular masses with bone destruction and heterogeneous density or signal intensity [18]. The growth pattern of maxillary sinus ACCs can be classified into expansile type with minimal bony defects and destructive type with extensive bony defects, and these tumors usually extend to the nasal cavity and, occasionally, to the retroantral fat pad, pterygopalatine fossa, or orbit [19]. ACCs show isointensity on T1WI and iso- to hyperintensity on T2WI, depending on the amount of cellularity (Figure 3). ACCs exhibit the greatest propensity for perineural spread, and the maxillary division of the trigeminal nerve is most commonly affected by sinonasal ACCs. These tumors sometimes easily extend into intracranial components including the cavernous sinus and the Gasserian ganglion, which are far away from the original site [20,21]. Furthermore, for the surgeons, it is often important to first evaluate on images whether the tumor is resectable or not and far away from vital structures. In cases with an advanced tumor, fluid collection and thickened mucosa caused by the isolated sinuses sometimes make it difficult to diagnose and stage the disease.

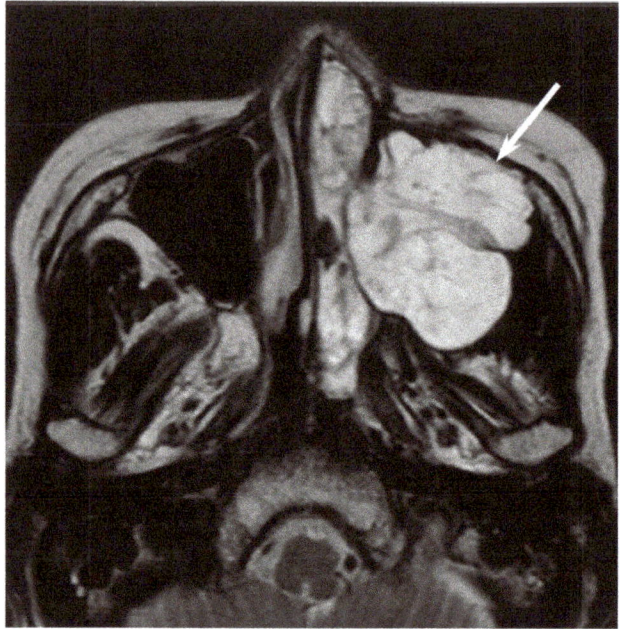

**Figure 3.** Adenoid cystic carcinoma of the left maxillary sinus and nasal cavity. T2-weighted image showing a well-demarcated, lobulated, heterogeneously and strongly hyperintense lesion (arrow).

*5.4. Sinonasal Undifferentiated Carcinoma*

Sinonasal undifferentiated carcinoma (SNUC) is a rare and highly aggressive malignancy, which accounts for approximately 3–5% of all sinonasal cancers. SNUC is a clinicopathologically distinct carcinoma of uncertain histogenesis with no glandular or squamous features. The median age at presentation is the sixth decade of life; the reported male-to-female ratio is 2–3:1. SNUC most commonly arises from the superior nasal cavity and the ethmoid sinus. SNUC usually presents as a rapidly enlarging tumor, and the majority of these patients presents with Stage IV disease. Orbital and intracranial invasion, nodal involvement, and distant metastasis are frequent findings. The recurrence rate is 42.3%. The time to recurrence ranges from 3 to 33 months; 32.1% of patients die of local disease, whereas 14.3% of patients die of metastatic disease [22].

Most SNUCs are larger than 4 cm in maximal diameter at presentation and have ill-defined margins [23]. The aggressive nature of the tumor is reflected in the bone destruction and invasion of adjacent structures, including the paranasal sinuses, anterior fossa, orbit, pterygopalatine fossa, parapharyngeal space, and cavernous sinus [23]. On CT, SNUCs usually appear as a noncalcified mass and show variable contrast enhancement and areas of central necrosis. On MRI, SNUCs show isointensity on T1WI, iso- to hyperintensity on T2WI, and exhibit heterogeneous enhancement on contrast-enhanced T1WI. Owing to the nonspecific imaging findings, it is typically difficult to distinguish between SNUCs and SCCs (Figure 4).

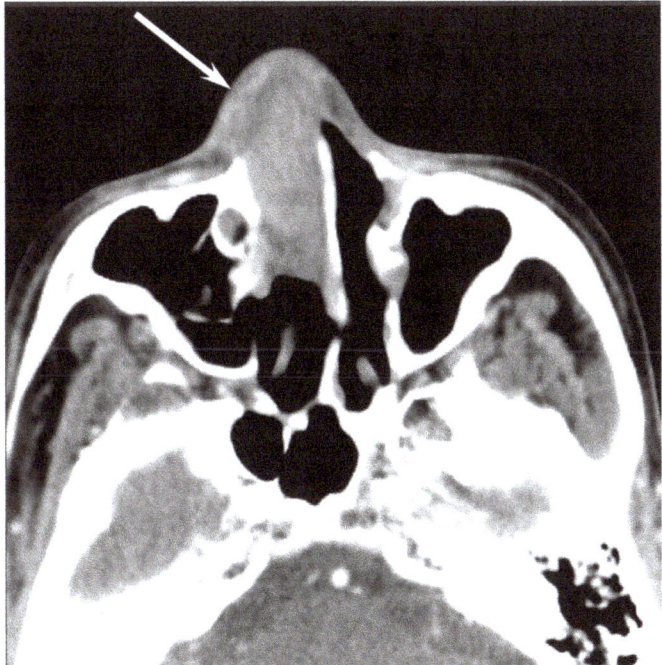

**Figure 4.** Sinonasal undifferentiated carcinoma of the right nasal cavity. Contrast-enhanced CT image showing an ill-demarcated, heterogeneously enhanced lesion (arrow).

## 5.5. Malignant Lymphoma

The head and neck region is the second most common site for extranodal lymphomas after the gastrointestinal tract. NHL is the second most common malignancy in the sinonasal tract after SCC. Patients classically present in the sixth to eighth decades of life; the reported male-to-female ratio is 2:1. Diffuse large B-cell lymphoma (DLBCL) most commonly arises from the paranasal sinuses; the maxillary sinus is the most common site of involvement, although DLBCL may arise from the nasal cavity. NK/T-cell lymphoma most commonly involves the nasal cavity and shows a predilection for occurrence in Asian and South American populations. B-cell lymphoma has a better prognosis than T-cell lymphoma.

On CT, sinonasal lymphomas frequently show both infiltrative or permeative bony invasion and exhibit varying degrees of regional bony destruction [12]. NHLs with permeative-type tumor invasion typically cross the sinus wall and exhibit remnants of sinus wall as a linear structure within the tumor (Figure 5) [24]. In contrast, bony resorption or remodeling caused by the lymphoma may also be accompanied by bone sclerosis [25]. NHLs usually show isointensity on T1WI and slightly hyperintensity on T2WI [11]. Although the signal intensity of NHLs is nonspecific, the ADC measurement helps differentiate these tumors from other malignancies. In the maxillary sinus, the ADC values of NHL ($0.61 \times 10^{-3}$ mm$^2$/s) were shown to be lower than those of SCCs ($0.95 \times 10^{-3}$ mm$^2$/s), which reflects the greater cellularity of NHLs [12]. Although NHLs usually appear as a homogeneously enhanced mass, necrotic areas within the tumor are occasionally observed in NK/T-cell lymphoma [26,27].

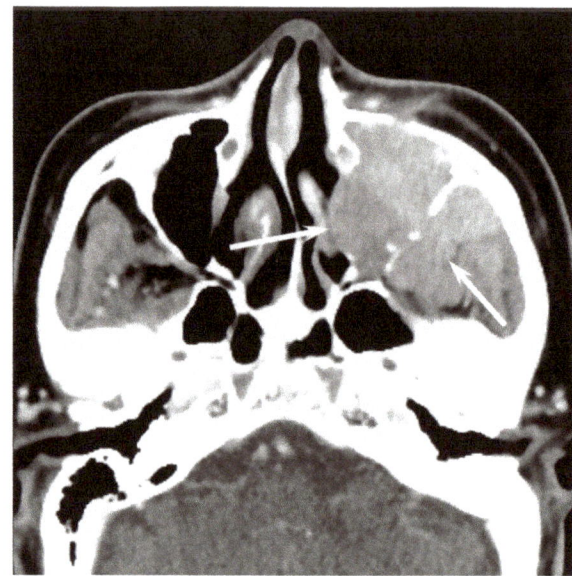

**Figure 5.** Diffuse large B-cell lymphoma of the left maxillary sinus. Contrast-enhanced CT image showing a homogeneously enhanced lesion accompanied by remaining sinus walls as a linear structure within the tumor (arrows).

*5.6. Extramedullary Plasmacytoma*

Extramedullary plasmacytomas (EPMs) (also referred to as extraosseous plasmacytomas) are characterized by soft-tissue monochronal plasma cell proliferation with no evidence of underlying multiple myeloma; these tumors account for 4% of all plasma cell tumors. EPMs usually occur in the sixth decade of life; the reported male-to-female ratio is 3–4:1. Approximately 80% of EPMs involve the head and neck region; the nasal cavity and paranasal sinuses are most commonly affected, followed by the nasopharynx, oropharynx, and larynx [28]. Regional recurrence or spread to other osseous sites may occur. Approximately 15% of the patients develop multiple myeloma [28]. The prognosis depends on the tumor size (>5 cm) and nodal involvement [29].

On CT, EMPs typically appear as well-defined, polypoid soft-tissue masses, which exhibit homogenous enhancement. Large tumors may show areas of necrosis, destruction of the adjacent bone, infiltration of the adjacent structures, and vascular encasement [30,31]. On MRI, EMPs show isointensity on T1WI, iso- to slight hyperintensity on T2WI, and exhibit variable enhancement on contrast-enhanced T1WI [30,31] (Figure 6). Because they are highly vascularized tumors, vascular flow void may be observed within the tumor.

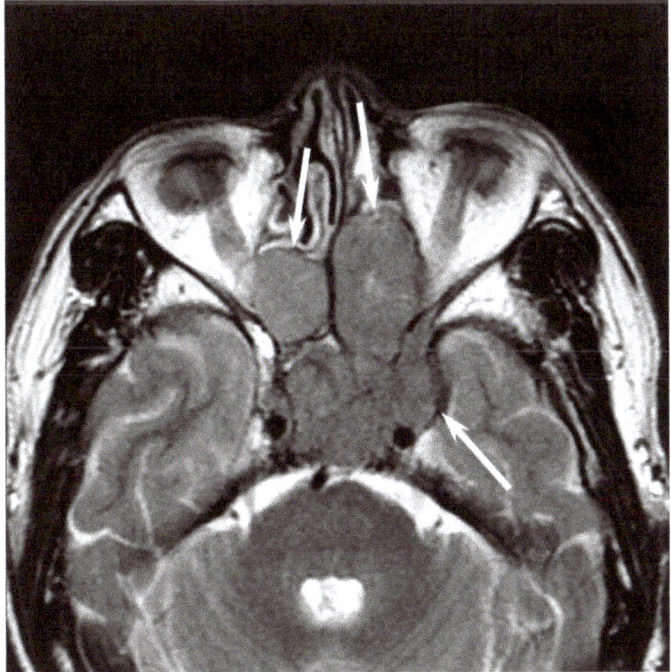

**Figure 6.** Extramedullary plasmacytoma of the bilateral nasal cavity. T2-weighted image showing a homogeneously isointense lesion (arrows).

*5.7. Olfactory Neuroblastoma*

Olfactory neuroblastomas (ONB) arise from the specialized sensory neuroepithelial (neuroectodermal) olfactory cells that are normally found in the cribriform plate, the superior turbinate, and the upper third of the nasal septum. ONBs account for 3% of all sinonasal tumors [32]. ONB may occur at any age, with a peak incidence in the fifth and sixth decades of life; the reported male-to-female ratio is 1.2:1. Direct tumor extension into the adjacent paranasal sinuses, cribriform plate, skull base, orbit, and intracranial cavity is frequently observed. Cervical lymph node metastasis (20–25%) and distant metastases (10–40%) develop over the course of the disease. The most frequent sites of distant metastasis are the lungs, liver, and bone. The most commonly used staging systems are the modified Kadish and Dulguerov classifications.

On CT, ONBs appear as a homogeneous, well-defined soft-tissue mass. Scattered speckled calcifications may be observed within the tumor. The tumor commonly extends into the ethmoid and maxillary sinuses, but rarely involves the sphenoid sinus. CT is essential for the evaluation of osseous involvement of the cribriform plate, fovea ethmoidalis, and lamina papyracea. On MRI, ONBs usually show hypointensity relative to the gray matter on T1WI and hyperintensity relative to the gray matter on T2WI [33]. These tumors demonstrate an avid and homogeneous enhancement except for occasional areas of necrosis or hemorrhage (Figure 7). When an intracranial extension is present, the peripheral or marginal cysts are a characteristic and specific feature of ONBs [34].

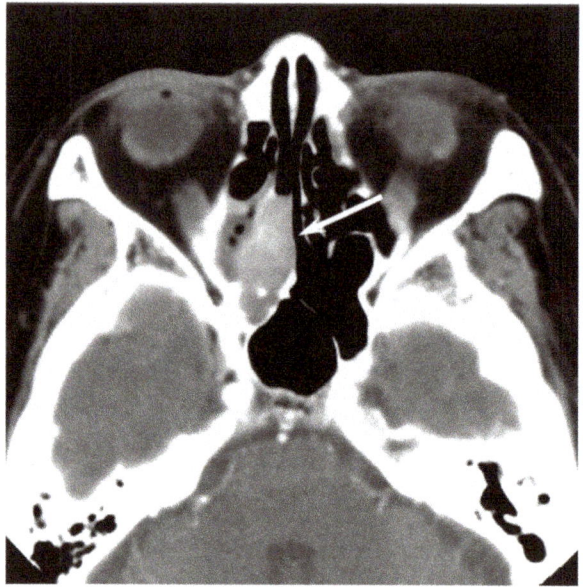

**Figure 7.** Olfactory neuroblastoma of the right nasal cavity. Contrast-enhanced CT image showing a homogeneously enhanced lesion in the right olfactory cleft (arrow).

*5.8. Malignant Melanoma*

Malignant melanoma (MM) originates from the pigment-producing cells (melanocytes) predominantly located in the skin. Sinonasal mucosal MMs account for 0.5–2% of all MMs and approximately 4% of all head and neck MMs. The age at occurrence may vary widely; the peak incidence is in the seventh decade of life. The tumor exhibits no gender predilection. The nasal cavity (including nasal septum, inferior and middle turbinates, and lateral nasal wall) is the second most common site for mucosal melanoma followed by the oral cavity. The paranasal sinuses are rarely affected; of these, the maxillary sinus is the most commonly affected. The occurrence of regional and distant metastases is relatively common (≥25% in most series) [35].

CT findings are nonspecific; however, CT is useful for the evaluation of the remodeling of the the surrounding bone or bony erosion [36]. On T1WI, sinonasal MMs that contain melanin or hemorrhage usually show iso- to hyperintensity relative to the gray matter; however, amelanotic melanoma may also show hypointensity (Figure 8). T1 shortening more often appears as a reflection of the paramagnetic effects associated with the products of hemorrhage rather than the presence of melanin [37]. On T2WI, sinonasal MMs typically show hyperintensity relative to the gray matter; however, melanotic melanomas may show iso- to hypointensity. MMs typically show a heterogeneous strong contrast enhancement owing to the rich vascular network.

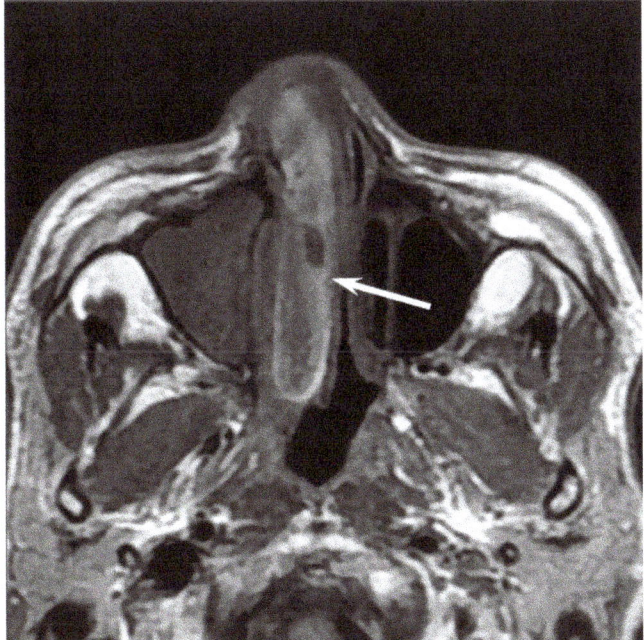

**Figure 8.** Malignant melanoma of the right nasal cavity. T1-weighted image showing heterogeneously hyperintense areas within tumor (arrow).

*5.9. Rhabdomyosarcoma*

Rhabdomyosarcoma (RMS) is a malignant mesenchymal tumor with skeletal muscle differentiation and is one of the most common pediatric soft tissue sarcomas, accounting for 3–5% of all malignancies in childhood. RMS is classified into embryonal, alveolar, pleomorphic, and spindle-cell subtypes. The mean age at diagnosis is 5–6 years, and 72–81% of patients are younger than 10 years; the reported male-to-female ratio is 1.3:1 [38]. Approximately 40% of all RMSs occur in the head and neck region; the most common sites are the orbit, nasopharynx, middle ear and mastoid, and sinonasal tracts. Embryonal RMS is the most common histopathological subtype occurring in the head and neck region and in the genitourinary system and is typically associated with a favorable prognosis.

The average diameter of head and neck RMSs (HNRMS) is 4.5 cm. Most of the HNRMSs have ill-defined margins with adjacent bony destruction and extension into the surrounding spaces [39,40]. On CT, HNRMSs appear as an isodense or slightly hypodense mass and show homogeneous enhancement on contrast-enhanced CT (Figure 9). Intratumoral calcification and hemorrhage rarely occur in HNRMS. On MRI, HNRMSs show isointensity relative to muscle on T1WI, and moderate hyperintensity relative to muscle on T2WI [39,40]. On contrast-enhanced T1WI, HNRMSs show various enhancement patterns; however, the majority of HNRMS shows moderate homogenous enhancement.

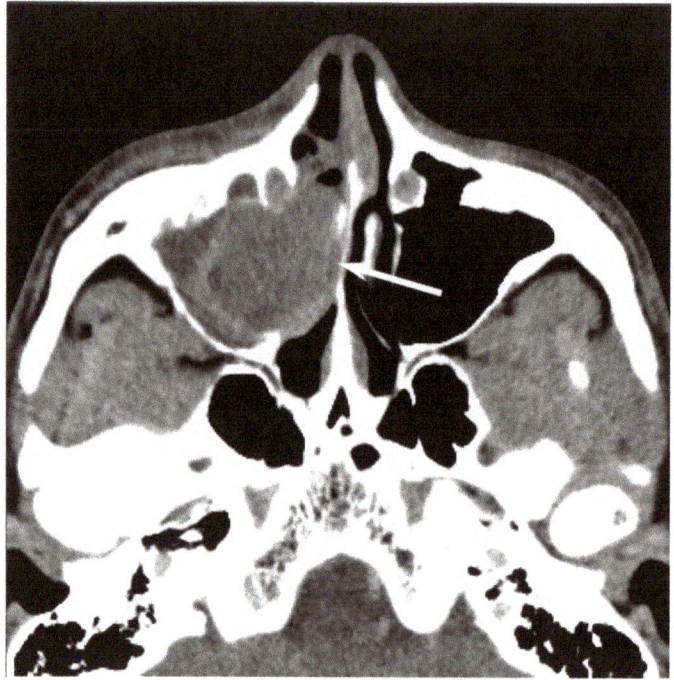

**Figure 9.** Rhabdomyosarcoma of the right nasal cavity. Contrast-enhanced CT image showing a homogeneously, slightly enhanced lesion (arrow).

*5.10. Malignant Peripheral Nerve Sheath Tumor*

Malignant peripheral nerve sheath tumors (MPNST) are highly aggressive malignant mesenchymal tumors that usually arise from peripheral nerves or cells of the peripheral nerve sheath and show variable differentiation toward one of the cellular components of the nerve sheath. MPNSTs account for approximately 5–10% of all soft tissue sarcomas, of which only approximately 8–16% occur in the head and neck region [41]. They occur mainly in adults; the age at presentation may vary widely, although the peak incidence is in the fifth decade of life. They are commonly associated with neurofibromatosis type 1 (NF1) but can also arise through sporadic mutation [41]. The cases associated with NF1 occur in younger patients (mean patient age in the third to fourth decades). MPNSTs may occur in the sinonasal tract, nasopharynx, oral cavity, and orbit. Approximately two thirds of the cases metastasize, usually hematogenously, to the lung and bone.

On CT, MPNSTs appear as a large, hypodense soft-tissue mass with infiltration of the adjacent structures. On MRI, 51% of MPNST on T1WI and 78% of MPNST on T2WI exhibit heterogeneous signal intensity [42] (Figure 10). Compared to neurofibromas, the peripheral enhancement pattern, perilesional edema, and intratumoral cystic change are characteristic MRI findings of MPNSTs [42]. Compared to non-neurogenic malignant soft tissue tumors, the intermuscular distribution, nodular morphology with a fusiform shape, location on the course of a large nerve, and homogeneity of the signal intensity and enhancement are characteristic MRI findings of MPNSTs [43].

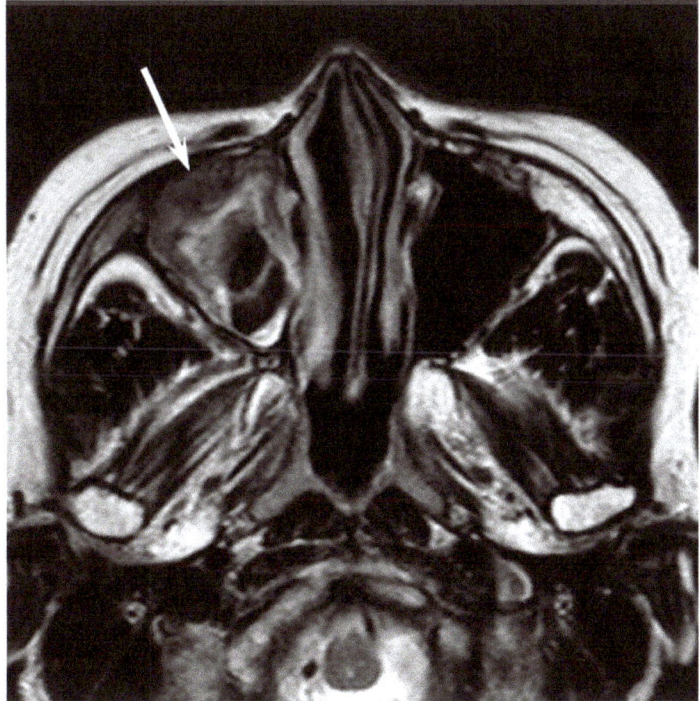

**Figure 10.** Malignant peripheral nerve sheath tumor of the right maxillary sinus. T2-weighted image showing a heterogeneously hypo- to hyperintense lesion (arrow).

## 6. Conclusions

Although the radiological differentiation of sinonasal malignancies is very difficult because of the similarity of imaging findings, the tumor location, growth pattern into adjacent bone, tumor homogeneity, internal signal intensity, contrast enhancement pattern, and DWI with ADC measurement may facilitate an adequate diagnosis. CT and MRI are useful tools for pretreatment evaluation of the characterization, localization, and distribution of malignant sinonasal tumors.

**Author Contributions:** M.K. reviewed the literature and wrote the first draft. H.K. reviewed the draft and revised the manuscript. H.T., M.K., A.M., H.A., and M.M. revised parts of the manuscript. All authors read and approved the final version of the paper.

**Conflicts of Interest:** The authors declare no conflicts of interest.

## References

1. Haerle, S.K.; Gullane, P.J.; Witterick, I.J.; Zweifel, C.; Gentili, F. Sinonasal carcinomas: Epidemiology, pathology, and management. *Neurosurg. Clin. N. Am.* **2013**, *24*, 39–49. [PubMed]
2. Turner, J.H.; Reh, D.D. Incidence and survival in patients with sinonasal cancer: A historical analysis of population-based data. *Head Neck* **2012**, *34*, 877–885. [PubMed]
3. Cooper, J.S.; Porter, K.; Mallin, K.; Hoffman, H.T.; Weber, R.S.; Ang, K.K.; Gay, E.G.; Langer, C.J. National Cancer Database report on cancer of the head and neck: 10-year update. *Head Neck* **2009**, *31*, 748–758. [CrossRef] [PubMed]
4. Razek, A.A.; Sieza, S.; Maha, B. Assessment of nasal and paranasal sinus masses by diffusion-weighted MR imaging. *J. Neuroradiol.* **2009**, *36*, 206–211. [CrossRef] [PubMed]

5. Sasaki, M.; Eida, S.; Sumi, M.; Nakamura, T. Apparent diffusion coefficient mapping for sinonasal diseases: Differentiation of benign and malignant lesions. *AJNR Am. J. Neuroradiol.* **2011**, *32*, 1100–1106. [PubMed]
6. Wang, X.; Zhang, Z.; Chen, Q.; Li, J.; Xian, J. Effectiveness of 3 T PROPELLER DUO diffusion-weighted MRI in differentiating sinonasal lymphomas and carcinomas. *Clin. Radiol.* **2014**, *69*, 1149–1156. [CrossRef] [PubMed]
7. Franchi, A.; Miligi, L.; Palomba, A.; Giovannetti, L.; Santucci, M. Sinonasal carcinomas: Recent advances in molecular and phenotypic characterization and their clinical implications. *Crit. Rev. Oncol. Hematol.* **2011**, *79*, 265–277. [PubMed]
8. Chowdhury, N.; Alvi, S.; Kimura, K.; Tawfik, O.; Manna, P.; Beahm, D.; Robinson, A.; Kerley, S.; Hoover, L. Outcomes of HPV-related nasal squamous cell carcinoma. *Laryngoscope* **2017**, *127*, 1600–1603. [CrossRef] [PubMed]
9. Kilic, S.; Kilic, S.S.; Kim, E.S.; Baredes, S.; Mahmoud, O.; Gray, S.T.; Eloy, J.A. Significance of human papillomavirus positivity in sinonasal squamous cell carcinoma. *Int. Forum Allergy Rhinol.* **2017**, *7*, 980–989. [PubMed]
10. Li, J.Z.; Gao, W.; Chan, J.Y.; Ho, W.K.; Wong, T.S. Hypoxia in head and neck squamous cell carcinoma. *ISRN Otolaryngol.* **2012**, *2012*, 708974. [PubMed]
11. Koeller, K.K. Radiologic features of sinonasal tumors. *Head Neck Pathol.* **2016**, *10*, 1–12. [CrossRef] [PubMed]
12. Kato, H.; Kanematsu, M.; Watanabe, H.; Kawaguchi, S.; Mizuta, K.; Aoki, M. Differentiation of extranodal non-Hodgkins lymphoma from squamous cell carcinoma of the maxillary sinus: A multimodality imaging approach. *Springerplus* **2015**, *4*, 228. [CrossRef] [PubMed]
13. Leivo, I. Sinonasal adenocarcinoma: Update on classification, immunophenotype and molecular features. *Head Neck Pathol.* **2016**, *10*, 68–74. [CrossRef] [PubMed]
14. Purgina, B.; Bastaki, J.M.; Duvvuri, U.; Seethala, R.R. A subset of sinonasal non-intestinal type adenocarcinomas are truly seromucinous adenocarcinomas: A morphologic and immunophenotypic assessment and description of a novel pitfall. *Head Neck Pathol.* **2015**, *9*, 436–446. [CrossRef] [PubMed]
15. Georgel, T.; Jankowski, R.; Henrot, P.; Baumann, C.; Kacha, S.; Grignon, B.; Toussaint, B.; Graff, P.; Kaminsky, M.C.; Geoffrois, L.; et al. CT assessment of woodworkers' nasal adenocarcinomas confirms the origin in the olfactory cleft. *AJNR Am. J. Neuroradiol.* **2009**, *30*, 1440–1444. [CrossRef] [PubMed]
16. Sklar, E.M.; Pizarro, J.A. Sinonasal intestinal-type adenocarcinoma involvement of the paranasal sinuses. *AJNR Am. J. Neuroradiol.* **2003**, *24*, 1152–1155. [PubMed]
17. Lupinetti, A.D.; Roberts, D.B.; Williams, M.D.; Kupferman, M.E.; Rosenthal, D.I.; Demonte, F.; EI-Naggar, A.; Weber, R.S.; Hanna, E.Y. Sinonasal adenoid cystic carcinoma: The M.D. Anderson Cancer Center experience. *Cancer* **2007**, *110*, 2726–2731. [CrossRef] [PubMed]
18. Eggesbo, H.B. Imaging of sinonasal tumours. *Cancer Imaging* **2012**, *12*, 136–152. [CrossRef] [PubMed]
19. Kato, H.; Kanematsu, M.; Sakurai, K.; Mizuta, K.; Aoki, M.; Hirose, Y.; Kawaguchi, S.; Fujita, A.; Ikeda, K.; Kanda, T. Adenoid cystic carcinoma of the maxillary sinus: CT and MR imaging findings. *Jpn. J. Radiol.* **2013**, *31*, 744–749. [CrossRef] [PubMed]
20. Gormley, W.B.; Sekhar, L.N.; Wright, D.C.; Olding, M.; Janecka, I.P.; Snyderman, C.H.; Richardson, R. Management and long-term outcome of adenoid cystic carcinoma with intracranial extension: A neurosurgical perspective. *Neurosurgery* **1996**, *38*, 1105–1112. [CrossRef] [PubMed]
21. Huang, C.C.; Lee, T.J. Radiology quiz case 2. Adenoid cystic carcinoma (ACC) of the sinonasal tract with perineural spread into the cavernous sinus. *Arch. Otolaryngol. Head Neck Surg.* **2008**, *134*, 11.
22. Xu, C.C.; Dziegielewski, P.T.; McGaw, W.T.; Seikaly, H. Sinonasal undifferentiated carcinoma (SNUC): The Alberta experience and literature review. *J. Otolaryngol. Head Neck Surg.* **2013**, *42*, 2. [CrossRef] [PubMed]
23. Phillips, C.D.; Futterer, S.F.; Lipper, M.H.; Levine, P.A. Sinonasal undifferentiated carcinoma: CT and MR imaging of an uncommon neoplasm of the nasal cavity. *Radiology* **1997**, *202*, 477–480. [CrossRef] [PubMed]
24. Yasumoto, M.; Taura, S.; Shibuya, H.; Honda, M. Primary malignant lymphoma of the maxillary sinus: CT and MRI. *Neuroradiology* **2000**, *42*, 285–289. [CrossRef] [PubMed]
25. Matsumoto, S.; Shibuya, H.; Tatera, S.; Yamazaki, E.; Suzuki, S. Comparison of CT findings in non-Hodgkin lymphoma and squamous cell carcinoma of the maxillary sinus. *Acta Radiol.* **1992**, *33*, 523–527. [CrossRef] [PubMed]
26. King, A.D.; Lei, K.I.; Ahuja, A.T.; Lam, W.W.; Metreweli, C. MR imaging of nasal T-cell/natural killer cell lymphoma. *AJR Am. J. Roentgenol.* **2000**, *174*, 209–211. [CrossRef] [PubMed]

27. Kim, J.; Kim, E.Y.; Lee, S.K.; Kim, D.I.; Kim, C.H.; Kim, S.H.; Choi, E.C. Extranodal nasal-type NK/T-cell lymphoma: Computed tomography findings of head and neck involvement. *Acta Radiol.* **2010**, *51*, 164–169. [CrossRef] [PubMed]
28. Alexiou, C.; Kau, R.J.; Dietzfelbinger, H.; Kremer, M.; Spieß, J.C.; Schratzenstaller, B.; Arnold, W. Extramedullary plasmacytoma: Tumor occurrence and therapeutic concepts. *Cancer* **1999**, *85*, 2305–2314. [CrossRef]
29. Straetmans, J.; Stokroos, R. Extramedullary plasmacytomas in the head and neck region. *Eur. Arch. Otorhinolaryngol.* **2008**, *265*, 1417–1423. [CrossRef] [PubMed]
30. Ooi, G.C.; Chim, J.C.; Au, W.Y.; Khong, P.L. Radiologic manifestations of primary solitary extramedullary and multiple solitary plasmacytomas. *AJR Am. J. Roentgenol.* **2006**, *186*, 821–827. [CrossRef] [PubMed]
31. Agarwal, A. Neuroimaging of plasmacytoma. A pictorial review. *Neuroradiol. J.* **2014**, *27*, 431–437. [CrossRef] [PubMed]
32. Broich, G.; Pagliari, A.; Ottaviani, F. Esthesioneuroblastoma: A general review of the cases published since the discovery of the tumour in 1924. *Anticancer Res.* **1997**, *17*, 2683–2706. [PubMed]
33. Yu, T.; Xu, Y.K.; Li, L.; Jia, F.-G.; Duan, G.; Wu, Y.-K.; Li, H.-Y.; Yang, R.-M.; Feng, J.; Ye, X.-H.; et al. Esthesioneuroblastoma methods of intracranial extension: CT and MR imaging findings. *Neuroradiology* **2009**, *51*, 841–850. [CrossRef] [PubMed]
34. Som, P.M.; Lidov, M.; Brandwein, M.; Catalano, P.; Biller, H.F. Sinonasal esthesioneuroblastoma with intracranial extension: Marginal tumor cysts as a diagnostic MR finding. *AJNR Am. J. Neuroradiol.* **1994**, *15*, 1259–1262. [PubMed]
35. Gore, M.R.; Zanation, A.M. Survival in sinonasal melanoma: A meta-analysis. *J. Neurol. Surg. B Skull Base* **2012**, *73*, 157–162. [CrossRef] [PubMed]
36. Wong, V.K.; Lubner, M.G.; Menias, C.O.; Mellnick, V.M.; Kennedy, T.A.; Bhalla, S.; Pickhardt, P.J. Clinical and imaging features of noncutaneous melanoma. *AJR Am. J. Roentgenol.* **2017**, *208*, 942–959. [CrossRef] [PubMed]
37. Escott, E.J. A variety of appearances of malignant melanoma in the head: A review. *Radiographics* **2001**, *21*, 625–639. [CrossRef] [PubMed]
38. Freling, N.J.; Merks, J.H.; Saeed, P.; Balm, A.J.; Bras, J.; Pieters, B.R.; Adam, J.A.; van Rijn, R.R. Imaging findings in craniofacial childhood rhabdomyosarcoma. *Pediatr. Radiol.* **2010**, *40*, 1723–1738. [CrossRef] [PubMed]
39. Zhu, J.; Zhang, J.; Tang, G.; Hu, S.; Zhou, G.; Liu, Y.; Dai, L.; Wang, Z. Computed tomography and magnetic resonance imaging observations of rhabdomyosarcoma in the head and neck. *Oncol. Lett.* **2014**, *8*, 155–160. [CrossRef] [PubMed]
40. Lee, J.H.; Lee, M.S.; Lee, B.H.; Choe, D.H.; Do, Y.S.; Kim, K.H.; Chin, S.Y.; Shim, Y.S.; Cho, K.J. Rhabdomyosarcoma of the head and neck in adults: MR and CT findings. *AJNR Am. J. Neuroradiol.* **1996**, *17*, 1923–1928. [PubMed]
41. Mullins, B.T.; Hackman, T. Malignant peripheral nerve sheath tumors of the head and neck: A case series and literature review. *Case Rep. Otolaryngol.* **2014**, *2014*, 368920. [CrossRef] [PubMed]
42. Wasa, J.; Nishida, Y.; Tsukushi, S.; Shido, Y.; Sugiura, H.; Nakashima, H.; Ishiguro, N. MRI features in the differentiation of malignant peripheral nerve sheath tumors and neurofibromas. *AJR Am. J. Roentgenol.* **2010**, *194*, 1568–1574. [CrossRef] [PubMed]
43. Van Herendael, B.H.; Heyman, S.R.; Vanhoenacker, F.M.; De Temmerman, G.; Bloem, J.L.; Parizel, P.M.; De Schepper, A.M. The value of magnetic resonance imaging in the differentiation between malignant peripheral nerve-sheath tumors and non-neurogenic malignant soft-tissue tumors. *Skelet. Radiol.* **2006**, *35*, 745–753. [CrossRef] [PubMed]

© 2017 by the authors. Licensee MDPI, Basel, Switzerland. This article is an open access article distributed under the terms and conditions of the Creative Commons Attribution (CC BY) license (http://creativecommons.org/licenses/by/4.0/).

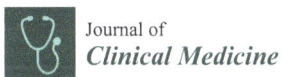 

*Case Report*

# Acute Encephalitis in an Adult with Diffuse Large B-Cell Lymphoma with Secondary Involvement of the Central Nervous System: Infectious or Non-Infectious Etiology?

Surinder S. Moonga [1], Kenneth Liang [2] and Burke A. Cunha [3,*]

1. Stony Brook School of Medicine, State University of New York, Stony Brook, NY 11790, USA; surinder.moonga@stonybrookmedicine.edu
2. Independent Scholar, 54 Catherine Street, New York, NY 10038, USA; liang.kenneth@outlook.com
3. Infectious Disease Division, NYU-Winthrop University Hospital, Mineola, NY 11501, USA
* Correspondence: bacunha@nyuwinthrop.org; Tel.: +1-516-663-2505; Fax: +1-516-663-2753

Received: 28 October 2017; Accepted: 18 November 2017; Published: 7 December 2017

**Abstract:** Both infectious and non-infectious etiologies of acute encephalitis have been described, as well as their specific presentations, diagnostic tests, and therapies. Classic findings of acute encephalitis include altered mental status, fever, and new lesions on neuroimaging or electroencephalogram (EEG). We report an interesting case of a 61-year-old male with a history of diffuse large B-cell lymphoma with secondary involvement of the central nervous system (SCNS-DLBCL). He presented with acute encephalitis: altered mental status, fever, leukocytosis, neuropsychiatric symptoms, multiple unchanged brain lesions on computed tomography scan of the head, and EEG showed mild to moderate diffuse slowing with low-moderate polymorphic delta and theta activity. With such a wide range of symptoms, the differential diagnosis included paraneoplastic and autoimmune encephalitis. Infectious and autoimmune/paraneoplastic encephalitis in patients with SCNS-DLBCL are not well documented in the literature, hence diagnosis and therapy becomes challenging. This case report describes the patient's unique presentation of acute encephalitis.

**Keywords:** neuropsychiatric presentation of encephalitis; paraneoplastic encephalitis; autoimmune encephalitis; infectious encephalitis; diffuse large B-cell lymphoma

---

## 1. Introduction

The substantial morbidity and mortality that is associated with encephalitis is well documented in the literature, although the specific etiology is not often well characterized. Among the identified etiologies, the most commonly described is of infectious nature, either through direct effects on the brain parenchyma or by post-infectious processes, including acute disseminated encephalomyelitis (ADEM) and acute hemorrhagic leukoencephalitis [1,2]. Viruses are the most common cause of encephalitis, with herpes simplex virus (HSV) being the most common [3]. Non-infectious etiologies are typically immune-mediated, divided between autoimmune pathogenic autoantibodies against surface neuronal antigens and paraneoplastic onconeural antibodies (most common Hu and Ma2) against intracellular neuronal antigens [4,5].

Boucher et al. revealed an estimated annual incidence of infectious encephalitis to be 1.5–7/100,000 [3]. A United Kingdom-based prospective surveillance study found the annual incidence of non-infectious autoimmune encephalitis to be 0.85/1,000,000 in children [6].

Per the International Encephalitis Consortium held in March 2012, the major criterion for the diagnosis of encephalitis includes altered mental status lasting >24 h without an otherwise identifiable cause [7]. Minor criteria for diagnosis include: temperature ≥ 100.4 °F (38 °C), new-onset seizure, new focal neurological abnormalities, cerebral spinal fluid (CSF) white blood cell (WBC) $\geq 5/\text{mm}^3$, acute lesion on neuroimaging, or abnormality on electroencephalogram (EEG) indicative of encephalitis [7]. In an EEG study of 52 patients with diagnosed encephalitis, 96.2% demonstrated generalized or focal slowing, 50% showed abnormal delta activity, and 46% of patients showed abnormal theta activity [8]. Overall, EEG rhythm disorder recordings were mild, moderate, and severe for 40.4%, 44.2%, and 13.5% of patients, respectively [8].

Not surprisingly, the neurologic manifestations of encephalitis are most commonly described in the literature; however, on rare occasions, psychiatric pathology can be the only clinical symptom marking the initial presentation of encephalitis, specifically in non-infectious, autoimmune encephalitis [9]. Psychiatric manifestations in non-infectious, autoimmune encephalitis have a well-documented association with autoantibodies against anti-N-methyl-D-aspartate receptor (NMDAR), α-amino-3-hydroxy-5-methyl-4-isoxazolepropionic acid receptor (AMPAR), and γ-aminobutyric acid receptor (GABAR) [10]. Symptoms of psychosis may include paranoid delusions and visual/auditory hallucinations; additionally, patients may also present with insomnia, confusion, and short-term memory loss, similar to delirium [10,11]. The CSF in these non-infectious cases may show lymphocytic pleocytosis and increased protein; further analysis of the CSF can show antibodies to the aforementioned autoantibodies [12]. An increased T2 signal of the medial temporal lobe on magnetic resonance imaging (MRI) or the complete absence of cerebral pathology can be seen on neuroimaging of patients with these autoantibodies [10].

We report an interesting case of acute encephalitis in a 61-year-old male with history of diffuse large B-cell lymphoma (DLBCL) with secondary involvement of the central nervous system (SCNS-DLBCL). Very few cases of encephalitis that are associated with DLBCL have been reported in the literature, and considerations of infectious versus non-infectious etiologies in this particular clinical scenario are not well addressed. Furthermore, previously documented cases of acute encephalitis in patients with DLBCL have not specified secondary lymphomatous central nervous system (CNS) involvement. Was the patient's presentation of altered mental status, fever, leukocytosis and neuropsychiatric symptoms secondary to infectious causes, or were non-infectious, paraneoplastic, or autoimmune processes responsible?

## 2. Case Report

A 61-year-old male presented to the Emergency Department (ED) with altered mental status and fever after a follow-up lumbar puncture (LP) one day prior. 18 h after the procedure, the patient's wife noted that he was "shaking in his wheelchair, mumbling to himself, unresponsive and staring into space". She recorded a home temperature of 99 °F. The patient has a past medical history of SCNS-DLBCL (diagnosed two years ago with right axillary lymph node biopsy and LP with CNS cytology, unknown location of primary tumor), associated with warm autoimmune hemolytic anemia, that has received multiple trials of chemotherapy and improved, but has not entered remission.

Of note, this patient was previously hospitalized two months ago for similar symptoms, including aphasia, lethargy, and right hemiparesis; he was found to have worsening SCNS-DLBCL involvement on computed tomography (CT) scan of the head. Imaging revealed significant left temporal lobe, left parietal lobe, and right occipital lobe lesions, with leptomeningeal involvement in the medial right parietal region. The patient clinically stabilized following whole brain radiation. A follow-up MRI (one month prior to this hospitalization) showed a marked improvement of CNS infiltration and disease. The patient saw his neuro-oncologist five days prior to hospitalization, who stated that the patient's neurologic symptoms, including his memory, had greatly improved. The patient's other medical problems include a urinary tract infection (UTI) that was diagnosed two weeks prior to admission (treated with cefadroxil) and likely steroid-induced hyperglycemia. The patient has never been diagnosed with any psychiatric disorder, has never taken any psychiatric medication, and has never been admitted to a psychiatric hospital. However, the patient's wife mentioned that he had been more isolative in the past few weeks, less talkative, and easily angered. She denies noting paranoia or any complaints of auditory/visual hallucinations from the patient.

On admission, the patient was febrile (102.1 °F, 38.94 °C) with sinus tachycardia (125 beats/min). His physical exam was notable for altered mental status (oriented to self only), generalized weakness, and unspecified aphasia. Pertinent negatives included: no neck stiffness, photophobia, vomiting, respiratory distress, recent trauma, or headache. Medications on admission included: dexamethasone 1 mg daily, long-acting insulin 11 units at bedtime, levetiracetam 500 mg twice/day, metformin 1000 mg daily, pantoprazole 40 mg daily, and ibrutinib 560 mg daily. The patient had no known drug allergies.

Admission laboratory results included: leukocytosis, WBC count = 16.6 K/μL (neutrophils 77%, stabs 3%, lymphocytes 17%, monocytes 9%), venous blood gas lactate of 3.3 mmol/L ($n$ = 0.5–2.2 mmol/L), and normal chemistry with the exception of elevated blood urine nitrogen (BUN 25 mg/dL, creatinine 0.8 mg/dL). Other laboratory results include: normal aspartate aminotransferase (AST) of 13 IU/L ($n$ = 4–36), normal alanine aminotransferase (ALT) of 13 IU/L ($n$ = 13–39), elevated C-reactive protein (CRP) of 76.98 mg/L ($n$ < 3), normal sedimentation rate (9 millimeters/h (MM/HR), $n$ < 20 MM/1HR), elevated ferritin (1593 ng/mL, $n$ = 14–235 ng/mL), normal thyroid stimulating hormone (TSH) (4.136 μIU/mL, $n$ = 0.36–5.80 μIU/mL), and thyroxine (T4) (1.27 ng/dL, $n$ = 0.89–1.76 ng/dL). Patient's urinalysis was positive for WBC > 182 ($n$ < 3/high power field (HPF)), 2+ urine protein, 1+ occult blood, 3+ leukocyte esterase, and positive nitrite. Patient's CSF analysis from LP two days prior was within normal limits.

The patient's concerning symptoms on evaluation necessitated repeat LP, which was performed one day after admission. CSF analysis was significant only for elevated protein (51 mg/dL, $n$ = 8–32 mg/dL) and appearance was non-xanthochromic and clear. The remaining CSF analysis showed 0/μL WBCs, 13/μL red blood cell (RBC), and 2.2 mmol/L lactic acid. CSF was negative for Cytomegalovirus polymerase chain reaction (PCR), Epstein Barr Virus PCR, HSV-1 PCR, HSV-2 PCR, Herpes 6 Virus IgG antibody and West Nile IgG/IgM. CSF cytology was non-diagnostic and flow cytometry was negative for the involvement of lymphoma. The patient was discharged before consideration arose to test his CSF for paraneoplastic or autoimmune antibodies. CSF culture with Gram stain showed no growth for three days.

CT scan of the head was reassuring, showing no significant changes from the patient's previous MRI, performed one month prior to this hospitalization. Unchanged lesions include: small inferolateral left temporal density, associated white matter low density, small medial right and left parietal occipital low densities, and a posterior cerebral white matter hypodensity (Figure 1). Patient's EEG result read: abnormal EEG due to mild to moderate diffuse slowing, with excess low-moderate voltage polymorphic delta and theta activity (Figure 2).

The patient's clinical presentation of acute altered mental status, fever, and generalized weakness, in combination with temporally related recent LP, abnormal EEG, and history of SCNS-DLBCL, suggests multiple different diagnoses, including acute encephalitis. This was added to the list of differential diagnoses, which included sepsis, meningitis, and delirium secondary to UTI. Therefore, the patient was treated with 1 dose of IV vancomycin 1 g and 2 doses at 1.5 g; 1 dose of IV meropenem 1 g and 4 doses at 2 g; and, 2 doses of oral (tablet) dexamethasone 1 mg. The patient also received 1 L of IV normal saline on admission.

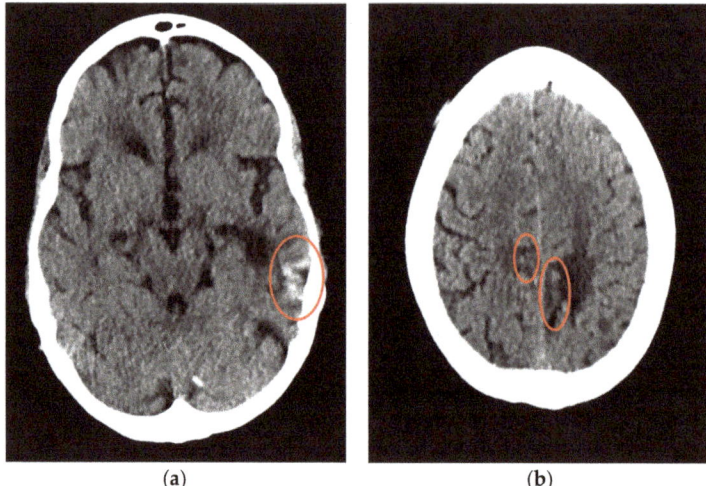

**Figure 1.** Computed tomography (CT) head of a 61-year-old male with SCNS-DLBCL presenting with acute encephalitis. (**a**) CT Head shows a small area of inferolateral left temporal density, which correlates with the blood products that were seen in patient's previous magnetic resonance imaging (MRI) associated with the temporal lobe lesion. There is associated white matter low density, which is similar to the non-enhancing signal on previous MRI; (**b**) CT Head shows a small area of medial left parietal occipital low density corresponds to the lesion and old blood seen on the MRI. It also shows a very small area of medial right parietal occipital low density corresponds to signal seen on the MRI.

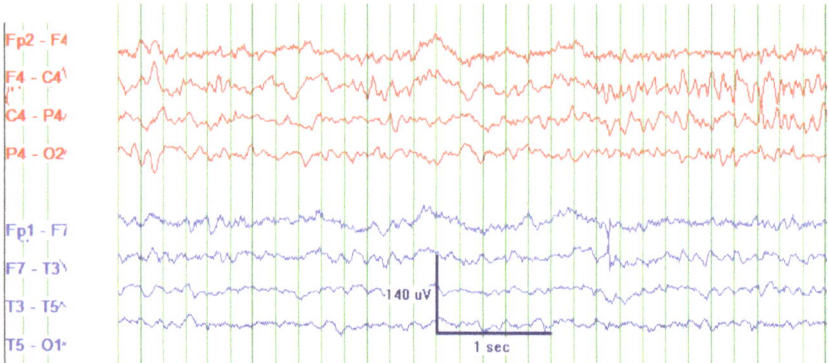

**Figure 2.** Electroencephalogram (EEG) of a 61-year-old male with SCNS-DLBCL presenting with acute encephalitis. Consistent with an abnormal EEG reading due to mild-moderate diffuse slowing. This specific frame shows excess low to moderate voltage (15 to 40 uV) polymorphic delta and theta activity. Interpretation of this EEG suggests mild to moderate diffuse cerebral dysfunction. Technical information: Electrodes were placed according to the 10–20 International Electrode System. Digital EEG was recorded using the Natus Digital EEG System and EEG was reformatted into multiple montages as needed.

Treatment resulted in resolution of fever and leukocytosis (98.3 °F and 4.7 K/µL WBC upon discharge). The patient was discharged appearing clinically stable; however, his neuropsychiatric impairments revealed on admission were unresolved. The patient remained disoriented to place and time, aphasic, and emotionally distressed by word recall disturbances. Initially, the patient's presentation was suggestive of memory impairment given his reluctance and anger toward questions that tested memory. Further examination with Montreal Cognitive Assessment (MoCA) score of 7/30 suggested profound memory loss and cognitive disturbances (Table 1) [13]. Additionally, the patient had several bizarre mannerisms in speech and behavior, sometimes speaking in paradoxes, e.g., "I am afraid, but I have no fear, is that not strange?" Mental status exam before discharge revealed: guarding throughout the interview, soft speech with regular rhythm and prosody, and blunted affect with anxious qualities. The patient appeared somewhat internally preoccupied and paranoid at times, although he specifically denied persecutory delusions and auditory/visual hallucinations. Motor behavior was significant for prominent psychomotor agitation. Overall, he demonstrated poor insight into his condition and poor judgment about the need for hospitalization, stating multiple times "there is no reason for me to be here, I am being held against my will."

**Table 1.** Patient Montreal Cognitive Assessment (MoCA) test assessment result of 7/30 with good effort.

| | MoCA |
|---|---|
| Visuospatial/executive function | 0/5, patient attempted a digital clock at first, could not put numbers on circle clock |
| Naming | 3/3 |
| Memory | Unscored, able to repeat 5/5 words in both 1st and 2nd trials |
| Attention | 2/2 for repeating digits forward and backward |
| | 0/1 attending to the letter A in a list (9 errors), and 0/3 serial 7's |
| Language | 2/2 repeating phrase |
| | 0/1 naming > 11 words that begin with the letter "F" in 1 min (named 3 words) |
| Abstraction | 0/2 |
| Delayed recall | 0/5 with no cue |
| | 0/5 with category cue |
| | 3/5 with multiple choice cue |
| Orientation | 0/6 (date, month, year, day, place, city) |
| Final score | 7/30 |

Score = $n$; $n \geq 26/30$ (normal), $n \leq 23/30$ (mild cognitive impairment), $n \leq 17/30$ (mild dementia), $n \leq 9/30$ (moderate dementia).

## 3. Discussion

Our patient with SCNS-DLBCL presented with symptoms of altered mental status, aphasia, fever, leukocytosis, and multiple neuropsychiatric symptoms. This clinical presentation yielded a wide differential diagnosis, including encephalitis, sepsis, meningitis, increased CNS tumor burden, and delirium. Appropriate procedural, imaging, and laboratory testing was performed. An MRI brain should have been considered to check for cerebral ischemia; however, this diagnosis was not on the differential at the time of admission. Though the patient presented after an LP, the absence of a stiff neck and negative CSF findings eliminated acute bacterial meningitis in the differential. Although the patient's presentation of dehydration and elevated CRP support the diagnosis of sepsis secondary to a UTI, the resolution of symptoms was not achieved with rehydration and the appropriate antibiotic therapy [14]. Regarding delirium, the patient had multiple risk factors, including underlying brain injury from his cancer and an active source of infection (UTI) [15]. Additionally, the disturbances in consciousness and diffuse slowing on EEG were consistent with delirium [16]. However, the clinical picture of 'waxing-waning' cognition and hypoactive/agitated states that classically characterizes delirium was not present in our patient [17].

Acute encephalitis was our diagnosis, given that our patient met the criteria of the International Encephalitis Consortium: major criteria of altered mental status and minor criteria of fever (102.5 °F), new abnormal EEG findings that were consistent with encephalitis and new focal neurological deficits, presenting as aphasia and psychiatric abnormalities on mental status examination [6]. We suggest that the patient's acute psychiatric presentation should be considered a focal neurological deficit, as it can be directly linked to the perturbations in the temporal lobe resulting in symptoms of fear, profound memory loss, and internal preoccupation [18–20]. Per the patient's neuro-oncologist, these symptoms were not present five days prior to our evaluation. Furthermore, the EEG findings of diffuse background slowing and abnormal delta/theta activity are indicative of encephalitis [7,8].

Extensive CSF analysis lowered infectious encephalitis on the differential. Additional CSF testing for Zika, chikungunya and dengue viruses was not performed. Acevedo et al. recommend multiplex real-time reverse transcription PCR (rRT-PCR) testing for patients in endemic areas presenting new neurological symptoms [21]. We believe that the acute change in fear, profound memory impairments, and mild internal preoccupation are suggestive of limbic encephalitis. However, we are not confident in labeling the patient with limbic encephalitis, given that temporal lobe inflammation is confounded by the patient's preexisting mass from SCNS-DLBCL in that region. The cost of ordering paraneoplastic/autoimmune autoantibodies tests is high, and testing all patients with SCNS-DLBCL with possible encephalitis may be impractical [22]. Therefore, we suggest a thorough examination of the neuropsychiatric symptoms of patients with SCNS-DLBCL presenting with acute encephalitis to prompt investigation of non-infectious etiologies.

## 4. Conclusions

In an adult with diffuse large B-cell lymphoma with secondary involvement of the central nervous system presenting with altered mental status, fever, and neuropsychiatric symptoms, it is imperative that clinicians consider encephalitis, both infectious and non-infectious etiologies.

**Acknowledgments:** The patient gave written consent for the publication of this case report. Publication of this report was conducted in accordance with the Declaration of Helsinki. Acquisition of the information for this case report was performed under the guidelines and standards of NYU-Winthrop University Hospital.

**Author Contributions:** S.S.M. and K.L. were responsible for the case report and literature review. S.S.M., K.L. and B.A.C. were involved in the editing and writing.

**Conflicts of Interest:** The authors declare no conflict of interest.

## References

1. Sonneville, R.; Klein, I.; de Broucker, T.; Wolff, M. Post-infectious encephalitis in adults: Diagnosis and management. *J. Infect.* **2009**, *58*, 321–328. [CrossRef] [PubMed]
2. George, B.P.; Schneider, E.B.; Venkatesan, A. Encephalitis hospitalization rates and inpatient mortality in the united states, 2000–2010. *PLoS ONE* **2014**, *9*, e104169. [CrossRef] [PubMed]
3. Boucher, A.; Herrmann, J.L.; Morand, P.; Buzele, R.; Crabol, Y.; Stahl, J.P.; Mailles, A. Epidemiology of infectious encephalitis causes in 2016. *Med. Mal. Infect.* **2017**, *47*, 221–235. [CrossRef] [PubMed]
4. Leypoldt, F.; Wandinger, K.P.; Bien, C.G.; Dalmau, J. Autoimmune encephalitis. *Eur. Neurol. Rev.* **2013**, *8*, 31–37. [CrossRef] [PubMed]
5. Rubio-Agusti, I.; Salavert, M.; Bataller, L. Limbic encephalitis and related cortical syndromes. *Curr. Treat. Options Neurol.* **2013**, *15*, 169–184. [CrossRef] [PubMed]
6. Guan, H.Z.; Ren, H.T.; Cui, L.Y. Autoimmune encephalitis: An expanding frontier of neuroimmunology. *Chin. Med. J. (Engl.)* **2016**, *129*, 1122–1127. [PubMed]
7. Venkatesan, A.; Tunkel, A.R.; Bloch, K.C.; Lauring, A.S.; Sejvar, J.; Bitnun, A.; Stahl, J.P.; Mailles, A.; Drebot, M.; Rupprecht, C.E.; et al. Case definitions, diagnostic algorithms, and priorities in encephalitis: Consensus statement of the international encephalitis consortium. *Clin. Infect. Dis.* **2013**, *57*, 1114–1128. [CrossRef] [PubMed]
8. Mei, L.P.; Li, L.P.; Ye, J.; Wang, Y.P.; Zhao, J.; Zhang, T. A special electroencephalography pattern might help in the diagnosis of antibody-positive encephalitis. *Chin. Med. J. (Engl.)* **2015**, *128*, 2474–2477. [PubMed]
9. Kayser, M.S.; Titulaer, M.J.; Gresa-Arribas, N.; Dalmau, J. Frequency and characteristics of isolated psychiatric episodes in anti-N-methyl-D-aspartate receptor encephalitis. *JAMA Neurol.* **2013**, *70*, 1133–1139. [CrossRef] [PubMed]
10. Lancaster, E. The diagnosis and treatment of autoimmune encephalitis. *J. Clin. Neurol.* **2016**, *12*, 1–13. [CrossRef] [PubMed]
11. Bost, C.; Pascual, O.; Honnorat, J. Autoimmune encephalitis in psychiatric institutions: Current perspectives. *Neuropsychiatr. Dis. Treat.* **2016**, *12*, 2775–2787. [CrossRef] [PubMed]

12. Lee, S.K.; Lee, S.T. The laboratory diagnosis of autoimmune encephalitis. *J. Epilepsy Res.* **2016**, *6*, 45–50. [CrossRef] [PubMed]
13. Saczynski, J.S.; Inouye, S.K.; Guess, J.; Jones, R.N.; Fong, T.G.; Nemeth, E.; Hodara, A.; Ngo, L.; Marcantonio, E.R. The montreal cognitive assessment: Creating a crosswalk with the mini-mental state examination. *J. Am. Geriatr. Soc.* **2015**, *63*, 2370–2374. [CrossRef] [PubMed]
14. Faix, J.D. Biomarkers of sepsis. *Crit. Rev. Clin. Lab. Sci.* **2013**, *50*, 23–36. [CrossRef] [PubMed]
15. Chae, J.H.; Miller, B.J. Beyond urinary tract infections (UTIS) and delirium: A systematic review of utis and neuropsychiatric disorders. *J. Psychiatr. Pract.* **2015**, *21*, 402–411. [CrossRef] [PubMed]
16. Koponen, H.; Partanen, J.; Paakkonen, A.; Mattila, E.; Riekkinen, P.J. EEG spectral analysis in delirium. *J. Neurol. Neurosurg. Psychiatry* **1989**, *52*, 980–985. [CrossRef] [PubMed]
17. Ali, S.; Patel, M.; Jabeen, S.; Bailey, R.K.; Patel, T.; Shahid, M.; Riley, W.J.; Arain, A. Insight into delirium. *Innov. Clin. Neurosci.* **2011**, *8*, 25–34. [PubMed]
18. Zhao, F.; Kang, H.; You, L.; Rastogi, P.; Venkatesh, D.; Chandra, M. Neuropsychological deficits in temporal lobe epilepsy: A comprehensive review. *Ann. Indian Acad. Neurol.* **2014**, *17*, 374–382. [PubMed]
19. Deutsch, S.I.; Rosse, R.B.; Sud, I.M.; Burket, J.A. Temporal lobe epilepsy confused with panic disorder: Implications for treatment. *Clin. Neuropharmacol.* **2009**, *32*, 160–162. [CrossRef] [PubMed]
20. Meador, K.J. Ictal fear: A predictor of surgical outcome. *Epilepsy Curr.* **2001**, *1*. [CrossRef] [PubMed]
21. Acevedo, N.; Waggoner, J.; Rodriguez, M.; Rivera, L.; Landivar, J.; Pinsky, B.; Zambrano, H. Zika virus, chikungunya virus, and dengue virus in cerebrospinal fluid from adults with neurological manifestations, guayaquil, ecuador. *Front. Microbiol.* **2017**, *8*. [CrossRef] [PubMed]
22. Mazonson, P.; Efrusy, M.; Santas, C.; Ziman, A.; Burner, J.; Roseff, S.; Vijayaraghavan, A.; Kaufman, R. The hi-star study: Resource utilization and costs associated with serologic testing for antibody-positive patients at four united states medical centers. *Transfusion* **2014**, *54*, 271–277. [CrossRef] [PubMed]

© 2017 by the authors. Licensee MDPI, Basel, Switzerland. This article is an open access article distributed under the terms and conditions of the Creative Commons Attribution (CC BY) license (http://creativecommons.org/licenses/by/4.0/).

MDPI  
St. Alban-Anlage 66  
4052 Basel  
Switzerland  
Tel. +41 61 683 77 34  
Fax +41 61 302 89 18  
www.mdpi.com

*Journal of Clinical Medicine* Editorial Office  
E-mail: jcm@mdpi.com  
www.mdpi.com/journal/jcm

www.ingramcontent.com/pod-product-compliance
Lightning Source LLC
LaVergne TN
LVHW070449100526
838202LV00014B/1694